DISEASE IN POP
IN TRANSI

Disease in Populations in Transition

ANTHROPOLOGICAL AND EPIDEMIOLOGICAL PERSPECTIVES

Edited by

Alan C. Swedlund

and

George J. Armelagos

Bergin and Garvey

New York • Westport, Connecticut • London

Library of Congress Cataloging-in-Publication Data

Disease in populations in transition : anthropological and
    epidemiological perspectives / edited by Alan C. Swedlund and George
    J. Armelagos.
        p.   cm.
    Includes bibliographical references.
    ISBN 0–89789–175–9 (lib. bdg. : alk. paper)
    1. Environmental health.   2. Human ecology.   3. Communicable
diseases.   I. Swedlund, Alan C.   II. Armelagos, George J.
RA565.D57   1990
614.4—dc20   89–18513

Library of Congress Catalog Card Number: 89–18513
ISBN: 0–89789–175–9

First published in 1990

Bergin & Garvey, One Madison Avenue, New York, NY 10010
An imprint of Greenwood Publishing Group, Inc.

Printed in the United States of America

The paper used in this book complies with the
Permanent Paper Standard issued by the National
Information Standards Organization (Z39.48–1984).

10 9 8 7 6 5 4 3 2 1

CONTENTS

PREFACE

The original impetus for this collection of essays was a meeting with the editors, Bruce Levin (University of Massachusetts), and R. H. Ward (University of Utah). We were discussing the evidence for and against the coevolution of human hosts and their pathogens in the course of history and the conversation turned to the broader issue of health transitions in human populations. It occurred to us that it would be of value to bring together a group of individuals with diverse interests in health and disease, to focus on populations in transition, and to incorporate both historical and contemporary perspectives. The intent was to see if we could collectively identify some common threads connecting populations that differ widely in space, time, and cultural manifestation.

The Wenner-Gren Foundation for Anthropological Research graciously agreed to support a conference on this topic, and it convened in Santa Fe, New Mexico, in the fall of 1985. In attendance at the conference were the senior authors of each of the chapters presented here. There was a great deal of discussion about epidemiological transitions during the week we were assembled. There was also considerable interest and concern regarding the effects of contact between human societies on health. While we may have left a lot of threads dangling, what we did accomplish was to begin asking the right questions. If this volume precipitates an increased or renewed interest in the effects of demographic and social change on the health of populations, then we will have achieved our most important purpose.

The papers presented at this conference were written and revised for this volume and thus represent original contributions by the authors. In the introduction George Armelagos and I try to bring some of the common themes and insights into sharper relief. In the brief conclusion we summarize the areas of consensus that grew out of the roundtable discussions.

In a project of this duration, and with this many contributors, there are numerous people to thank. We would like to especially thank those contributors and co-authors who were not in attendance but who have shared their hard work without the offsetting reward of being in Santa Fe in October. We would like to thank the several student assistants, among them: Anne Grauer, Robin Macks, Dylan Scott, Charlene Rheaume, Janelle Bisacquino, Megan Donnelly, and Robert Paine. We also express our deep appreciation to the people of Bergin & Garvey Publishers for their patience and encouragement, most notably to editors Ann Gross and Deborah Klaum. Finally, our most heartfelt thanks go to Nina Watson, former Conference Coordinator, and Lita Osmundsen, former Director of the Wenner-Gren Foundation. Through their considerable efforts and finely honed skills we were able to work very long, and very hard, and very enjoyably toward the completion of this project.

DISEASE IN POPULATIONS
IN TRANSITION

INTRODUCTION

Alan C. Swedlund and George J. Armelagos

Societies in transition are frequently faced with new settings and/or new pathogens which require a response in order for the affected group to thrive or survive. The adaptive responses that such societies make in the face of transition is a neglected topic in the current literature. Several volumes have appeared over the past decade (e. g., Logan and Hunt 1978; Foster and Anderson 1978; Stanley and Joske 1980; Rothschild 1981; Romanucci-Ross et al. 1983; Chakraborty and Szathmary 1985; Cohen and Armelagos 1984; Janes et al. 1986) that deal with selected aspects of the health and disease of human populations. This volume is an outgrowth of our growing recognition that many human populations are undergoing rapid change today, a recogniton that leads us to question the nature of transitions in both historical and prehistoric populations. In this book a group of investigators identify topics and present original research on aspects of disease in populations in transition. These researchers first came together in the fall of 1985 to discuss various common concerns and issues. The articles were subsequently revised and rewritten for this book.

Recent articles on health in acculturated versus traditional populations (Wirsing 1985; Dennett and Connell 1988) reflect a similar duality of positions, as do controversies about other sociocultural and biocultural phenomena. That is (quite possibly harking back to the classical theories of Hobbes, Rousseau, and others), we see shifting positions regarding whether health (or life) was basically "nasty" or "nice." Recently the prevailing notions have been that traditional societies have sustained themselves, perhaps for eons, in a state of homeostatic balance with their disease environments. While they may experience moderate, and perhaps on occasion even high, levels of infectious disease, they are relatively healthy populations with adequate nutrition in most circumstances (see Wirsing 1985). Contact with the outside world and "acculturation" are likewise seen as variously positive or negative in their impact, with much of the recent work emphasizing that, along with the medical technology that accompanies many contact situations, there are also many disruptive and negative impacts.

This book reflects a related but distinctive trend in the study of health and disease. On the one hand it strives to move forward from the notion of groups living in one state as opposed to another (e.g., acculturated versus nonacculturated), and accepts the likelihood that groups have always had an impact on each other; the colonial and modern periods just intensify the interactions. This approach acknowledges that groups often move from one set of conditions to another, but it is intended to deemphasize the concept of pristine populations becoming acculturated ones. While we may be able to reconstruct what a precontact, traditional society might have been like, the growing body of evidence suggests that virtually all of the populations studied by anthropologists have had ongoing outside contact for a long period of time. On the other hand, it is our purpose to make transitional periods a focal point of interest, whether the changes in a group's ecological context are cultural or biotic. In addition, whether transitions are the exception or the rule, they do present conditions that challenge any group's ability to respond to disease. Thus, we believe they are significant from the standpoint of improving our understanding of disease in human evolution and contemporary variation, and this approach, in turn, is relevant to understanding issues of public health.

It is also our intention to take a broad approach to questions about the diseases affecting populations in transition. This comes with some natural pitfalls. For example, highly disparate populations and varying research questions are addressed here. We see this volume as a beginning to understanding the problems rather than a synthesis. We encouraged a broad perspective by our selection of contributors and their respective paradigmatic frameworks.

We will briefly outline some of the definitional problems, connecting threads, and larger issues addressed by the various authors. We will discuss some of the broader frameworks or models that emanated from our discussion (see Preface), and we will highlight some of the contributions made by the authors, with particular attention to themes raised in more than one chapter.

TERMS AND DEFINITIONS

The notion of a population in transition, be it cultural or epidemiological, is admittedly vague and imprecise. What constitutes a transition? How do we identify its beginning and end points? Are not populations constantly in flux? Moreover, while mortality as an event has a certain precision and definiteness to it, the concepts of morbidity and disease are very imprecise and interpretations vary. The authors of these chapters have spent considerable time discussing these definitional problems and sorting out the various implications.

Although genetic epidemiologists might have a very different concept of disease than, say, social anthropologists studying sorcery, certain generalizations and broad models are still possible. Conversely, in the United States alone, the National Institutes of Health and other private and public agencies fund literally thousands of projects on health and disease. The majority of these studies bear fruit regardless of whether the various investigators agree on a common definition of disease. Therefore, we wish to tread carefully along the path between the chasm of particularization and the abyss of overgeneralization. We want to acknowledge the difficulties in defining some of our most fundamental concepts and terms without becoming incapacitated by doing so.

One simple way to view the spectrum of disease etiology is to envision those diseases that are entirely genetic on one extreme and those that are exclusively environmental on the other. A careful consideration of those diseases most interesting to epidemiologists quickly reveals that the extremes are rarely the provinces in which the answers lie. For example, most cancers are regarded as being environmentally induced, but carcinogenesis is also clearly a genetic process. Infectious disease is certainly of environmental origin, but the immune system of potential hosts shows genetic variability. Phenylketonuria is a Mendelian inborn error of metabolism, but its expression and clinical symptoms are environmentally mediated, and so on. From this we conclude that the primacy of any one component of causality should thus depend more on the purposes of the analysis and the control of effects and interactions than on any concept of a pure etiology of a disease (see Weiss and Szathmary herein).

Ethnomedical Model of Disease

In anthropology there are two distinct models used to understand human disease interactions. Cultural anthropologists have traditionally used an ethnomedical model to interpret the cultural response to disease (Armelagos et al. 1978; Fabrega 1975; Hughes 1968; Wellin 1978). In the ethnomedical model a major concern is a society's definition of disease. Defining a disease is a critical undertaking since it is evidence that a society perceives a threat and is ready to mobilize its resources to challenge it. Whether a disease is viewed as originating supernaturally, or as a part of nature, can provide insights into a society's cosmology and worldview. The ethnomedical perspective can also be used to develop an understanding of how a society mobilizes its social resources to contain the disease threat. In this way, the basic features of the social system are revealed as the group organizes itself to control the disease (Fabrega 1975).

Ecological Model of Disease

The ecological model, the other anthropological framework for the study of disease, basically involves the analysis of the biological response to disease. This model, used extensively by biological anthropologists, is derived from epidemiology. The epidemiological model originally was concerned with the interaction of the variables—the host, the pathogen, and the environment. There are a number of problems with this simplistic approach to the study of disease. Turshen (1977), for example, argues that the epidemiological model is bourgeois since it obscures the real elements in the spread of disease. By focusing on the pathogen as the major cause, the model does not consider the sociocultural factors which affect pathogen transmission. Her solution to this shortcoming would be to abandon the model and move to a political-economic interpretation of the disease process. Criticisms of the model have taken another and independent route. Medical anthropologists are aware of the shortcomings of the model but have been interested in modification to expand its use. These researchers want to modify the variables to encompass a broader interpretation of the disease cause and impact.

While these variables were useful in early epidemiological research, they have been modified into a broader ecological model in recent years. For example, the model has been modified so that the concept of host is expanded to consider the population rather than the individual as the unit of study. This represents an important change in perspective which may have resulted from the influence of epidemiology and population biology on human disease ecology. This view also allows us to move beyond the clinical perspective and to consider disease in an ecological context.

Now the ecological model is no longer restricted to the study of pathogens as the only source of disease. Following Audy and Dunn (1974), there has been a shift to consider a broader range of insults as the source of disease. Insults include factors which adversely affect the ability of the host-population to adapt successfully to the environment. They include pathogens, toxins, physical forces which cause trauma, chemical pollutants, and even psychological factors. Disease is defined in this context as the lowering of an individual's or a population's ability to cope with its environment. Health is defined as an individual's or a population's continuing ability to rally from insults. Health and disease are considered to be a continuum and not an either/or situation (Audy and Dunn 1974:329).

The most significant change in the ecological model is the change in perception of the environment. The original view of the environment was restricted to consider the biotic, climatic, topographic, and geographic factors which may influence disease. Marston Bates (1953) and Jacque May (1960) argue that this conception of the environment is too limiting and must include the cultural system as a part of the human-disease interaction. Culture is comprised of the technology (the way in which energy and resources are extracted from the environment), the social organization (how the society maintains and reproduces itself), and ideology (ideas, attitudes, and beliefs). The cultural system often acts as an effective barrier, buffering the population from the insults that emanate from the environment. There is, however, the possibility that cultural systems can be the source of insults. The technology, social organization, and ideology may create insults that affect the health of the population. Liberally interpreted, and with a few caveats regarding its origins and purposes, we maintain that the ecological model can serve as a general construct for organizing the major elements in the disease process. Much more important, however, is what we do with it once we can place the insult, host, and environment into neatly delineated categories. The questions asked and the approaches taken are where the real utility of a descriptive model is tested. Furthermore, Turshen's (1977) criticisms can be addressed. There is nothing inherent to the ecological model that prevents a consideration of political and economic spheres of influence.

TRANSITIONS

What constitutes a transition? In this volume we are concerned with populations undergoing transitions with respect to their disease environment, events that significantly change their risk factors through changes in the population, the pathogen, or the environmental context. We believe we can identify certain long-term transitions that are important to the human condition. These transitions are difficult to specify temporally and are perhaps most interesting on a theoretical level regarding the coevolution and adaptation between pathogen and host. Episodes within this continuous transition can be important. For example, debate about the attenuation of the plague and/or the tubercle bacilli in European populations historically is a case where specifying the precise time frame is difficult, and probably irrelevant, but general periods within the long transition can be identified.

Somewhat easier to identify are short-term and relatively rapid transitions when populations undergo dramatic epidemiological processes in periods that are much more accurately specified. These are usually marked by a precise event or series of events, and the end of the transition can be quantitatively defined by stabilizing disease or mortality rates or by a new demographic regime (see Jorde et al. herein). Short-term transitions are often characterized by the introduction of new pathogens, new therapies, environmental modification, or demographic changes brought about by contact with outside groups or technologies. A major focus of the discussions at this conference was on contact situations in colonial and development periods.

Major transitions in this history of human disease have been identified. McKeown (1976), McNeil (1976), and many others have developed broad perspectives on the transition in the western world to modern levels of infectious disease rates. Omran (1971), in a widely cited paper, presented his notion of the "Epidemiological Transition." In his view the period in the late nineteenth and early twentieth centuries underwent a change in disease incidence and experience unparalleled in human history. This was the transition from a predominance of infectious diseases to one of chronic and degenerative diseases, as has occurred in many parts of Europe and North America. Two common assumptions of his model (and so interpreted by others) are that the transition would move rapidly throughout the rest of the world and the morbidity and mortality from infectious diseases would be greatly reduced.

This view of medical positivism has required substantial modification, since we have witnessed the continuation of severe epidemics and widespread infant mortality from the dyad of undernourishment and common infections of the pneumonia/diarrhea complex. The deaths of millions each year from a combination of starvation and the major infectious diseases like malaria, cholera, and the common pneumococcal and diarrheal infections should give us pause regarding the progress made. Furthermore, some health professionals have viewed the rising AIDS epidemic as a dramatic contradiction to our view that we now have, or can ever have, control over infectious disease.

Even if we accept Omran's Epidemiological Transition as circumscribed for the western world, it should certainly not be seen as the first human epidemiological transition. As Armelagos argues in Chapter 7, a major transition undoubtedly occurred in the millennia when many human populations were turning from gathering to horticulture. Approximately 10,000 years ago the distribution, density, and subsistence patterns of many human populations in both the Old and New World began to change in significant ways as a function of agricultural intensification.

Prehistoric Epidemiological Transition

For four million years, human disease ecology probably remained fairly stable. *Homo sapiens*, as gatherer-hunters, maintained relatively small population sizes and low population densities. Changes in the disease pattern would have varied as human groups moved into new environmental zones or shifted their subsistence strategies. The major problem with infectious disease would have been zoonotic infections contracted from the animals that were eaten. Such diseases would vary with the animals that were being exploited. Since gathering and hunting has been the major source of subsistence until the domestication of plants and animals, zoonotic diseases were correspondingly the major source of infectious disease. It has been assumed that the zoonotic diseases would not have been a major selective force since the small population size and the distance between the groups precluded the spread of any infections that developed.

The first epidemiological transition would have begun with the development of primary food production, about 10,000 years ago. Agriculture would have dramatically altered the disease patterns in human populations. The decrease in mobility that occurs as people become more sedentary so as to care for their fields and to protect their stores of food is responsible for a new disease ecology. Sedentism increases the likelihood that pathogens and parasites carried by animals may be also transmitted to humans. Human-to-human spread of disease is also more likely since group members remain in closer contact, and meanwhile the accumulation of human waste becomes a source for the spread of disease. Contamination of water is also a frequent problem in sedentary groups.

The major factor in the first epidemiological transition was the increase in population size and density. As sedentary populations grew, the potential for infectious disease grew with them. The increase in human populations based on agricultural subsistence continued with the development of urban centers. While the potential for large-scale epidemics remained, the large urban population centers provided the potential for the endemicity of infections. For perhaps the first time in human history, there were populations of sufficient size and density for infectious diseases to be present at all times.

So, at the very least, we may refer to two major epidemiological transitions in the past, and perhaps there is a third, a modern epidemiological transition resulting from the widespread contact between the "developed" and "less-developed" worlds. This transition has probably been envisioned by most health professionals as a phase of Omran's model and an extension of colonial involvement in other nations. However, there are many simultaneous processes going on in the Third World today that do not fit the classic model. On the one hand, there are the large-scale operations of many international and national agencies to modernize the health care systems of the less-developed countries. These activities run the gamut of public health measures and family planning efforts. Simultaneously, however, there are the opposing effects of social and environmental disruption, the introduction of many environmental contaminants through manufacturing involving hazardous and toxic materials, heavy use of pesticides and fertilizers, the dumping of unwanted wastes, and the destabilization of local institutions that have traditionally been intentionally or incidentally involved in human welfare. In brief, the efforts to "modernize" the traditional regions of the world have no doubt been accompanied by some modest progress and some noteworthy regression in terms of standards of health and well-being.

Contexts for Analysis

The chapters in this book cover a broad assortment of populations and topics. Anticipating that all-too-common refrain of the cynical reviewer, "the papers are uneven and do not fit together into a logical context," we would like to elucidate the organizing principles behind each section of the volume. Some of the controversies, alternative hypotheses, and tensions that develop between the chapters are not necessarily the best elements around which to organize a book. Rather, we have selected three general categories that formed the basis for the topics addressed at the Wenner-Gren Conference. These are: I. Genetic and Evolutionary Perspectives, II. Infectious Disease and Nutrition in Temporal Perspective, and III. Social Epidemiology. The categories are neither inclusive nor mutually exclusive as regards the content of the chapters, but they do highlight the major topic of interest for each author's contribution. From these sections the reader should be able to glean information on the current debates surrounding the various topics and on how the data from various groups correspond to the prevalent hypotheses.

In each section there is usually a predominant theoretical posture evident and also a set of variables, or etiological model, that is deemed most important. In the genetic and evolutionary section we see an emphasis on genetic explanations and evolutionary questions. The coevolution of human and pathogen genotypes is, as noted, the most interesting issue here. In the second section there is less emphasis on explicit theory and much implicit interest in the relationship between infection and nutrition in mortality, particularly infant mortality. There is also a diachronic perspective in which papers deal with prehistoric, historical, and contemporary populations. Several authors take up the issue of proximate causes in morbidity and mortality versus the broader, ultimate causalities which condition the presence or absence of disease and risk factors. Finally, in the social epidemiology section, these environmental and biological factors are broadened to maximize inference on sociocultural, economic, and political affects or effects.

Cross-cutting the topics emphasized in each section are various models and paradigms that may be more abstract than the first-order questions with which the authors deal or which logically follow from the differing paradigmatic orientations of the authors themselves. One such example would be the contrast between a biomedical perspective that is clearly present in, say, Jorde et al., Chapter 10, with the more ethnomedical perspective of Lindenbaum in Chapter 16 on kuru. Neither perspective validates or invalidates the other; instead, the problem being investigated lends itself more to one view than the other; often elements of both approaches are present in a single, empirical context. Several authors are concerned with the concept of pathogen-insult-stress and the adaptive response that may be elicited, whether evolutionary or behavioral, short-term or long-term. The adaptation model has a long tradition in human biology and social anthropology, and it is one that needs to be questioned rigorously and tested often (Goodman et al. 1988). There is also the cross-cutting thread of how human institutions cause significant variability and complexity to disease relationships. There is a general consensus that the formal models employed by many population biologists are only the roughest approximations for what happens in human cultures. However, the recognition that complex etiological factors are the norm for diseases affecting human populations does not deter us from an informed view (and some faith) that these patterns can be unraveled and understood.

CONTRIBUTIONS

Genetic and Evolutionary Models

A longstanding concern of human biologists and geneticists has been the role of infectious disease in evolution. Haldane's (1949) now-classic paper posited that disease should be considered a very significant selective agent in humans. Also, we have tended to view human evolution through a framework that sees local populations becoming adapted to their particular disease environment. As population growth and migration occur, groups move or are displaced into new environments where novel pathogens may affect that population. Derek F. Roberts, in Chapter 1, on genetics and change, presents an introductory lesson on the mechanisms of population genetics and their role in relation to genetic and nongenetic diseases. An understanding of heredity and the distribution of genetic alleles in neighboring populations is fundamental to an appreciation of the impact of genetic diseases today and of how the human population may have evolved in response to infectious diseases.

Catharina Svanborg-Eden and Bruce R. Levin provide a very valuable perspective in Chapter 2; an immunologist and a population geneticist, respectively, they make their observations from the pathogens' point of view. Perhaps too often in human biology the attractiveness of the adaptational model seduces us into a less critical appraisal of the outcomes of coevolution and prompts us to overestimate the potential genetic responses the human population is capable of making. These two authors elucidate which of the infection-resisting mechanisms present in humans is most capable of responding, and they evaluate how the various properties of bacteria, viruses, and other pathogens may contravene those mechanisms. The result is a very tempered view of disease-mediated selection in humans and points to the significant role of environmental factors.

John Barrett follows with a brief but important note regarding another methodological issue in our attempts to identify the role of evolutionary factors in infectious disease. He presents a simple exercise to demonstrate the sampling problems in detecting natural selection in human populations. Sample size becomes a formidable problem when one considers the kinds of controls necessary and the types of populations with which anthropologists and human population biologists normally deal. To what extent can we hope to find statistically significant evidence for selection using the conventional approaches common today?

Francis Black, in Chapter 4, "Infectious Disease and Evolution of Human Populations," investigates disease and evolution in Amerindian populations. He discusses the findings he, his colleagues, and others have made among South American tribal populations over the last several years. In addition to providing a survey of some of the more important infectious diseases and the genetic diversity at the loci that are important immunologically, he also provides germane commentary on the postcontact period. He reviews the impact of some of the diseases brought by European populations, their relative pathogenicity in "virgin soil" populations, and also considers diseases possibly originating in the New World. His comments on the observation that New World populations show no major deficiencies in their immune defenses to European diseases is significant empirical evidence of the points made by Svanborg-Eden and Levin.

Emöke Szathmary and Kenneth Weiss share the same interest in a constellation of noninfectious, chronic diseases in Amerindian populations. Frequently, late-onset diabetes, gall bladder disease, and obesity have been found in association and noted to be common in at least some Native American populations. These clinical findings have been associated with only preliminary speculations on their possible genetic etiology. Szathmary and Weiss have been at the forefront of current research to ascertain more carefully the potential genetic associations with these diseases and to evaluate the "thrifty gene" hypothesis (Neel 1962). Did Amerindian populations, perhaps during their long waves of migration from Asia, across the Bering land bridge to North America, undergo selection for metabolic gene(s) which, under modern, high-fat diets, compromise their health? What are the roles of environment and modernization in the "New World Syndrome?" While these two authors differ somewhat in their etiological views, both regard a genetic component as highly probable and suggest research designs for current and future work.

Infectious Disease and Nutrition

Infectious disease has been the primary agent of mortality in human history, but the diseases and their impacts have varied in time and place. George Armelagos presents a review of disease in prehistory, focusing on two skeletal populations, one from North America and the other from Sudanese Nubia. Armelagos's time frame is the First Epidemiological Transition from gathering-hunting to agriculture. He argues, based partly on evidence provided by several other researchers, that agriculture came with considerable costs to health. That there were offsetting conditions which contributed to population growth cannot be disputed, but agriculture no longer connotes "progress" the same way it once did, at least with regard to the health of the human population.

Luis Vargas considers the major transitions occurring prehistorically, historically, and during this century in a single nation — Mexico. His use of ancient accounts of the Conquest provides graphic and literary testimony to one of the most significant transitions in the New World. This episode also suggests to us how far-reaching the impact of colonialism was in Latin America, Africa, and elsewhere. Remote societies contacted during the last century by health officials and anthropologists must have felt the effects of this earlier contact. Vargas also reminds us of one of the very significant side effects of modernization on indigenous societies, namely, the impact of "western" processed foods on what may be a more balanced and affordable native diet.

Alan Swedlund and Lynn B. Jorde, K. Pitkänen, James H. Mielke, J. O. Fellman, and A. W. Eriksson provide case studies from two historical populations, nineteenth-century United States and Finland. Swedlund discusses the evidence for a secular trend in infant mortality in the United States, with particular emphasis on western Massachusetts. We can follow the transition from early commercial agriculture to industrialization in a semirural area of the eastern United States. During this transition the distribution of infant mortality tends to shift somewhat along cause-specific and socioeconomic lines. Mortality actually shows some evidence for increase at certain times, contradicting our notions of "progress" during the nineteenth century. And he also notes the parallels that can be drawn between the experience of the United States 100 years ago and the less-developed countries today.

Jorde et al., present the epidemiological history of a specific disease, smallpox, from the mid-1700s to the early 1900s in two parishes on the Finnish mainland. This period covers several changes in the demographic history of the region as well as the all-important era of introduction of smallpox vaccination. Using time-series analysis the authors show how the incidence and seasonality of smallpox changed over this 170-year period. Through this case study we can witness the earliest phases of one of the more dramatic examples in which medical intervention led to major reductions in deaths from an infectious disease.

Francisco Salzano brings us back into the present with a discussion of parasitic disease in South American tribal populations. Parasitic diseases are a major cause of infection in tropical environments and were also more important in temperate environments historically. Salzano relates the various modes of transmission for the major parasites and provides a compendium on the incidence of specific parasites in several South American groups. He briefly outlines some of the measures taken by government agencies and those measures which should be taken in the near future. One especially important discovery noted is that some of the infectious micro-organisms infecting these groups may already show antibiotic resistance.

Jere Haas provides a broad survey of research on the association between nutrition and growth and their impact on infant and child morbidity and mortality. He offers a good summary of the current trends in assessment procedures for growth and nutrition deprivation, with accompanying data from Mexico City and Indonesian children. Low birthweight is perhaps the single best predictor of high-risk infants throughout the world today, yet we are still in the early stages of assessment of the ethnic distribution of birthweights and their causes. A major objective of Chapter 12 is thus to relate some of the criteria that are going into the development of international growth standards.

Social Epidemiology

In Chapters 13 and 14, Henry Harpending, Patricia Draper, and Renee Pennington, and also Geoffrey A. Harrison and David A. Jennner, look at aspects of our social behavior in light of hypotheses regarding the human evolutionary legacy. Harpending et al., citing Wilson (1974), refer to our "phylogenetic constraints" resulting from Darwinian evolution. Harrison and Jenner, citing Boyden (1970, 1972), refer to our potential "phylogenetic maladjustment." The former refers to the theory that our behavior — in this case, parental care of children — is conditioned by selective factors in past evolution that would tend to optimize the number of offspring to the environmental conditions in which a group subsists. The latter refers to a set of hard-wired behaviors, such as the "fight-or-flight" response, and how the physiological mechanisms associated with these behaviors can be problematic in the modern world.

Harpending, Draper, and Pennington present a cross-cultural perspective on social support in the form of parental care of children. They present what they observe to be a common phenomenon in many societies, the tendency to nurture infants with intensity through their most precarious, first year or two, and then to reduce that care dramatically at an age at which further parental investment will not significantly affect the survivorship of the child. The level of parental care and the age at which it is attenuated or terminated should be predictable, according to Harpending et al., given information on the ecology and demographic structure of the group. They acknowledge that child care is a learned behavior, but that it must logically fall within the "phylogenetic constraints" of our past evolutionary experience.

Harrison and Jenner are concerned with the physiological and behavioral responses populations will make in the transition from traditional to westernized experience or in fully westernized populations. They have been looking for some years now at the level of catecholamine hormones (adrenaline and noradrenaline) excreted in urine and in other indicators of stress, such as patterns of sleep. The two study populations referred to here are Samoans from Tokleau and rural and city-dwelling residents of Oxfordshire, England. Objective measures of stress and psychological well-being are very difficult to define and assess, and products like the catecholamines and corticosteroids offer opportunities for such measures. In general, Harrison and Jenner find support for their hypothesis that modernization leads to higher indices of stress, using the hormonal data and other behavioral indicators. They suggest that the fight-or-flight response, allegedly very adaptive in past human evolution, does definitely take its toll in the modern world.

Stephen Kunitz approaches the questions of stress, health, and social support from a very different and nongenetic perspective. He reviews the recent literature on the purported effects of social isolation on morbidity and mortality in western, Japanese, and transitional-traditional groups (Navaho). Kunitz is particularly concerned with the definitional problems in measuring social support cross-culturally and the kinds of cultural assumptions that are made in this area of research. He reviews the historical development of the concepts of stress and social support in the United States and England over the last fifty or more years. This is an effective reminder of a chapter in the origin and development of the biomedical model. Does social support affect health? Undoubtedly it does, but the causality is by no means simple, according to Kunitz (see also Carey and Thomas 1987; Goodman et al. 1988); how a society is organized (kin-based or non-kin-based) and how social support is defined are all important in assessing its impact on health.

Shirley Lindenbaum, in Chapter 16 on theories of pathogenesis among the Fore of New Guinea, takes us within the belief system of a transitional culture and demonstrates how their views on the origins of illness have changed through the colonial and into the modern period. Lindenbaum shows how traditional concepts of sorcery can change through time and accommodate trauma, infectious diseases, and psychosocial disease as the incidence and impact of these illnesses changes. Lest we feel too smug about their indigenous belief systems, she relates this period of transition to the experiences in Europe and the United States with witchcraft in the sixteenth and seventeenth centuries. There is a lesson here with broad implications for other societies undergoing rapid change.

The last three chapters in this section mesh quite closely with each other as they all deal with infant mortality in the same general region of the Eurasian continent. Kalish Malhotra discusses mortality in India; Barry Edmonston and Shirley Lindenbaum discuss research in the neighboring country of Bangladesh. These chapters, taken together, also furnish a comprehensive picture of analyses at national, community, and intracommunity levels. Malhotra's general survey of major causes of infant and childhood mortality in India covers the experience of the last twenty or so years. He notes that, although infant mortality has been reduced dramatically, the rates are still comparatively high, especially in some of the more rural and depressed districts. Major diseases such as malaria, cholera, and plague have responded to government programs, but mortality from pneumonia and diarrheal infections is still very serious. Malhotra points to some of the variables strongly associated with infant mortality — age and education of mother, health facilities, and sanitation.

Edmonston has examined detailed data on 240 communities in Bangladesh. His approach is much more formalized, and interested in the relative contributions of a host of independent variables to the distribution of infant mortality in these communities. He focuses on established explanatory variables such as level of female education, sanitation, health facilities, and agricultural development. His analysis of variance design shows significant associations between the level of mortality and years of female education, and the level of health facilities is much more weakly associated. Little evidence for effects of sanitation or agricultural development is found, but the author suggests that the homogeneity and generally low levels of development in Bangladeshi communities afford little opportunity for significant differences in infant mortality to emerge.

Finally, Shirley Lindenbaum, in Chapter 19, again takes us within a culture by analyzing the educational attainment of 700 women in two communities in Bangladesh. She conducted intensive interviews with fifty-one men and thirty-nine women from these two communities. Here we see the strong, positive association between women's educational attainment and infant survivorship. But, most importantly, by interviewing the men and women in these villages she is able to establish the myriad ways education improves the chances of infants.

Whether it is the very objective fact that educated women are more likely to take their infant to a health clinic at an earlier stage of an illness, or the more elusive fact that educated women enjoy higher status and may have more confidence in the presence of health practitioners and others, Lindenbaum convincingly demonstrates the complex effects of education.

These, then, are some of the major issues addressed in this book. This summary of some of the key points and issues is intended to give the reader a road map through the chapters in the next three sections, to give a sense of the linkages that were being formed during the Symposium. We will return to an overview of the chapters in our conclusions.

REFERENCES

Armelagos, G. J., A. Goodman, and K. Jacobs. 1978. The ecological perspective in disease. In *Health and the Human Condition,* M. Logan and E. Hunt, eds. North Scituate, Mass.: Duxbury Press.

Audy, J. R., and F. L. Dunn. 1974. Health and disease. In *Human Ecology.* F. Sargent II, ed. Amsterdam: North Holland Publishing Co.

Bates, M. 1953. Human ecology. In *Anthropology Today.* A. L. Kroeber, ed. Chicago: University of Chicago Press.

Boyden, S.V. 1972. Ecology in relation to urban population structure. In *The Structure of Human Populations.* G. A. Harrison and A. J. Boyce, eds. Toronto: Oxford University Press.

Boyden, S. V., ed. 1970. *The Impact of Civilization on the Biology of Man.* Toronto: University of Toronto Press.

Carey, J., and R. B. Thomas. 1987. Social influences on morbidity and mortality patterns: A case from Peru. Paper presented at the Annual Meeting of the American Association of Physical Anthropologists. New York.

Chakraborty, R., and E. Szathmary, eds. 1985. *Diseases of Complex Etiology in Small Populations: Ethnic Differences and Research Approaches.* New York: Alan R. Liss.

Cohen, M. N., and G. J. Armelagos, eds. 1984. *Paleopathology at the Origins of Agriculture.* Orlando, Fla.: Academic.

Dennett, G., and J. Connell. 1988. Acculturation and health in the highlands of Papua New Guinea. *Current Anthropology* 29(2):273–99.

Dunn, L. 1968. Epidemiological factors: Health and disease in hunter-gatherers. In *Man the Hunter.* R. B. Lee and I. DeVore, eds. Chicago: Aldine.

Fabrega, H. 1975. The need for an ethnomedical science. *Science* 189:969–75.

Foster, G. M., and B. G. Anderson, eds. 1978. *Medical Anthropology.* New York: Wiley.

Goodman, A., R. B. Thomas, A. C. Swedlund, and G. J. Armelagos. 1988. Biocultural perspective on stress in prehistoric, historical, and contemporary population research. *Yearbook of Physical Anthropology* 31:169–202.

Haldane, J. B. S. 1949. Disease and evolution. Supplement to *La Ricerca Scientifica* 19:68–76.

Hughes, C. C. 1968. Ethnomedicine. In *International Encyclopedia of the Social Science,* vol. 10. New York: Free Press/Macmillan.

Janes, C. R., R. Stall, and S. Gifford, eds. 1986. *Anthropology and Epidemiology.* Boston: D. Reidel.

Logan, M., and E. Hunt, eds. 1978. *Health and the Human Condition.* North Scituate, Mass.: Duxbury Press.

McKeown, T. 1976. *The Modern Rise of Population.* New York: Academic.

McNeil, W. H. 1976. *Plagues and Peoples.* New York: Anchor.

May, J.M. 1960. The ecology of human disease. *Annals of the New York Academy of Science* 84:789–94.

Neel, J. V. 1970. Lessons from a "primitive" people. *Science* 170:815–22.

———. 1962. Diabetes mellitus: A "thrifty" genotype rendered detrimental by "progress"? *American Journal of Human Genetics* 14:353–62.

Omran, A. R. 1971. The epidemiological transition. *Milbank Memorial Fund Quarterly* 49:509–38.

Romanucci-Ross, L., D. E. Moerman, and L. R. Tancredi, eds. 1983. *The Anthropology of Medicine.* S. Hadley, Mass.: J.F. Bergin and Praeger Publishers.

Rothschild, H. 1981. *Biocultural Aspects of Disease.* New York: Academic.

Stanley, N. F., and R. A. Joske, eds. 1980. *Changing Disease Patterns and Human Behavior.* London: Academic Press.

Turshen, M. 1977. The political ecology of disease. *The Review of Radical Political Economics* 9(1):45–60.

Wellin, E. 1978. Theoretical orientations in medical anthropology: Change and continuity over the past half-century. In *Health and the Human Condition.* M. Logan and E. Hunt, eds. North Scituate, Mass.: Duxbury Press.

Wilson, E. O. 1974. *Sociobiology: The New Synthesis.* Cambridge, Mass.: Harvard University Press.

Wirsing, R. 1985. The health of traditional societies and the effects of acculturation. *Current Anthropology* 26:203–22.

I GENETIC AND EVOLUTIONARY PERSPECTIVES

1 GENETICS AND CHANGE

Derek F. Roberts

To appreciate the genetic effects of the changes that occur in populations in transition, a few definitions should be established. Every existing human population can be regarded as a continuing entity occupying a particular space. It has a definite demographic structure, sex composition, age composition, which fluctuates with time, but which can be described at any given moment. A population can be characterized statistically, and distinguished from other populations, by the use of parameters, its group attributes (e.g., birth rates and death rates, means and variances of metrical characters, territorial density, gene frequency). These variables are meaningless relative to any individual. The population is permanent in relation to the individuals composing it, for the individual is born into the population, which exists before his arrival and continues to exist after his death. Most important for our purposes, a population has a heredity, and it is this, its genetic characteristics, with which we are particularly concerned.

GENETIC CONSTITUTION

Each population has a genetic constitution, in simple terms a pool of genes that are, as it were, held in trust by the individuals making up the population at any one time. Every individual born receives a sample of the gene pool from his parents, half from the father and half from the mother, and then passes on half of them to each of his children for subsequent transmission in their turn. For each of the many characters that are under the control of a pair of genes at a particular locus on a chromosome, for example some blood groups or red cell enzyme types, the number of individuals possessing it in the population (or a sample of it) can be counted, that is to say, the phenotype frequency can be obtained and from this the frequency of a given gene in the population can be calculated. The population gene pool at any given moment can thus be specified in terms of the gene frequencies, the total gene pool being the array of gene frequencies over all loci. This, then, is a definition of the genetic constitution of the population, the total gene pool, the array of gene frequencies over all loci.

There is another way in which the genetic constitution of a population can be defined that is applicable when the pedigree of the population is known. Instead of the array of gene frequencies at a given time, it is specified in terms of the contributions to it from particular ancestors. These "probable ancestral contributions" constitute the so-called PACK method. If, say, there are six founding ancestors, one has two children and another three, and there are nine offspring in the first filial generation, then the contribution of those two ancestors to the gene pool of that generation is one-ninth and one-sixth respectively. The difference is due to their differential fertility. The probability that an autosomal allele present in a grandparent is present in any one grandchild is one quarter, and that ancestor's contribution likewise to the total second filial generation will depend on the number and fertility of immediate descendants. The genetic constitution of any generation of descendants can therefore be specified in terms of the contributions to it from particular ancestors. Now in real human populations generations overlap, and the one individual can belong to several different generations simultaneously, with respect to the same ancestor, but the same principle can be applied for any group of individuals of known descent. Thus, the genetic constitution of a population at any given time can be specified in terms of the probable ancestral contributions.

These two definitions of genetic constitution can be employed for different purposes. Using the first definition, the positions of populations in relation to each other can be compared, either by considering the allele frequencies at a given locus one at a time and mapping or plotting them along a unidimensional scale; or by multivariate comparison by means of a measure of genetic distance. These frequencies can be employed in assessments of the amount of admixture and, on certain assumptions, its rate. The second definition is particularly valuable in tracing secular variation within a population by calculating the probable ancestral contributions at a series of points in time. For this shows how the genetic constitution of the population so defined varies over the period and can be used to help identify the factors responsible.

GENETIC STRUCTURE

Genetic structure is a different concept. Whereas genetic constitution as defined above is concerned essentially with individual loci, genetic structure concerns the way in which genes are distributed and combined within populations. As such, it is concerned not with gene frequencies, but with measures of gene relationships — correlations between uniting or adjacent gametes (E), coefficients of inbreeding (F), coefficients of kinship (Phi), the parameters of the decline in kinship with distance (a, local kinship; b, systematic migration pressure; d, distance), rate of decay of heterozygosity, linkage, and linkage disequilibria. For all these, factors are of relevance that do not enter the simple concept of genetic constitution — effective population size, population distribution, population density, clines, assortative mating, migration, marriage systems.

The idea of genetic structure seems to have developed from the work first of Wahlund (1928), who explored the consequences of population subdivision, Dahlberg (1929), who developed the concept, and Wright (1931), who investigated the mathematical theory. Few human populations can be regarded as a homogeneous social entity, but within most there exist some boundaries to breeding. The boundaries may be geographical or social in nature, so that every individual has his own circle, within which it is probable that he will marry, and the population is therefore made up of many such circles, overlapping with each other, minor subpopulations, or isolates. They rarely coincide with actual geographically defined communities except, perhaps, in reproductively sequestered island populations such as the descendants of the Bounty mutineers on Pitcairn Island or in small religious communities such as the Dunkers, but it is to these isolated populations that the word "isolate" of recent years has come to be particularly applied, and not to segments within larger populations. These contrasting situations may be viewed as a matter of degree, the effectiveness of isolating mechanisms between those within and those without the isolate, and in practice it is usually clear how the term is being used.

All these subdivisions, and the departures from random mating that they produce, affect the distribution and evolution of genes within the population, and the existence of such a population structure is of considerable importance in population genetics. The size of the population, important in the evolutionary process, is considerably smaller than may appear at first sight. Instead of the large population there is a series of smaller units. In the absence of differential selection, mutation, and assuming random mating within each isolate, this division would lead merely by chance processes to genetic differentiation of the isolates, extreme if they are totally cut off from each other, less so according to the degree of migration. The variance due to drift (negligible in a large population but large in a small one) in one generation is compounded with the passage of generations, and the gene frequencies of the isolates become more and more divergent, even though the gene frequency for the total population as a whole remains unchanged. When isolation is partial, the rate of divergence depends on the amount of gene flow.

With the passage of time the gene frequencies become so divergent that more and more genes become either lost or fixed. A second consequence then is that, since the smaller numbers increase the probability of fixation at a given locus, division into isolates makes for greater genetic uniformity with each isolate. There are limits, either gene loss or fixation, beyond which random dispersion cannot go, and the rapidity with which these limits are attained in a given isolate depends on its size, initial gene frequency, and amount of gene flow. Again, however, the gene frequency in the total population remains unchanged.

A third consequence is that there is a tendency to increased homozygosity within the population as a whole. Within each isolate the genotype frequencies are those expected from the changed gene frequencies; as the isolates drift apart in gene frequencies, their genotype frequencies are correspondingly divergent. As the gene frequencies for each isolate assume extreme values with the approach of fixation, there is a diminution in the number of heterozygotes, since heterozygotes are most numerous when gene frequencies are at intermediate values. In the population as a whole, the frequency of heterozygotes is less than expected from the overall gene frequencies by an amount related to the gene frequency variance among isolates. In other words, there is a departure of the genotype frequencies of the total population from those expected from Hardy-Weinberg relationships. For those loci at which more than a single pair of alleles is available, the greater the number of coexisting alleles at a locus the more rapid the rate at which some are lost or fixed (Kimura 1955), so that the population subdivision is particularly effective in restricting the number of coexisting alleles in an isolate. Indeed, the rate of decrease in genetic variation in a population with many isolates varies with their number (Maruyama 1970).

It is not only the genotype frequencies that are affected by the existence of isolates; there is greater opportunity for another random variable to take effect, namely the establishment of new mutants, structural chromosomal and DNA rearrangements, changes in linkages and linkage groups. The concept of population structure is central to Sewall Wright's (1931) shifting balance theory of evolution and, just as in this the fixation of individual alleles is important for establishing differentiation, so too is the fixation of new linkage groups and chromosomal structure.

Following the early work, especially that of Wright, the concept of genetic structure has been much developed by Malecot (1948), Morton (1969), Harpending (1974), Jacquard (1974), and many others. Today comprehensive description of a population's genetic structure may utilize the relationships among alleles, loci, chromosomes, gametes, individuals, aggregates of individuals, sib pairs, families, genealogies, social classes, and geographical and other subpopulations.

THE EFFECTS OF CHANGE

Genetic Constitution

We are now in a position to examine the effects of change. The effects of the factors of gene frequency change were well worked out in the early days of classical population genetics by Haldane (1930), Fisher (1930), and Wright (1931), and the types of process that they envisaged are those that apply in differing degrees to populations in transition. The arrival of an occasional individual may bring new ideas which affect the way of life of the population but may have relatively little effect on the gene pool. It will depend on whether he marries into the population and on the number of his offspring; unless he is more fertile than the average, the chance of survival of any gene that he introduces is remote, rather like the chance of survival of a new mutant. If, however, there is a succession of new arrivals who enter the recipient population rather like recurrent mutation, they will influence the recipient gene pool in the direction of the migrants. When a number of newcomers arrive together and intermarry with the locals, the genetic effects will be those described by the several models of admixture (e.g., Roberts and Hiorns 1962). Their arrival, moreover, is likely to introduce new diseases and new ways of exploiting the environment and so disturb any balance that there may be among the preexisting selective factors and the original gene frequencies. Hence, the processes that affect gene frequency remain essentially the same as in nontransitional populations, but their tempo differs. The newcomers may not be intentionally destructive. They may, for example, bring improved health facilities and health care, yet these certainly disturb any preexisting selective balance. In such circumstances a major effect is likely to occur in child survival, and this will mean a change in the relative contributions of selection through mortality and selection through differential fertility, as is suggested by the comparison of different types of populations by Spuhler (1963). The process is self-limiting — as the population size increases, a whole new array of selection pressures comes into operation.

If, however, the immigrants and the indigenes keep themselves largely apart, there may be appreciable effects on gene frequencies in a particular territory, not by the accepted processes of gene frequency change but by population replacement. This is well illustrated in Fiji (Roberts and Mohan 1976). Had it been technically and physically possible in 1870 to examine the ABO blood groups of all the inhabitants of the Fiji Islands, the survey likely would have shown the blood group B gene to be present at a frequency of about 9 percent. Such a survey today would give double that frequency, about 18 percent. A change of gene frequency as great as this in any other species would suggest the operation of natural selection; by analogy one might suppose that individuals with the B gene were endowed with improved survival conditions on Fiji, more successful fertility, or a combination of both. The explanation, however, lies elsewhere. It is due to population replacement. The coming of the European brought disaster to Fiji. With the introduction of firearms, the nature of native warfare changed, and, to a society geared to a relatively harmless system of strife, the new barbarism brought losses impossible to assess. Enormous numbers of men, women, and children of all ages died, many of the victims being of the age groups of the greatest reproductive potential. A second effect of European contact was the scourge of epidemic disease. This was particularly heavy on the Fijians, who, by reason of their geographical isolation, possessed little immunity to the more usual infections of the outer world. The first Fijian epidemic is thought to have occurred about 1791–92, followed by an outbreak of dysentery in 1802–3, both with devastating mortality. In 1874–75 measles swept through the almost totally susceptible native population, reputedly causing the deaths of one-quarter of the population. There were other subsequent epidemics, and mortality rates exceeded fertility until 1905.

But in 1879 a first group of Indian indentured laborers arrived to work in the sugar industry, and though these and the others that followed them also succumbed to the epidemics, many did not. Superimposed on the increasing numbers of Indian immigrants were the demographic effects of their lower age at marriage than among the Fijians, the higher proportion married, the higher birthrates, and their lower mortality. As a result, there was partial replacement of the indigenous, presumably adapted, gene pool by that of an alien population. The demographic differences between the two populations are a direct reflection of the cultural differences between them and their recent cultural history. The changes in gene frequency in the Fiji Islands after the initial Indian immigration have been due primarily to interpopulation differential mortality and fertility. There is no evidence that they are selective or that they make for increased fitness and increased adaptation of the population to the Fijian environment. They are not due to differences in the adaptive value of the individual biological characters; it was the whole population which was favored, and so the characters of all its component members, irrespective of whether they are biologically advantageous or disadvantageous.

Another way in which transition will affect genetic constitution is through the change in population size. A formerly stable population that suffers a sudden reduction in size, say by an epidemic disease after contact from outside or some other calamity, is going to develop a bottleneck situation. A typhoon on the island of Puka-Puka in the late eighteenth century swept away all the population except seventeen (Beaglehole and Beaglehole 1938), and the population lost all its genes for tall stature (Hulse 1957). This particular bottleneck was obviously an extreme, but similar phenomena occur time and time again. The genetic effect is difficult to establish if one assesses genetic constitution in terms of gene frequencies. One would need to have foresight to know that a change was going to occur, hindsight to know that it had finished. However, the effects are easily demonstrable by the PACK method. The population of Tristan da Cunha suffered a severe bottleneck in 1856 and 1857 when there was emigration of some two-thirds of the population, and again in 1885–91 when fifteen adult males were drowned in an accident at sea and the departures of their widows and children subsequently diminished the population to approximately half its size. In the first bottleneck the primary effect was to deprive the population of eight of its nineteen founder ancestors and a recent arrival, so that instead of the genes from twenty ancestors that were present in the gene pool in 1855, at the end of 1857 there were contributions from only eleven ancestors. Second, there was a change in their relative contributions. Genes from two of the principal contributors were among those that completely disappeared. The contribution of ancestor 1 was halved, that of ancestors 3 and 4 more than doubled. Four ancestors (nos. 3, 4, 9, and 10) now contributed 60 percent of the genes in the new population compared with their previous total of less than 29 percent. The profile of the ancestral contributions altered appreciably as a result of this first bottleneck. In the second bottleneck, again all the contributions (some 8 percent) were lost from four relatively recent arrivals, and there was a change in the proportional contributions of the remainder. Ancestors 3 and 4 again increased their contribution by about one-half, while that from ancestor 22 doubled and ancestor 10 was halved. If populations in transition, then, undergo massive reduction in size, their genetic resources diminish, and there is appreciable reduction in the genetic variability in the population. The early ethnological literature is full of accounts of depopulation (e.g., Rivers 1922), and the resulting impoverishment of the gene pools can only be imagined.

In a situation of changed population size, there is also alteration in the rate of change of genetic constitution as a result of genetic drift, as originally defined in terms of the random nature of the gametes that are transmitted. But there is one other effect that accompanies the increase in population that follows a bottleneck, and that is the retention of new variability. In a population which is in a state of numerical equilibrium, that is to say the average survival in each filial generation is two per pair of parents, the retention of a new mutation occurring as an isolated event is very unlikely. Of all such new mutations, 99.7 percent will be lost within a hundred generations if the mutation is neutral, and 97 percent even if it has a 1 percent selective advantage. To account for the accumulation of genetic variability, it seems that one has to postulate expansion of the population. If the total population is expanding, then all new mutants have a lower probability of extinction. If a few individuals contribute more than average numbers of children to each successive generation, then the mutant alleles they carry will tend to be retained. A transitional state that results in a great expansion of population size can be expected to lead to the retention of more mutants in the population, and if these mutants are deleterious, then the genetic load will proportionately increase. It has been suggested that the proportion of deleterious recessives in modern Europeans is unduly high on account of their (recent) expansion in numbers.

Genetic Structure

The Fijian example may be seen as a dichotomized genetic structure of recent origin. Such structuring may have quite pronounced public health implications. In the United Kingdom the presence of the Cypriot immigrant community with its high incidence of thalassemia led to the development of research and a successful antenatal diagnostic service. There was a similar program for Tay-Sachs disease in the Jewish communities of the Baltimore region. But there are some interesting examples of the direct effect of change on genetic structure. In a long-established population, with the destruction of the balance that exists, some of the first things to change are established custom, the long-established laws, the marriage laws governing choice of spouse, and therefore those elements of the genetic structure that are dependent on the mating pattern will themselves change. This may also occur following situations of bottleneck. On the island of Tristan da Cunha, for example, though a steady increase in the mean inbreeding level was inevitable, the first exodus boosted the levels of both the mean autosomal and the mean sex-linked inbreeding coefficients, for there were fewer members of the opposite sex of suitable age to marry. When the father of the first inbred individual wanted to marry in 1854, there were only seven women of marriageable age on the island (excluding his own sisters), and five of these were his first cousins, of whom he chose one of his own age. But after the first exodus, by the time of the third consanguineous marriage in 1871, there were no nonrelatives. Indeed, there were no other women available on the island, and neither were there at the time of the fourth consanguineous marriage in 1876.

The second exodus likewise produced a small change in the level of the mean autosomal inbreeding coefficient but a pronounced diminution in the mean sex-linked coefficient. These episodes of population size reduction also affected mean kinship in the population. The first exodus doubled the mean kinship coefficient between all members of the population and greatly reduced the number of pairs of individuals on the island who were not related to each other, that is, the percentage of zero coefficients. The second exodus did likewise but on a much smaller scale. These effects on genetic structure on Tristan are presumably due in large part to the fact that the emigrants were members of particular families, that is, it was family groups that emigrated. But such changes in the inbreeding level also occur in a mainstream population in transition, as shown by examples from the north of England.

A major type of transition that has occurred repeatedly is agriculture giving way to industry. How this affected the genetic structure in a south Northumberland parish is well illustrated (Roberts 1980). Previously the farming parish communities remained fairly constant in genetic constitution, with little immigration from outside. The little gene flow that there was tended to be essentially local — mainly within a parish, a little between adjacent parishes, and very little from more distant regions — so the total population consisted of small, local, partially isolated units. Whickham, today a suburb of Newcastle, was a rural community from Saxon times, maintaining an essentially subsistence livelihood in the traditional pattern of rural life until the agrarian revolution. This reached Whickham in 1672, when the first of the divisions of the common fields occurred. But the shape of things to come was foreshadowed as early as the mid-fourteeth century when mention was first made of the local coal, which was extracted on a small scale as a family and domestic industry until the sixteenth and early seventeenth centuries. Then, during the seventeenth century, the coal industry saw great expansion, coal extraction and export made a major contribution to the economic wealth of the region. The Industrial Revolution arrived in the 1690s, when ironworks were established in Whickham parish.

During the early eighteenth century the parish flourished, and then, with the working out of the local coal, the heavier industries moved to the less accessible coal seams downriver, toward the deeper waters capable of accommodating the larger ships bringing iron ore in from outside. A distinct ecological progression can be traced, from the simple colonist-style farming of the early Saxons, through the peasant farming of medieval times, followed by the development, slow at first, of domestic extractive industry and, subsequently, of larger manufacturing industry initially using local and then imported material, and finally its decay.

For present purposes, it is the middle part of the progression that is of interest, the transition from farming to industry. Records are available from 1580 onward. The numbers of marriages and baptisms per year suggest a stable, slowly increasing population from 1580 to 1700. There were, of course, quite pronounced fluctuations about the general level, associated with disasters, but in the first decades of the eighteenth century the annual number of marriages and baptisms rose above the previous peak levels, reaching a maximum about 1750. This period of greater increase in numbers coincided with the period of growth and prosperity of the iron factory. At the time of its foundation there were few skilled workmen in the parish, and men were brought in from elsewhere, an immigration which played an important part in the increase in total population size to the mid-eighteenth century.

Levels of the inbreeding coefficients were calculated by isonomy from 1579 to the mid-eighteenth century. There is a slight increase in the first fifteen years, compatible with a fairly stable or slowly growing population, and there is a slight positive nonrandom component at this period, but the general level actually varies little before the mid-seventeenth century. Then the period 1662 to 1686 shows a distinct fall, as does the period 1687 to 1711, and the level continues to remain low until 1787 to 1811, when it reaches its lowest point. The values are much below those observed in rural communities in mid-Northumberland. Whickham is unlikely to have been as isolated initially as the mid-Northumberland parishes, on account of its situation on an important waterway, its relative proximity to a city, and its situation on a major line of communication between that city and its hinterland. The coming of the Industrial Revolution, bringing as it did immigration from outside the locality, altered the characteristic marriage pattern, destroyed the partial isolation of the locality, and reduced the mean inbreeding level of the population to a tenth of what it was earlier. There is no doubt that the genetic structure of the Whickham population was profoundly altered by the coming of major industry and the associated population movement and increase.

An interesting example in a population undergoing twentieth-century transition is that in the French Pyrenees studied by Serre et al. (1985). The Pyrenean village Arthez-d'Asson, situated at the mouth of the Ouzom valley, until the eighteenth century was a peripheral hamlet of Asson, a large village situated six kilometers out in the plain. It obtained its religious autonomy in 1743 and its civil independence in 1787. The evolution of the population was traced by a derivative of the PACK method, and the history may be divided into three periods. After the first six generations, the period of establishment of the village, the second period, from the seventh to eleventh generation (end of the eighteenth century and the nineteenth), was one of stability. The third period (the twentieth century) saw an important rural exodus out of the valley toward the plain and the towns, and an increase in village exogamy. Over the whole history the mean inbreeding levels steadily increased, until in the latest generation it is one of the most inbred populations in France. The method of analysis allowed the separation of the total consanguinity into close (marriage between close relatives) and remote consanguinity. In the most recent generation there is a remarkable increase in remote consanguinity, and the pedigree analysis shows that the new genes that were apparently coming in from outside were in fact derived from the original gene pool and had been absent elsewhere for only a few generations. Thus some of the gene flow from outside, instead of increasing genetic heterogeneity, is in fact quite the reverse.

CONCLUSION

Population transitions can affect genetic constitution and genetic structure in a variety of ways. Gene frequencies may alter as a result of new arrivals, new selective pressures, or random changes resulting from calamities; there may be loss or enhancement of genetic variability, according to the direction of change in the population size. But perhaps equally, if not more, sensitive is genetic structure. One may detect changes in inbreeding levels, affecting the distribution and incidence of recessive and polygenic disorders; changes in kinship levels, affecting dominants; changes in the distance and gene pools from which incoming genes are drawn; and disturbance of linkage disequilibria and of coadapted gene complexes. As yet, relatively little effort has been devoted to tracing such processes and their effects, but, as evidenced here, methods are available and have been evaluated. The examples given suggest that continued efforts along these lines would be worthwhile.

REFERENCES

Beaglehole, E., and P. Beaglehole. 1938. Ethnology of Puka-Puka. *Memoirs of the Bishop Museum* 150.

Dahlberg, G. 1929. Inbreeding in man. *Genetics* 14:421–54.

Fisher, R. A. 1930. *Genetical Theory of Natural Selection.* Oxford: Clarendon.

Haldane, J. B. S. 1930. A mathematical theory of natural and artificial selection. VI. Isolation. Proceedings of the Cambridge Philosophical Society. 26:220–30.

Harpending, H. 1974. Genetic structure of small populations. *Annual Review of Anthropology.* 3:229–43.

Hulse, F. S. 1957. Some factors influencing the relative proportions of human racial stocks. Cold Spring Harbor Symposia on Quantitative Biology. 22:33–45.

Jacquard, A. 1974. *The Genetic Structure of Populations.* New York: Springer-Verlag.

Kimura, M. 1955. Stochastic processes and distribution of gene frequencies under natural selection. *Cold Spring Harbor Symposia on Quantitative Biology.* 20:33–53.

Malecot, G. 1948. *Les mathematiques de l'heredite.* Paris: Masson et Cie.

Maruyama, T. 1970. Rate of decrease of genetic variability in a subdivided population. *Biometrica* 57:229–311.

Morton, N. E. 1969. Human population structure. *Annual Review of Genetics* 3:53–74.

Rivers, W. H. R. 1922. *Essays on the Depopulation of Melanesia.* Cambridge: Cambridge University Press.

Roberts, D. F. 1980. Inbreeding and ecological change; an isonymic analysis of a Tyneside parish over three centuries. *Social Biology* 27:230–40.

Roberts, D. F., and R. W. Hiorns. 1962. The dynamics of racial intermixture. *American Journal of Human Genetics* 14:261–77.

Roberts, D. F., and M. Mohan. 1976. History, demography and genetics: the Fiji experience and its evolutionary implications. *Journal of Human Evolution* 5:117.

Serre, J. L., L. Jakobi, and M. C. Babron. 1985. A genetic isolate in the French Pyrenees: Probability of origin of genes and inbreeding. *Journal of Biosocial Science* 17:405.

Spuhler, J. N. 1963. The scope for natural selection in man. In *Genetic Selection in Man.* W. J. Schull, ed. Ann Arbor: University of Michigan Press.

Wahlund, V. S. 1928. Zusmmensetzung von Populationen und korrelationsercheinungen vom standpunkt der vererbungslehre aus betrachtet. *Hereditas* 11:65–106.

Wright, S. 1931. Evolution in Mendelian populations. *Genetics* 16:97–159.

2 INFECTIOUS DISEASE AND NATURAL SELECTION IN HUMAN POPULATIONS: A CRITICAL REEXAMINATION

Catharina Svanborg-Eden and
Bruce R. Levin

Infectious disease has been proposed as a major selective force in evolution, as well as an important factor maintaining genetic variation within and between populations. Charles Darwin, in 1871, stated that "New diseases and vices have in some cases proven highly destructive; and it appears that a new disease causes much death until those most susceptible to its destructive influences are gradually weeded out." In the position paper of the disease and evolution school, J. B. S. Haldane (1949) presented compelling arguments for infectious diseases as agents of natural selection, in view of their role as major causes of mortality and reduced fertility in natural populations of higher organisms. He also proposed disease-mediated selection as a general mechanism maintaining biochemical variation in populations, an interpretation that has been championed and expanded upon by B. Clarke (1976, 1979). Selection mediated by infectious disease has also been postulated as the mechanism responsible for the evolution and maintenance of sexual reproduction in eukaryotes (Hamilton 1982).

The significance of infectious disease as a cause of mortality and morbidity certainly provides it with the potential for being a strong selective force in human populations. The 1346–1350 epidemic of bubonic plague is considered responsible for killing nearly one-third of the population of Europe. The 1918–1919 influenza epidemic was responsible for more than 20 million deaths (McNeill 1976). It has been argued that until relatively recent times, mortality due to infectious disease in densely populated urban areas was so high that cities could not maintain their populations without immigration from the countryside (McNeill 1976). This may still be the case in recently urbanized parts of the world. And, worldwide, enteric and respiratory tract infections are the major cause of infant mortality. Collectively, infectious disease (including parasitism) remains the dominant cause of mortality and morbidity in young adults (Pio 1985; Shann 1986).

The proposition is compelling that infectious disease has been a major force in human evolution and is responsible for maintaining genetic variation within and between human populations. However, the theory of disease-mediated selection has limitations that have not been adequately considered, and some of the modest empirical evidence put forth in support of these propositions has inferential problems. In this chapter we describe these theoretical limitations, outline the requirements for an unqualified empirical demonstration of disease-mediated selection, and consider how well existing evidence fits these requirements. We propose that current information on the molecular mechanisms of infectious disease suggests systems where the potential role of disease-mediated selection may be evaluated.

THEORETICAL CONSIDERATIONS

Conditions for Effective Disease-Mediated Selection

An agent of natural selection is effective when it overrides the influence of stochastic factors (genetic drift and founder effects) in determining the genetic structure of populations. For infectious disease to act as an effective agent of directional or balancing selection, the following criteria must be met.

1. There is inherited variation in susceptibility to disease within populations.

2. This inherited variation is determined by one gene or a few major genes acting alone or collectively in a largely additive manner.

3. There is relatively little nongenetic (environmental) contribution to variation in the likelihood or magnitude of infection or the physiological response to it.

4. Variation in susceptibility to disease is manifest prior to the termination of reproduction (during ages of high reproductive value; Fisher 1958).

5. There are differences in the rates of mortality and/or fertility among susceptible and resistant individuals (selection coefficients much greater than the reciprocal of the population size; Crow and Kimura 1970).

6. The population encounters the infectious agent(s) continuously or at frequent intervals.

We conjecture that in humans, (1) there are only a few situations where the conditions for effective disease-mediated selection will obtain; and (2) much of this selection will be for evolutionary stasis, that is, the purging of mutations that reduce the effectiveness of the already-evolved defenses. Our view of these constraints on disease-mediated selection is based on a consideration of the nature of infection and resistance, upon which we now expand.

Infection and Levels of Resistance

The establishment and maintenance of a parasite population is the end result of a sequence of interactions between the parasite and its host. At each step in the infectious process, the persistence of the parasite is challenged by one or more of the host defenses. The balance between the host and the parasite may be altered by defects in host resistance and/or by special virulence of the parasite. Virulence can be defined as the sum of the properties permitting the parasite to proceed through the infectious process uninterrupted by host defenses. A resistant host, on the other hand, is able to interrupt an infection at an earlier stage than a sensitive one. Neither virulence nor resistance is an all-or-none phenomenon. In hosts that are highly susceptible or have compromised defenses, avirulent and commensal organisms can be pathogenic. The same disease condition, by all diagnostic criteria, may result from the interaction of highly virulent organisms with a resistant host, or of avirulent organisms with a highly susceptible host. Resistance to infection can be rationalized into two major categories: exposure and host defenses. Individuals may vary in the extent of exposure to micro-organisms and in the effectiveness of their defenses following exposure. Theoretically, all of this variation could have a genetic component and be subject to disease-mediated selection.

Disease-Mediated Selection Operating on Variation in Exposure

The diversity and density of pathogens in the environment depends primarily on geographic and temporal factors and the densities of the host populations. Consequently, the species of parasites and pathogens and the levels of exposure to them can be expected to vary among populations in different geographic areas, as well as within populations in single locales. For humans, these exposure rates would be greatly influenced by age, sex, and a variety of cultural factors, such as living conditions and socioeconomic status. Access to clean water is probably the single most important factor contributing to variation in exposure to enteric pathogens and waterborne parasites. Population density would play a critical role in the rate of exposure to droplet and airborne viruses and other microbes (Anderson and May 1982).

While we cannot formally rule out the possibility that there are inherited components to some of the cultural factors contributing to the variation in rates of exposure to parasites, such as the desire to drink clean water or to live in uncrowded areas, we would not want to champion such a hypothesis. Furthermore, even if there were genetic components to this variation, the conditions outlined above for infectious disease to be an effective selective agent make it unlikely that this type of genetic variation will serve as good fodder for natural selection.

Disease-Mediated Selection Operating on Variation in the General and Specific Host Defenses

Given access to a host, a parasite has to traverse a gauntlet of general (nonimmune) and specific (immune) defenses before it can establish its population. Among exposed hosts, two components of the nonimmune defenses represent the major barrier to infection: skin and mucous membranes. In the absence of trauma or vectors (e.g., biting insects), microparasites such as protozoans, bacteria, and viruses rarely penetrate the skin. Mucosal membranes line the portals of entry that are heavily exposed to parasites, like those of the respiratory and gastrointestinal tracts. These serve as habitats for the "normal" flora, which, by competition for space and resources and by the production of allelopathic substances (such as bacteriocins), inhibit the growth of pathogenic microbes and act as a blockade against pathogens penetrating into the underlying tissue. Contributing to the mucosal barrier function are mechanical factors (flow secretions, peristalsis, ciliary movements) and antibacterial substances (e.g., mucus, lactoferrin, peroxidase). Parasites that make it past the skin or mucosal membranes encounter the tissue elements of the nonimmune defense system. Included among these are fixed and migrating phagocytic cells, iron-binding proteins, bactericidal compounds in the serum, complement, acute phase reactants, and others.

Although populations may vary in the specific parasites and pathogens they encounter and the overall magnitude of their parasite burden, frequent confrontations with wide varieties of micro- and macroparasites is a general feature of all populations. For this reason, it seems unlikely that disease-mediated selection would lead to variation in the generalized nonimmune defenses within or between human populations. Furthermore, because of the compensatory nature of the different nonimmune defenses, a mutation leading to a modest increase in effectiveness of one component is unlikely to engender a substantial fitness advantage. On the other hand, mutations completely destroying the function of one or more component of the nonimmune host defense system are likely to engender a substantial disadvantage.

The nonimmune defenses may be highly specific and, as such, provide potential mechanisms for disease-mediated selection. For example, pathogenic microbes may overcome elimination (due to competition with the normal flora or mechanical factors) by attaching to components of the mucosal membrane. Attachment can be highly specific and involve the binding of bacterial surface components to receptors on epithelial cells or their products. Thus, selection would favor phenotypic differences that could be attributed to variation in single genes, such as parasites with specific attachment sites and hosts with altered receptors. If parasites and pathogens with this capacity to bind to specific receptors have limited geographic ranges, such selection could result in inherited interpopulation variation in the susceptibility to diseases caused by these organisms. It is also conceivable that disease-mediated selection on receptor site variation could maintain stable polymorphisms, for example, if the heterozygoses for the variant receptor have an advantage.

Disease-Mediated Selection Operating on Variation in the Immune Response

The immune system differs from the nonimmune defenses in that it is adaptive: its effectiveness increases after exposure to microbial antigens, cross-reacting antigens, or polyclonal stimulators, in other words, the phenomenon of immunity. The mucosal surfaces have a specialized immune system — IgA antibodies — that are secreted in molecular form and are capable of operating in seemingly inhospitable environments, such as the stomach and large intestine. These IgA antibodies bind to and aggregate microbes and toxins. Parasites that traverse the skin or mucosal membranes — generally an extremely small minority of those to which the host is exposed — confront circulating antibodies of the immune system. These protect the host by, (1) directly blocking viruses and toxins from binding to host cells; and (2) marking bacteria and other parasites for phagocytosis, lysis by complement, and discovery by marauding microphages. In addition, specific classes of immune system cells, sensitized "T" cells, kill "target cells" that bear foreign antigens, such as protozoans and fungi, as well as host cells that are infected with viruses (Amman and Fudenberg 1976).

The immune system responds to a diverse array of parasites and pathogens by a form of somatic cell evolution called "clonal selection" (Jerne 1974) which, to a large extent, precludes the need for germ-line evolution. As a consequence of acquired immunity to parasites and pathogens, the intensity of selection favoring specific resistance to those organisms is likely to be weak. Thus, even if there were major gene mutations that increased specific resistances, selection for them would only be effective if the immune system were ineffective in controlling that parasite or pathogen. While mutations that augment the general effectiveness of the immune system would be favored by disease-mediated selection, for the same reasons given for the generalized nonimmune defenses, we would not expect this selection to lead to genetic variation within or between populations. On the other hand, we would expect that mutations impairing the immune system would be under intense negative selection due to the action of infectious disease.

The immune system is open to at least one major form of disease-mediated selection. As a consequence of the need to distinguish self from foreign, it offers little protection against parasites that mimic host antigens. If such mimicking parasites represent a significant cause of mortality or reduction in fertility, selection would favor host mutations that alter the primary antigens involved in the recognition of self. As hosts with these novel antigens become more common, parasite selection would be increasingly directed at mimicking them. As these parasite mutants increased in frequency, selection in the host population would then favor mutants with other rare self-recognition antigens. The net effect of this mutual frequency-dependent process would be the stable maintenance of polymorphisms at the loci coding for these self-recognition antigens. This type of selection was proposed by Haldane (1949) and Clarke (1976) as a general mechanism for maintaining biochemical diversity and by Bodmer and Bodmer (1978) for the maintenance of allelic diversity observed at histocompatibility loci.

EMPIRICAL EVIDENCE FOR DISEASE-MEDIATED SELECTION

Evidence for the action of infectious disease as an agent of natural selection can be obtained from studies of genetic variation within or between populations. It is our feeling that at this time the only compelling evidence for this selection is from studies of within-population variation, and, when considered critically, the magnitude of this evidence is modest at best.

Evidence for Disease-Mediated Selection from Studies of Within-Population Variation

Disease-Mediated Selection Against Occasional Variants

Populations may maintain one functional phenotype with respect to resistance to many infectious agents. The physiological basis for these disease-resistant phenotypes may be attributed to a single host resistance factor or a number of factors. Regardless of the genetic basis of the resistance, occasional sensitive variants would be subject to increased mortality and morbidity due to disease and, as such, would be selected against. One interpretation of this is that the predominance of the resistant phenotypes is not coincidental (a spandrel, in the sense of Gould and Lewontin 1979) but rather the consequence of past and present disease-mediated selection. There are a number of examples of this type of evidence for disease-mediated selection in humans.

1. Complement defects. Complement is a cascade of serum factors which operate in a sequential and additive manner. The end point of the action of complement is the death of the complement-fixing cells, to which it adheres. This may be achieved through one of three pathways: the classical pathway, where complement factor C1 binds to antibody molecules and lyses the antibody-coated cell; the alternative pathway, where the complement component C3 is activated directly; or the properdin system with resulting lysis (Cooper 1976). Individuals lack-

ing complement factors C1, C4, and C2 are subject to immune complex disease. Individuals lacking complement factors C3 to C9 have an increased risk of death due to meningococcal or gonococcal septicemia (Ammen and Fudenberg 1976).

2. Immunodeficiencies. Severe combined immunodeficiency is a condition in which infants are born without the cells required for a specific immune response. This results in early death due to infection.

Hypogammaglobulinemia signifies the absence of all immunoglobulin classes or the production of low levels of these antibody molecules. This disease occurs in early onset (X-linked, Vogel and Motulski 1987) and late onset forms and results, for example, in a generalized susceptibility to respiratory tract infections with encapsulated bacteria.

Deficiencies in single antibody classes, for example, the IgG subclasses of IgA, have a less clear relationship to susceptibility to infection than deficiencies in multiple classes of immunoglobulin molecules. Nevertheless, individuals with inherited deficiencies in single antibody classes appear to be more liable to infection than normal individuals. For example, IgA-deficient individuals have an increased susceptibility to traveler's diarrhea and a higher incidence of late onset autoimmune diseases (Hanson, Soderstrom and Oxelius 1976). Presumably, the modest deleterious effects of IgA deficiency are a consequence of compensatory production of other components of the host defenses (e.g., secretory IgM).

As would be predicted from population genetic theory, the frequencies of these complement and immunological defects in the population are inversely related to the liability to infections (the intensity of selection). Severe combined immunodeficiency and late complement factor defects are rare, and it seems reasonable to assume that their occurrence can be explained by a balance between mutation and intense disease-mediated selection against individuals with these defects. IgA deficiency, on the other hand, occurs in about one in 600 individuals and is the most prevalent immunodeficiency.

Disease-Mediated Selection Operating on Standing Genetic Variation (Genetic Polymorphisms)

Individuals within populations may vary in their susceptibility to infectious disease. If this variation has a genetic basis, disease-mediated selection may (or may not) be responsible for maintaining the polymorphism. The methodological problem is to eliminate nongenetic factors so as to obtain evidence for the action of this selection. For this the following criteria must be met:

1. The etiological agent of the disease has been identified.
2. Infections due to this pathogen can be differentiated from other diseases with similar symptoms.

3. The genetic basis of the variation in susceptibility is known, and the phenotype can be assessed independently of the disease.

With this background, population data can be used to ascertain whether selection operates on the disease-associated phenotype. If this selection does operate, then among populations there could be a correlation between the incidence of the disease and the frequency of the genotypes at the loci involved. And, within populations, there should be differences in mortality, morbidity, and/or fertility associated with that phenotype and disease. Unfortunately, correlative evidence is not sufficient, and the direct demonstration of fitness differences is not an easy task. Whether or not exposure to the disease will have a demonstrable effect on the relative fitness of individuals depends on the mode of inheritance of that phenotype, the incidence of the disease, and other factors affecting mortality and fertility. Furthermore, even when there are substantial fitness differences among genotypes of single loci (the best case), the sample size needed to demonstrate those differences may be too great to make that direct demonstration feasible (see Chapter 3 by J. Barrett herein).

Sickle Cell Anemia

By far the best known example of this type of evidence for disease-mediated selection is the sickle cell, HbA-HbS polymorphism in humans. The genetic basis of this hemoglobin difference is well understood: alleles of a single structural gene. The frequency of the near-lethal HbS allele is directly related to the incidence of falciparum malaria, an endemic disease attributable to infections by a single protozoan species, *Plasmodium falciparum*. Among populations there is a direct correlation between the incidence of this type of malaria and the frequency of the HbS allele. And, most critically, among individuals exposed to this parasite within a population, HbA/HbS heterozygotes have higher rates of survival than HbA/HbA homozygoses (Allison 1954).

While some details of the processes responsible for the fitness advantage of sickle heterozygoses are not known, the basic mechanism is understood. At low oxygen tensions there are reduced survival rates for *Plasmodium falciparum* infecting HbA/HbS erythrocytes, relative to the rates for those infecting HbA/HbA erythrocytes (Friedman 1978), and HbS has a detrimental effect on the parasites' capacity to invade and multiply in red cells (Pasvol, Weatherall, and Wilson 1978). Although it is not essential to the hypothesis of disease-mediated selection, the fitness advantage of the HbA/HbS heterozygote in the presence of falciparum malaria provides a sufficient explanation for the maintenance of this polymorphism.

While there is evidence for the association of other genetically well-characterized hemoglobin polymorphisms with the incidence of malaria (Livingstone 1958; Flint et al. 1986), to our mind, none is as strong as that for sickle cell. In fact, we are unaware of any other examples of disease-mediated selection operating on standing genetic variation that come as close as sickle cell to fulfilling the criteria listed above. Perhaps if there were such examples, the sickle cell story wouldn't be told so often as the example of disease-mediated selection and also as the example of heterosis maintaining genetic polymorphisms.

Bacterial Attachment

While not compelling as the sickle cell story, there is some emerging evidence for disease-mediated selection derived from studies of the molecular mechanisms of infectious disease. Pigs offer an elegant example of this type of evidence for disease-mediated selection. Since this example is probably not well known by the readers of this volume, some expansion seems warranted.

Neonatal diarrhea in piglets results in loss of up to 20 percent of newborn animals. The virulence of the *E. coli* bacteria causing the diarrhea has been shown, by genetic techniques, to depend on the combination of attachment to the epithelial surface of the intestinal tract and production of a toxin (Smith and Halls 1972). Susceptibility is inherited as an autosomal recessive trait (Sellwood et al. 1975) and is determined by the presence of receptors in the intestine. *E. coli* attach to the intestinal lining of the susceptible piglets but not to that of the resistant phenotypes (Sellwood et al. 1975). The progeny of susceptible sows that have recovered are less likely to succumb to this infection than those of heterozygous sows. Vaccination of heterozygous sows results in protection of the piglets by production of antiadhesive antibodies in the milk of the sow. At this juncture, it is not clear how the susceptible phenotype is maintained.

Parallel phenomena of inherited variation in the capacity of pathogens to adhere to mucosal surfaces in humans may also reflect the action of disease-mediated selection. The *E. coli* causing urinary tract infections, and especially those responsible for acute pyelonephritis, bind to receptors in the uroepithelial cells (Leffler and Svanborg-Eden 1980, 1986). The receptors have been identified as glycolipids of the globo series with the common disaccharide Gal. α 1–4 Gal β (Lomberg et al. 1986). These structures are antigens in the P blood group system (P1, P2, and $\bar{p}$). Individuals of blood group P1 express the three structures; P2 individuals lack the P1 and have less of the P antigen. The P1 individuals comprise approximately 75 percent of the population and P2 approximately 25 percent. Individuals of the $\bar{p}$ blood group phenotype lack a glycosyl transferase required to add Gal. α 1–4 Gal β to glycolipid and glycoprotein oligosaccharide. Cells from $\bar{p}$ individuals thus lack functional receptors for attaching *E. coli*. The frequency of $\bar{p}$ individuals is extremely low — about 75 known cases in the world. Since acute pyelonephritis was a lethal disease prior to the advent of antibiotics, and $\bar{p}$ individuals are somewhat resistant to this disease, one might have expected to find the $\bar{p}$ blood group to be in higher frequency. There is, however, likely to be selection against the $\bar{p}$ allele in the following way: women of the $\bar{p}$ blood group who carry fetuses of the P1 or P2 antigen phenotypes have an increased frequency of abortions, a potential case of selection against the heterozygote.

The low frequency of individuals of the $\bar{p}$ blood group precludes a direct evaluation of the relative morbidity and mortality (fitnesses) of the P1, P2, and $\bar{p}$ alleles due to selection mediated by urinary tract infections. On the other hand, there is indirect evidence for this character being under disease-mediated selection. Individuals of the P1 blood group phenotype have about an elevenfold higher relative risk of attracting recurrent kidney infections compared to P2 individuals (Lomberg et al. 1981). An additional blood group parameter, secretor state, which determines the density of the P blood group receptors on epithelial cells, is similarly overrepresented (Lomberg et al. 1986).

Familial Variation in Susceptibility to Cholera

Controlling for the contribution of environmental factors may well be the major obstacle to obtaining evidence for a causal association between disease and the fitness of genotypes. One way to control for these environmental effects is to examine the progress of a disease among individuals living together, such as members of the same family. One example of family data providing evidence for disease-mediated selection comes from a recent investigation by Glass et al. (1982).

As part of the study of a cholera epidemic in Bangladesh, the ABO blood group of the population was recorded for infected and uninfected people. Individuals exposed to cholera were examined familywise for the severity of infection. Infected individuals of blood group O had a hospitalization rate of about 60 percent – significantly greater than the approximately 30 percent hospitalization rate for infected family members of other blood groups. Although no mechanistic explanation has been given, it seems reasonable to postulate that blood group O individuals have more mucosal receptors for the V. cholerae – a testable hypothesis.

It is interesting that the frequency of blood group O in Bangladesh is one of the lowest so far described (Mourant et al. 1976). On the other hand, it is important to resist the temptation of assuming this, or other disease-mediated selection, is responsible for maintaining the ABO blood group polymorphism.

Histocompatibility Loci

The histocompatibility loci of the HLA complex seem to have a part in almost every recent review of the genetic basis of susceptibility to noninfectious as well as infectious disease in humans. On à priori grounds these loci appear to be particularly good candidates for the operation of disease-mediated selection. They are extremely polymorphic, play a prominent role in the generation of immunity, and have been proposed, although not shown, to serve as receptors for parasites and pathogens. As a consequence of their role in the recognition of self, they would also be good subjects for parasite mimicry. In either case, there would be selection at the HLA for alleles coding for novel antigens. Nevertheless, despite extensive study, evidence that infectious disease is responsible for selection at the HLA loci is limited and, in our opinion, very much weaker than for the preceding examples.

In their treatise on histocompatibility, Snell, Daussett, and Nathenson (1976) cite three lines of evidence which they interpret to be inconsistent with the receptor hypothesis. First, in spite of the extreme polymorphism of the HLA system, many common viruses, such as influenza, are able to infect almost everyone. Second, the adsorption and replication of two RNA viruses (ECHO virus and measles virus) and two DNA viruses (herpes virus and adenovirus) on fibroblasts typed for HLA were found to be unrelated to HLA type, although there is some recent evidence for an association between HLA haplotype and symptomatic measles (R. Anderson, personal communication). Finally, three enteroviruses (poliovirus, Coxsackie B3, and ECHO virus 11) are able to replicate on man-mouse hybrid cells that have lost their HLA antigens.

Snell, Daussett, and Nathenson (1976) discuss a variety of observations they interpret as support of the mimicry hypothesis for histocompatibility systems. Antigens derived from bacteria either cross-react with the transplantation antigens of rodents and rabbits or induce hypersensitivity to skin allografts of the same kind as that resulting from pretreatment with allogenic material. Snell, Daussett, and Nathenson (1976) also cite evidence that the M1 protein from *Streptococcus pyogenes* has a structural similarity with human HLA antigens. Although the number of bacterial species capable of producing these mimicking antigens appears to be limited, their existence certainly suggests that this form of disease-mediated selection may be occurring at the HLA loci. On the other hand, we are unaware of any direct evidence that parasite and pathogen mimicry cause differential survival or reproduction of individuals of different HLA types.

Variation Between Populations

Geographically and racially distinct populations vary in the incidence and the severity of infection. High infection frequency and severe symptoms have been used to define susceptibility of populations, whereas low infection frequencies or modest clinical signs have been equated with resistance. It is possible that interpopulation variation in susceptibility to infectious disease reflects underlying genetic differences that may be under disease-mediated selection.

Unfortunately, except in situations where populations differ in the frequencies of alleles of well-characterized loci, inferences about a genetic basis for interpopulation variation are necessarily limited, for any phenotype. In the case of susceptibility to infectious disease, we consider this line of evidence to be particularly weak. A plethora of environmental and cultural factors—such as climate, living conditions, and sanitation—would have a profound effect on the species and densities of parasites and pathogens among host populations. Interpopulation variation in culture, nutrition, and hygiene will greatly affect the rate at which individuals are infected and the course of the disease among infected individuals.

An additional level of complication is conferred by the immune system and what can be called immunological sophistication. Immune-mediated resistance to infection is a function of both natural and induced immunity. The induction of immunity is exposure dependent. The lack of immunity in an unexposed population cannot be equated with genetic susceptibility, and increased resistance in a previously exposed and immune population cannot be equated with resistance.

As a consequence of immunological processes, one would expect substantial interpopulation variation in the frequency and severity of endemic and novel diseases. The overall immunity of individuals to infectious agents and the apparent resistance of populations is likely to be directly related to the number of distinct species of parasites that induce an immune response. Cross-reacting antigens or idiotypes (Jerne 1974; Bona 1980) could produce in individuals a partial and possibly complete immunity to parasites and pathogens they have never encountered. Thus, differences in the diversity and density of parasites and pathogens among populations may influence their susceptibility to infectious disease due to variation in immunological sophistication rather than to genetic factors.

Genetic Diversity and Susceptibility to Disease

There is a tradition of assuming a direct relationship between the genetic diversity maintained in a population and its collective fitness (Dobzhansky 1951, 1963) and evidence for a positive correlation between the heterozygosity and the fitness of individual organisms (e.g., Mitton and Grant 1984). Although the physiological basis of this association between fitness and heterozygosity has yet to be elucidated, theoretically there are mechanisms that could account for it (Clarke 1976, 1979; Turelli and Ginzberg 1983). There is, in fact, a positive correlation between the estimated genetic diversity of human populations and their susceptibility to infectious disease (see Chapter 4 by Francis Black herein).

In spite of the appeal of these arguments and correlative data, we see this diversity-susceptibility association as weak evidence for the operation of disease-mediated selection. Almost all of the caveats associated with inferences for a genetic basis for phenotypic differences among populations still apply. While variation in overall genetic diversity can be considered "a well-characterized genetic difference," in the absence of a mechanism to account for the association of the studied marker with disease, one cannot extract cause from correlation. Furthermore, the same processes that reduce the genetic diversity of populations — small population size and founder effects — would also reduce the diversity of parasites and pathogens maintained in those populations and thus their immunological sophistication.

CONCLUSION AND IMPLICATIONS

We challenge the proposition that selection mediated by infectious disease is a major factor in the evolution and maintenance of genetic variability in human populations. We conjecture that in recent and contemporary human populations, the primary effect of infectious disease as an agent of natural selection is to maintain already-evolved defenses.

Three constraints prevent infectious disease from serving as an effective agent of natural selection.

1. Most variation in the frequency of infections can be attributed to environmental factors.

2. An array of host defenses is general in its action and overlapping in its functions.

3. The specific immune defenses are adaptive at the somatic level and, as such, reduce the intensity of (and need for) selection leading to germ-line evolution.

Empirical evidence for the operation of disease-mediated selection in humans (and other species) is modest at best. Some of this evidence supports the proposition that selection is for evolutionary stasis — the persistence of already-evolved defenses — rather than the evolution of new ones. There are few unequivocal examples of disease-mediated selection operating on standing genetic variation in human populations. The dearth of this evidence is particularly apparent when infectious disease (parasitism) is suggested as the primary factor responsible for maintaining genetic variation within populations (the motivation for many studies of the association between the incidence of disease and allelic polymorphisms). While there are examples of differences in susceptibility to infectious disease among human populations, we are unaware of any cases where these differences have a demonstrated genetic base, much less an origin in the differential operation of disease-mediated selection.

Lest our subtlety fool the reader, our position in this issue is largely heuristic. We accept the proposition that infectious disease has been and remains the major cause of morbidity and mortality in human populations, that is, is a very reasonable candidate as an agent of selection. Unlike most evolutionary questions, where evidence for the operation of natural selection can only be drawn from historical considerations, the action of disease-mediated selection can be studied in extant populations. Even in the best case — as is clearly illustrated by single gene selection (see Chapter 3 herein) — the sample size necessary for a direct demonstration of disease-mediated selection may be too large to be practical for studies of human populations.

For this reason, we believe that the study of disease-mediated selection should focus on situations where this selection would be likely. Studies of the mechanisms of virulence and resistance suggest two general classes of phenotypes that are likely candidates for the operation of disease-mediated selection: (1) host-determined characters critical to the infectious process that can be modified by changes at single loci (called "resistance factors"), like the receptor sites for adherence of bacteria and adsorption of viruses, and metabolic defects in cells that inhibit the survival and reproduction of intracellular parasites; and (2) host antigens (and idiotypes) that contribute to the recognition of self that may be mimicked by micro-organisms.

Although with realistic sample sizes it may not be possible to demonstrate disease-associated differences in mortality or fertility among genotypes at specific loci, it may be possible to obtain statistically significant data for differential susceptibility and morbidity. It is our feeling that the most promising source of this data is from within population studies in which control for environmental factors can be obtained, as in the family study of cholera morbidity and the ABO blood group (Glass et al. 1982). It may also be possible to estimate the intensity of disease-mediated selection from the rates of morbidity and mortality associated with rare deficiencies in one or more host defenses and the effects of medical intervention on those rates.

NOTE

We wish to thank George Armelagos, John Barrett, David Gordon, Dillon Scott, and Alan Swedlund for their comments, and those who support BITnet for providing an interuniversity computer network. Funds for this research were provided by the Swedish Medical Research Council, the Swedish Board for Technical Development, the Lundberg Foundation (CS-E), and the U.S. National Institutes of Health, GM33782 (BRL).

REFERENCES

Allison, A. C. 1954. Protection afforded by sickle cell trait against malarial infection. *British Medical Journal* 290–94.

Amman, A. J., and H. H. Fudenberg. 1976. Immunodeficiency diseases. In H. H. Fudenberg, D. P. Stites, J. L. Caldwell, and J. V. Wells, eds. *Basic and Clinical Immunology*, Los Gatos, Calif.: Lange Medical Publications.

Anderson, R. M., and R. M. May. 1982. Directly transmitted infectious disease: control by vaccination. *Science* 215:1053–60.

Bodmer, W., and J. Bodmer. 1978. Evolution and function of the HLA system. *British Medical Bulletin* 34:309–16.

Bona, C. A. 1980. Inverse fluctuations of idiotypes and anti-idiotypes during the immune response. In *Regulation of Immune Response Dynamics*. I. C. Delisi and J. T. J. Hiernaux, eds. Boca Raton, Fla.: CRC Press.

Clarke, B. C. 1979. The evolution of genetic diversity. *Proceedings of the Royal Society of London*, Ser. B. 205:453–74.

———. 1976. The ecological genetics of host-parasite relationships. In *Genetic Aspects of Host-Parasite Relationships*. A. E. R. Taylor and R. Muller, eds. Oxford: Blackwell.

Cooper, N. R. 1976. The complement system. In *Basic and Clinical Immunology*. H. H. Fudenberg, D. P. Stites, J. L. Caldwell, and J. V. Wells, eds. Lange Medical Publications.

Crow, J. F., and M. Kimura. 1970. *Introduction to Population Genetic Theory*. New York: Harper and Row.

Darwin, C. 1871. *The Descent of Man and Selection in Relation to Sex.* Reprinted 1960, New York: Modern Library, Random House.

Dobzhansky, T. 1963. *Mankind Evolving.* New York: Columbia University Press.

————. 1951. *Genetics and the Origin of the Species.* 3d ed. New York: Columbia University Press.

Fisher, R. A. 1958. *The Genetical Theory of Natural Selection.* New York: Dover Press.

Flint, J., A. V. S. Hill, D. K. Bowden, S. J. Openheimer, P. R. Sill, S. W. Serjeantson, J. Bana-Koiri, K. Bhatia, M. P. Alpers, A. J. Boyce, D. J. Weatherall, and J. B. Clegg. 1986. High frequencies of thalassemia are the result of natural selection by malaria. *Nature* 321:744–49.

Friedman, M. J. 1978. Erythrocyte mechanism of sickle cell resistance to malaria. *Proceedings of the National Academy of Sciences* USA 75:1994–97.

Glass R. I., J. Holmgren, C. E. Haley, M. R. Khan, A. Svennerholm, B. J. Stoll, K. M. Belayet Hossain, R. E. Black, M. Yunus, and D. Barua. 1982. Predisposition for cholera of individuals with O blood group: Possible evolutionary significance. *American Journal of Epidemiology* 121:791–96.

Gould, S. J., and R. C. Lewontin. 1979. The spandrels of San Marco and the Panglossian paradigm: A critique of the adaptionist programme. *Proceedings of the Royal Society of London.* Ser. B. 205:581–98.

Haldane, J. B. S. 1949. Disease and evolution. Supplement to *La Ricerca Scientifica* 19:68–76.

Hamilton, W. D. 1982. Pathogens as a cause of genetic diversity in host populations. In *Population Biology of Infectious Disease.* R. M. Anderson and R. M. May, eds. New York: Springer-Verlag.

Hanson, L. A., T. Soderstrom, and V. A. Oxelius. 1976. *Immunoglobulin Subclass Deficiencies.* Monographs in Allergy. Basel: Karger.

Jerne, N. K. 1974. Towards a network theory of the immune system. Annales Immunologie Institute de Pasteur 125C.:373.

Leffler, H., and C. Svanborg-Eden. 1986 Glycolipids as receptors for *E. coli* lectins and adhesins. In *Microbial Lectins*, D. Mirelman, ed. New York: Wiley.

————. 1980. Chemical identification of a glycosphingolipid receptor for *E. coli*, attaching to human uroepithelial cells and agglutinating human erythrocytes. *FEMS Microbiology Letters* 8:127–34.

Livingstone, F. B. 1958. Anthropological implications of sickle cell gene distribution in West Africa. *American Anthropologist* 60:533–62.

Lomberg, H., B. Cedergren, H. Leffler, B. Nilsson, A. S. Carlstrom, and C. Svanborg-Eden. 1986. Influence of blood-group on the availability of receptors for attachment of uropathogenic *E. coli. Infection and Immunity* 51:919–26.

Lomberg, H., C. Svanborg-Eden, H. Leffler, and B. Samuelsson. 1981. P1 blood-group and urinary tract infection. *Lancet* 1:551–52.

McNeill, W. H. 1976. *Plagues and People.* New York: Anchor Press.

Mitton, J. B., and M. C. Grant. 1984. Association among protein heterozygosity, growth rate and developmental homeostasis. *Annual Review of Ecology and Systematics* 15:479–99.

Mourant, A., E. Ada, C. Koepec, and K. Diomaniewska-Sobczak. 1976. *The Distribution of Human Bloodgroups and Other Polymorphisms.* 2d ed. London: Oxford Press.

Pasvol, G., D. J. Weatherall, and R. J. M. Wilson. 1978. Cellular mechanism for the protective effect of haemoglobin S against *P. falciparum* malaria. *Nature* 274:701–03.

Pio, A. 1985. Acute respiratory infections in developing countries: An international point of view. *Pediatric Infectious Disease* vol. 5:179–83.

Sellwood, R., R. A. Gibbons, G. W. Jones, and J. M. Rutter. 1975. Adhesion of enteropathogenic *E. coli* to pig intestinal brushborders: The existence of two pig phenotypes. *Journal of Medical Microbiology.* 8:405–11.

Shann, F. 1986. Etiology of severe pneumonia in developing countries. *Pediatric Infectious Disease.* 5:247–52.

Skamene, E. 1985. Genetic control of host resistance to infection and malignancy. *Progress In Leucocyte Biology,* vol. 3. New York: Allan R. Liss.

Smith, H. W., and S. Halls. 1972. The production of oedema disease and diarrhea in weaned pigs by the oral administration of *E. coli*: Factors that influence the course of experimental disease. *Journal of Medical Microbiology* 1:243–50.

Snell, G. D., J. Daussett, and S. Nathenson. 1976. *Histocompatibility.* New York: Academic.

Sussman, M. 1985. The virulence of *E. coli*. Published by the Society for General Microbiology. 12–13:53. New York: Academic.

Turelli, M., and L. Ginzberg. 1983. Should individual fitness increase with heterozygosity? *Genetics* 104:191–209

Vogel, F., and A. G. Motulsky. 1987. *Human Genetics: Problems and Approaches.* Berlin: Springer-Verlag.

3 THE DETECTION OF SELECTIVE DIFFERENCES IN POPULATIONS

John A. Barrett

If any papers deserve the epithet of "classic," they are J. B. S. Haldane's of 1949 and, to a lesser extent, his 1954 essay, in which he postulates that interactions between hosts and parasites or pathogens may lead to the maintenance of biochemical polymorphisms in the host and "probably in the parasite also" (Haldane 1949). Perhaps because of the beautiful, logical symmetry of Haldane's hypothesis, there has tended to be an uncritical acceptance of his proposition despite a lack of supporting data.

Mathematical models based on Haldane's ideas have suggested that stable equilibria or stable limit cycles in phenotype, genotype, and gene frequencies of both host and parasite could be maintained by selection of the form that he envisaged, depending on the genetic assumptions built into the model (for examples, see Jayakar 1970; Yu 1972; and Clarke 1976). This suggests that differential survival or reproductive success as a consequence of parasitic infection or infectious disease should, in principle, be detectable.

However, the problem of detecting natural selection, from whatever cause, is a recurrent problem in evolutionary biology. When the biology of the organism permits genotype or phenotype frequencies to be determined over several generations, regression techniques can often provide good estimates of selective differences even when the sample sizes in any one generation are relatively small. With long-lived species — long-lived, that is, with respect to the duration of the average research grant — detection of relative survival rates (selection operating through differential mortality) can be problematical.

In this short chapter I do not attempt to provide a rigorous treatment of the problem of estimating selective differences in human populations but merely draw attention to the fact that the sample sizes required to detect even relatively large selective differences are often beyond the scope of most studies. Reed

(1975) commented on this problem with respect to the ABO blood groups when he pointed out that most studies carried out up to that time were incapable of detecting selective differences of the order 10–20 percent. For a more comprehensive treatment of the problems of estimating selective differences, the reader should consult Wright (1977) and Manly (1985).

DIRECT AND INDIRECT APPROACHES

In order to detect the effects that infectious disease may have on the genetic composition of a population, two approaches may be adopted, the direct and the indirect.

The direct approach estimates the proportions of different genotypes or phenotypes in samples before and after an epidemic to detect differential mortality. A similar approach could be adopted for diseases which may have their main effect on lifetime reproductive output, but the estimation and sampling procedures are more complex in populations with overlapping generations, such as humans.

The indirect approach estimates the proportions of different genotypes or phenotypes within samples of affected and unaffected individuals within the same population and thus estimates differential susceptibility. How this differential susceptibility translates into differential mortality or reproductive success will depend on the severity, aetiology, and epidemiology of the disease. However, the assumption is that differential susceptibility does produce differences in fitness, but the fitness effect may be one or two orders of magnitude less than the differential susceptibility may suggest, depending on the proportion of the population as a whole that is affected by the infectious organism. For example, one phenotype may be 10 percent more susceptible than another, but if only 1 percent of the less susceptible type is affected then the evolutionary effect will be considerably less than if 10 percent of the less susceptible type is affected.

Basic Model

The simplest technique for detecting such effects is by use of the contingency X^2 test in which the proportions of different genotypes or phenotypes in two or more samples are compared. The simplest case is for two phenotypes and two samples. Let the two phenotypes be H and h:

	H	h	
Sample 1	A	B	A + B
Sample 2	C	D	C + D
	A + C	B + D	N

$$X^2 = \frac{(AD - BC)^2}{(A + B)(C + D)(A + C)(B + D)} \qquad (1)$$

with one degree of freedom.

We can also write the relative frequencies within each sample as:

$$p = \frac{A}{A + B} \qquad\qquad q = \frac{B}{A + B}$$

$$p' = \frac{C}{C + D} \qquad\qquad q' = \frac{D}{C + D}$$

For simplicity, let the two samples be of equal size, viz.

$$A + B = C + D = n$$

The contingency table can now be written as:

	H	h	Totals
Sample 1	pn	qn	n
Sample 2	p'n	q'n	n
Totals	n(p + p')	n(q + q')	2n

and the expression for X^2 becomes, after some rearrangement:

$$X^2 = \frac{2n (p - p')^2}{(p + p')(q + q')} \qquad (2)$$

Direct Measurement of Mortality

In this approach the proportions of the two phenotypes are estimated before and after an epidemic. One of the phenotypes, say h, has a lower survival rate, say 1 - s, relative to H. Hence the proportions can be written as:

	H	h
Sample at t	p	q
Fitnesses	1	1 - s
Sample at t'	p' = p / (1 - qs)	q' = q(1 - s) / (1 - qs)

Substituting these values into (2), we obtain

$$X^2 = \frac{2n\,(pqs)^2}{(2p - pqs)\,[2q - qs(1 + q)]} \qquad (3)$$

This can be rearranged to yield

$$n = \frac{X^2\,(2p - pqs)\,[2q - qs\,(1 + q)]}{2(pqs)^2} \qquad (4)$$

If we know the value of s and have estimates of p and q, we can estimate the sample size n required to give a X^2 of a certain value when a contingency test is carried out on the data.

For a X^2 test to be significant at the 5 percent level on a 2 x 2 contingency table, X^2 must be greater than 3.84. Thus, by substituting this value in (4) above we can obtain an estimate of the minimum sample sizes required to detect a significant difference in relative survival for any stated combination of relative fitness and phenotype frequency, viz.

$$\hat{n} = \frac{3.84\,(2p - pqs)\,[2q - qs\,(1 + q)]}{2(pqs)^2} \qquad (5)$$

Table 3.1 shows the values of $\hat{n}$ required to detect a relative fitness difference, s, with a probability of 95 percent when p, the frequency of the fitter phenotype, takes values between 0.9 and 0.1.

Since the sample sizes required are proportional to $1 / (pqs)^2$, it follows that the sample sizes required increase substantially if the phenotype frequencies are unequal or the selective differences are small. Thus, to detect a relatively large difference in survival rate of about 10 percent, s = 0.1, requires sample sizes of the order of 2,500 to 10,000, depending on the frequencies of the phenotypes. If the h phenotype is very common and H, the fitter phenotype, is rare, say 1 percent of the population, then sample sizes of the order of 66,400 (66,399.5) will be required to detect a fitness difference of 10 percent. (A fitness difference of 10 percent is very

TABLE 3.1
Minimum Sample Sizes Needed to Detect Selection.
Direct Approach, 5 Percent Level of Significance.

	Values of p		
s	0.1	0.5	0.9
0.5	140	67	241
0.25	924	374	1163
0.1	7,375	2,771	8,024
0.05	31,781	11,679	33,112

TABLE 3.2
Minimum Sample Sizes Needed to Detect Differential Susceptibility.
Indirect Approach, 5 Percent Level of Significance.

	Values of p		
t	0.1	0.5	0.9
0.5	617	190	436
0.25	1,880	620	1,592
0.1	9,764	3,385	9,048
0.05	36,559	12,908	35,160
0.01	865,316	310,278	858,456
0.005	3,437,263	1,234,950	3,423,576

large and will produce rapid evolutionary change. The fitness difference between the typical and melanic forms of Biston betularia was of this order.)

Indirect Approach by Estimation of Relative Susceptibility

Suppose that the data consist of two samples, one of affected individuals and one of unaffected individuals.

Let phenotype h have an increased probability of contracting the disease, say $(1 + t)$, relative to H. The proportions in the two samples can be written as

	H	h
Sample 1 (unaffected)	p	q
Sample 2 (affected)	$p' = p/(1 + qt)$	$q' = q(1 + t)/(1 + qt)$

Following the same procedure as before, we obtain

$$\hat{n} = \frac{3.84 \, (2p + pqt) \, [2q + qt \, (1+q)]}{2 \, (pqt)^2} \tag{6}$$

Values of $\hat{n}$ are shown in the body of Table 3.2. Note that such estimates often only detect the relative susceptibilities which may be somewhat larger than the differences in relative fitness.

DISCUSSION

Large sample sizes are required to detect even reasonably large differences in survival rate or susceptibility. Although this analysis makes the simplifying assumption that the sample sizes are equal, having unequal sample sizes makes little difference to the analysis because the ability of the X^2 test to detect differences in the proportions in the two samples is determined primarily by the size of the smaller sample. Therefore, the values quoted in Tables 3.1 and 3.2 can be taken as minimum estimates for the smaller sample size.

For example, from Table 3.1, it can be shown that sample sizes of 11,679 are required to detect a selective difference of 5 percent, if $p = 0.5$. Therefore, sample sizes of 11,500 should not detect a significant difference between the two samples.

	H	h	Totals
Sample 1	5,750	5,750	11,500
Sample 2	5,897	5,603	11,500
	11,647	11,353	23,000

$$X^2 = 3.76 \text{ with one degree of freedom}$$

This value is not quite significant at the 5 percent level, at which the critical value is 3.84.

If we now double the size of Sample 1, we obtain:

	H	h	Totals
Sample 1	11,500	11,500	23,000
Sample 2	5,897	5,603	11,500
	17,397	17,103	34,500

$$X^2 = 5.011 \text{ with one degree of freedom } 0.05 > p > 0.025$$

For a significance level of 2.5 percent, $X^2 = 5.024$, with one degree of freedom. The net effect of doubling the size of Sample 1 is to make the difference between the two samples only just detectable. In other words, by surveying an extra 11,500 individuals in Sample 1, a difference has only just been detected. On the other hand, increasing the size of both samples by just 200–300 would have had the same effect; increasing both samples to 15,240 would have produced the same X^2 with a total sample size 12 percent smaller. From a practical point of view, it is obvious which strategy is more efficient in time and resources.

REFERENCES

Clarke, B.C. 1976. The ecological genetics of host-parasite relationships. In *Genetic Aspects of Host Parasite Relationships.* vol. 14. *Symposia of the British Society for Parasitology.* A. E. R. Taylor and R. Muller, eds. Oxford: Blackwell Scientific Publications.

Haldane, J. B. S. 1954. The statics of evolution. In *Evolution as a Process.* J. Huxley, A. C. Hardy, and E. B. Ford, eds. London: Allen & Unwin.

———. 1949. Disease and evolution. Supplement to *La Ricerca Scientifica* 19:68–76.

Jayakar, S. D. 1970. A mathematical model for the interaction of gene frequencies in a parasite and its host. *Theoretical Population Biology* 1:140–64.

Manly, B. F. J. 1985. *The Statistics of Natural Selection.* London: Chapman and Hall.

Reed, T. E. 1975. Selection and blood group polymorphism. In *The Role of Natural Selection in Evolution.* F. M. Salzano, ed. New York: Plenum.

Wright, S. 1977. Evolution and the Genetics of Populations. vol. 3. *Experimental Results and Evolutionary Deductions.* Chicago: The University of Chicago Press.

Yu, P. 1972. Some host-parasite interaction models. *Theoretical Population Biology* 3:347–57.

4 INFECTIOUS DISEASE AND EVOLUTION OF HUMAN POPULATIONS: THE EXAMPLE OF SOUTH AMERICAN FOREST TRIBES

Francis L. Black

Because mutation is inherent in DNA and RNA replication, pathogens evolve continuously to improve or maintain their reproductive potential. At the same time, every host population continuously changes to better defend itself against pathogen caused diseases. Although the rate of change in DNA base sequences is at least approximately uniform (Sibley 1984), this uniformity does not mean that evolution proceeds at a steady pace. New germ line mutations are only expressed with a new generation, and the time between successive generations varies from a matter of minutes in viruses and bacteria to a quarter-century in humans. Moreover, evolution is only made possible by mutation; it is driven by changes in selective pressures. Some species living in stable environments have changed little over many millions of years, while others have gone through periods of very rapid change. The major cultural transitions in human history must have been associated with rapid changes in the circumstances surrounding transmission of infectious agents and in the secondary effects of disease on host survival. Hence, each cultural transition would have been associated with periods of accelerated evolutionary change both in disease agents and in human biology.

Because of these continuous, though variably paced, processes of evolution, two races of one species that have been separated long enough to acquire distinctive characteristics would also have distinctive sets of pathogens and, to some extent, distinctive defenses. If the two races come again into contact, each race will be exposed to a set of pathogenic agents to which they may be poorly adapted in their cultural and genetic defenses. In order to investigate this phenomenon we have studied the effects of contact between the people of the Americas and those of the Old World. This reassociation has been going on for almost 500 years now, but in the Amazon forest there are still groups of people who have been very little affected by it until now. These groups are rapidly being brought into contact with the larger melded culture by a process of deliberate "pacification" carried out by the government of Brazil, as well as by penetration of their forest reserves by oil companies and other developers.

This being a natural laboratory, it does not provide a simple test of the effects of exchanging pathogens. This time of contact is also a time of major cultural transition for the forest people. While almost all these tribes have some horticulture, their garden plots have been small and dispersed, their population density has been very low — less than one person per ten square kilometers — and their gene pool divided into tribal groups of, at most, a few hundred persons. (I will refer to these predominantly endogamous groups as tribes, although several may share cultural characteristics and one may include one or several villages.) It is obvious that we cannot study these people before the contact occurs, but only as soon as possible afterward. In three instances we have been able to collect specimens within three months of initial regular direct contact. With data from these three tribes, and from studies conducted after more extended contact, we have extrapolated backward to try to determine the precontact situation and the full effect of the meeting of races.

COEVOLUTION OF HOST AND PARASITE

When trying to determine the role of evolution of parasite and host in human history we must seek to learn: the frequency of appearance of new agents of human disease; the relative time scales of pathogen and human genetic change and, in humans, the relative roles of mutation versus diffusion of advantageous genes; and the trend of agent evolution, whether to greater or lesser virulence.

Appearance of New Diseases

The influenza pandemics of 1919, 1957, and 1968 were each caused by viruses that were new to most people alive at the time, but they were probably not new to human history. The viruses represented reassortments of genetic elements that had persisted in animal reservoirs, with genes that conferred efficiency in infecting humans. They were not therefore new in an evolutionary sense. At least three other diseases, which do seem to have been new, caused pandemics during the last three decades. The first of these was ECHO 9, which swept all age groups during the late 1950s with a relatively mild disease that appeared as aseptic meningitis in adults and erythema in children (Nihoul, Quersin-Thierry, and Weynants 1957). The virus of this disease may have arisen by an increase in virulence and basic reproductive rate of a preexisting innocuous virus of humans. Then in the late 1970s, acute hemorrhagic conjunctivitis caused by enterovirus 70 swept the tropical parts of the world. Enterovirus 70 seems to have arisen from a virus endemic in livestock of western Africa (Kono et al. 1981). Finally, in this decade acquired immune-deficiency syndrome (AIDS) has appeared. It is caused by a new virus, HLV1, which is related to viruses that infect monkeys, although not closely related to any that have been studied (Essex et al. 1985). The first two diseases of this group spread around the world in a few years, and, although I believe they were new to mankind, humans were able to mount good immune responses. The rapid spread and good immunity meant that the viruses very soon ran out of potential hosts. The diseases have not persisted in epidemic form, although nonepidemic ECHO 9 is occasionally isolated, as before the pandemic. AIDS virus has moved more slowly and promises to be with us for a long time. It now seems that a few people carry the virus for many years without disease, but that in most humans the virus destroys the immune system and ultimately causes death. This death comes slowly, and the virus has a period of several years in which to pass to a new host. Unless we can develop some medical or sociologic defense, the conflict between humans and AIDS virus will be protracted. A worst-case scenario, but one that must have occurred often in evolutionary history, is that those of us with defenses that can be overwhelmed by the virus will die off and be succeeded by descendants of persons who can control the infection.

The pattern of ephemeralism exhibited by two of three new disease agents may be characteristic. The traits needed for persistence of an infectious agent are different from those needed for rapid spread in inexperienced populations, and the proportion of new disease agents that possess both sets of characteristics will be relatively small. Over a period of millennia, however, a large number of new diseases can accumulate. During the last four millennia the human population has grown manyfold, and the size of the individual social units into which it is divided has also become greater. Many of those diseases which we traditionally considered childhood infection, smallpox, measles, and rubella for example, can only maintain themselves in social groupings of several hundred thousand persons and must therefore have evolved since urbanization began. In any smaller population they would have quickly killed or immunized all available hosts and failed to persist.

Relative Rates of Evolution of Mammals and Infectious Agents

The rates of pathogen and host evolution in response to selective forces created by their interaction have been most systematically studied in the instance of myxoma and the *Oryctolagus* rabbit of Australia (Fenner and Ratcliffe 1965). Myxomavirus is a member of the pox group and a common natural pathogen in the *Sylvilagus* rabbit of South America, where it causes a mild disease. During the 1950s it was transferred intentionally to Australia in a largely successful attempt to control the rabbit population. There, it initially caused very close to 100 percent mortality, and by the end of the third year, large parts of the country were cleared of rabbits. However, even in the second year many virus isolates showed diminished virulence and permitted more than 1 percent of infected laboratory rabbits to survive. By the third year most strains of virus killed only 70 to 95 percent of the animals infected. Moreover, whereas rabbits rarely lived longer than two weeks after infection with the original strain, those infected with the modified strains regularly remained alive and contagious for three weeks or more. Some virus strains were isolated which killed less than 50 percent of infected animals, but the lesions caused by these strains usually healed more quickly and they never became dominant. Spread of the virus from one warren to another seems to be by mechanical transmission on the proboscides of mosquitoes, and the rapidly healing lesions did not provide an adequate source of virus for continuous transmission. It was only after several years that changes in resistance of the rabbit population to a standard strain could be detected. A strain of virus that killed 90 percent of the rabbits collected in the first year of the epidemic killed only 60 percent of the rabbits collected in the sixth year. The difference in rate of evolution between virus and rabbit can logically be attributed to differences in genetic complexity and differences in generation time. The human generation time is twenty times that of the rabbit, and we would evolve, at best, at one twentieth the rate of the rabbit.

Sources of Host Change: New Mutation versus Diffusion

Single-base change mutations characteristically occur at a rate of about 10^{-6} per generation, and therefore in any large population there should exist at least one copy of every possible single-step variant. Nevertheless, in human history, as in the Australian rabbits, favorable selective pressure seems to be very slow in bringing new traits to the fore. The situation is most clearly illustrated in the case of hemoglobin S and resistance to malaria. Although this trait derives from a single-base change, it seems to have arisen only twice in Africa and once in India. It has spread partly by population displacement and partly by diffusing ahead of other characteristics of the original carriers, into surrounding areas. It attained high frequencies in the African rain forest belt and substantial frequencies in southwest Asia. However, it has never been found in Amerinds unmixed with Africans and does not seem to occur in southeast Asia, populations which it could not easily penetrate by diffusion. Falciparum malaria exacts a heavy toll in these other areas, and yet no independent focus of hemoglobin S has been recognized.

DIRECTION OF EVOLUTION OF PATHOGENS

The question as to whether pathogens can be expected regularly to evolve toward lower pathogenicity has generated considerable discussion. B. R. Levin et al., draw attention to a model for pathogen evolution in which decreased virulence is tied to reduced amounts of the pathogenic agent (Levin et al. 1982). According to this model, evolution could carry the agent in either direction—toward increasing or decreasing pathogenicity. In the example of myxoma the most virulent strains were not successful because they soon destroyed all the rabbits in their reach, but the highly attenuated strains also failed to gain ascendancy because the lesions they caused healed quickly and virus from them had little time in which to find new hosts. The history of myxoma in Australia is, however, still quite short; in South American rabbits the virus is more temperate. It seems that pathogenicity and infectiousness are only loosely associated, and that, with some regularity, extended periods of evolution select strains which permit the host to remain infectious for the longest possible time, that is, close to a normal life span. As described in the following sections, this seems to have been the most common host-pathogen relationship in the relatively stable ecological association which existed in American populations before contact with the Old World.

INFECTIOUS DISEASES IN ISOLATED NEW WORLD SOCIETIES

Method for Determining Disease Prevalence in Periods Prior to Sample Collection

Immunological techniques permit us to reconstruct infectious disease histories for any population group back to the date of birth of the eldest surviving members. Infections, with a few exceptions, elicit an immune response in each survivor that includes the appearance of some antibodies which persist for the survivor's lifetime. By testing for these immunological changes we can tell if a person has ever been infected with a particular disease. Positive reactions indicate that the relevant infectious agent was present in the population after the youngest responder was born. Negative reactions in all members of a population younger than a particular age cutoff indicate that the agent has been absent throughout that period.

This process is illustrated in the example of hepatitis A, the more acute, waterborne form of hepatitis, in the Parakanã of Bom Jardim (Jacobson and Black, 1986). Beginning in 1927 both these Parakanã and an Asurini group were involved in raids on the railway which paralleled a turbulent stretch of the lower Tocantins River (Arnaud 1961). The locale of these raids has recently been inundated by a reservoir behind the world's fourth largest dam. After a period of about ten years of raiding, the Parakanã disappeared back into the forest, while the Asurini settled on a reserve just below the site of the present dam. In the early 1980s, the Parakanã were both victims and perpetrators of a series of raids, and the National Indian Foundation (FUNAI) set out to bring them into its fold. A team led by Luis Montero succeeded with one group in December 1983 and with another in March 1984. We were able to study both groups in June of 1984 and found that everybody over fifty years of age had antibody to hepatitis A, but nobody younger had it. Apparently the virus got into the tribe fifty years ago when they were raiding but did not persist and had not been encountered again in a half-century of living in the forest. Among the Asurini, on the other

TABLE 4.1
Infectious Diseases among Indigenous Amazon Populations According to Endemicity.

Introduced	Zoonotic	Endemic
Smallpox	Yellow Fever	Herpes Type 1
Measles	Mayaro Fever	Infectious Mononucleosis
Rubella	Oropuche Fever	Cytomegalo Disease
Mumps	Toxoplasmosis	Hepatitis B
Influenza A and B	Leishmaniasis	Ascaris
Parainfluenza	Trichinosis	Hookworm
Poliomyelitis	Tetanus(?)	Whipworm
Malaria	Malaria	Amoebiasis
Hepatitis A		Treponemal Infection
Dengue		Syphilis (?)
Common Cold		
Respiratory Syncycial Disease		
Rotovirus Diarrhea		
Dipphtheria		
Scarlet Fever		
Whooping Cough		

hand, all ages have been infected. The virus must be a frequent visitor, if not permanently endemic, in their settled village.

Exogenous Diseases

As shown in Table 4.1, many of the most important infectious diseases, smallpox, measles and influenza among them, behave like hepatitis A in that antibody, if present at all, is present only in persons above a specific age cutoff. This has been discussed fully in earlier publications (Black, Hierholzer, Pinheiro, et al. 1974; Black 1982).

Several diseases of this group, measles and rubella for example, must have developed in their modern form since the migration of the ancestors of these tribes to the New World, because they require such large populations for their perpetuation that they cannot persist in groups of the size that existed 20,000 years ago. The other diseases of the group, even though they may have existed at that time in settled populations, could not have been carried by the intercontinental migrants. They spread so rapidly, while inducing substantial immunity in persons who survive infection, that they quickly exhaust the supply of susceptible persons in any small group of humans. They still pose no continuing threat to forest tribes that maintain their isolation, but they have persisted in the Central American and Andean populations since they were introduced by the Spanish.

Special mention needs to be made of tuberculosis and malaria because they are two of the most serious diseases of the contact and postcontact periods. Even though the agents of both diseases can persist for many years in an infected person, they seem not to have been endemic in Amerinds before initiation of contact. The situation is clearer with tuberculosis. Nutels (1968) found that its prevalence increased rapidly after contact, and the curve needed only to be extrapolated a short distance to indicate that the disease had probably been absent before contact. All strains of malaria, also, seem to be of Old World origin, but at least one has become endemic in South American monkeys and reaches isolated tribes independently of contact with other humans. As Livingstone (1958) noted in Africa, until steel tools also reach a tribe and permit the clearing of larger gardens, malaria seems to remain at low levels of endemicity. The serious problems with malaria come with cultural changes of the transition. Malaria must have been left behind by migrants from the Old to New World, because the anopheline mosquito, an essential vector of the disease, could not tolerate the environmental changes along the route. Whether tuberculosis evolved after the migrants left the Old World, or was left behind en route, I cannot tell.

Endemic Diseases

Although many diseases seem to have been foreign to New World peoples, others are so broadly distributed among them that it seems probable they were common long before contact was established. We find antibody to the agents of these diseases in all except the youngest members of every tribe. In every case the incubation period is long, and immunity fails to eliminate the agent from the body. Some of these infections cause serious disease when they infect adults or children carried *in utero*, but they are essentially innocuous in early childhood and, in the populations we have studied, 100 percent cumulative attack rates are regularly found by an early age. Although the agents of infectious mononucleosis, chronic viral hepatitis, and congenital cytomegalovirus disease are prevalent in all tribes, we have never seen the more serious manifestations of the infections in the Amazon tribes. Thus, the outcome of long-term association between infectious agent and Amerindian people has regularly been attenuation of the disease.

Diseases Originally Unique to New World Populations

Our study method is not well suited to identification of diseases which were confined to the New World before contact. It is most unlikely that such diseases would have been limited to the remaining isolated tribes, and any diseases of the major New World populations would long since have spread to the rest of the world, if possessed of that capacity. The disease most commonly cited in this category is syphilis, which was first recognized in Europe near the time and place of Columbus's return (Crosby 1972). We have found evidence of a common infection among the Kayapo which is acquired at puberty and cross-reacts specifically with *Treponema pallidum*, the cause of syphilis but is not associated with acute, chronic, or congenital symptoms (Lee et al. 1978). It is tempting to think that this might be the form a spirochetal pathogen would evolve into over a long period in a stable environment, but such a hypothesis presumes that long-term association does lead to attenuation and that the spirochete, when transferred to hosts of another race, temporarily assumed very high levels of pathogenicity.

There has been discussion of why relatively few diseases were transmitted from Amerinds to Old World people. By the time of initial Viking and Columbian contacts, the major population centers of the New World were sufficiently large to sustain the most demanding viruses. The New World populations had attained this level more recently, however, and the total population of the New World was probably less than a tenth of the Old. Perhaps on a per capita, per year basis the exchange of new diseases was not imbalanced.

Zoonotic Diseases

The particular tribes we have studied do have infectious diseases that are not common among us, but these are diseases which have a reservoir in forest animals and do not cycle freely in human populations. This turns out to be a relatively small group of agents, and the particular diseases involved depend on the local ecology. In some of the populations we have studied there is evidence of high yellow fever and leishmaniasis infection rates. With leishmaniasis we have seen less evidence of pathology among the Indians than we expected on the basis of disease seen in Caucasians who ventured into the territory. The indigenous populations may have cross-reacting immunity derived from infection with related nonpathogenic agents, but why would not the interlopers be infected by the same sequence? It is tempting to speculate that the Indians of the forest may have been selected for resistance to *Leishmania braziliensis* during the course of a long history of exposure.

GENETIC CHARACTERISTICS OF SOUTH AMERICAN FOREST TRIBES

Characteristics Derived From the Founding Stock

Only small bands could initially have passed each of the successive bottlenecks along the route from Asia to South America, and they could carry only a fraction of the gene pool that existed behind them. These pioneers would then have multiplied to obstruct the passage of subsequent waves. The

TABLE 4.2

Genetic Traits Not Found in South American Lowland Indians.[1]

System	Missing Alleles	Frequency in:	
		Europeans	Blacks
ABO	A_1, A_2, B	.34	.34
Kell	K	.05	.00
Hemoglobin	All except A	.04	variable
G-6-PD	All except B	.002	.20
6PGD	B,C	—	—
Esterase A1-3	All unusual	—	—
Adenylate Kinase	All except 1	—	—
Adenosine Deaminase	All except 1	.089	.017
Gm	All except 1, 17; 21 1, 2, 17; 21 & 1, 17; 5, 13	.625	.993
HLA A	All except 2, 24, 28, 31	.41	.63
HLA B	All except 35, 39, 40, 51, 53, 62	.63	.69
HLA C	2,5,6,8	.33	.24
HLA DR	1, 3, 5, 7, 9, 10	.42	.50

[1] Values for comparison frequencies in Europeans and Blacks for blood groups and enzymes are taken from the tables of Mourant, Kopec, and Domaniewska-Sobczak (1976), the Gm data are taken from the work of van Loghem (1984), and the HLA data from Baur and Danilovs (1982). The European values are those for Portuguese or the geographically closest available population, and the data for Blacks are from former Portuguese colonies where possible.

descendants of these people possess only a subset of the genes possessed by North American Indians, who in turn possess only a subset of the traits common in the northeast Asian races. They carry no unique trait in high frequency, although there are some rare geographically localized "private polymorphisms" that seem to represent relatively recent mutations that have not been subject to strong selective pressure.

Although the South American race cannot be characterized by any unique trait, it lacks so many common polymorphisms it is relatively easy to recognize admixture with other races. Some of the absent genes are listed in Table 4.2. The frequencies given in the last column can be used to estimate the chance of missing admixture. If several systems are used together, this chance becomes very small. The fact that the South Americans do not carry A1, A2, or B of the ABO system provides a handy marker. They have only three of many possible IgG allotypes, and one of those is rare. However, we have found the HLA system most valuable for characterizing the race and distinguishing different groups within the race. Only four of eighteen recognized distinct antigens controlled by the A locus occur in the South American lowland Indians, only six of thirty-seven alleles at the B locus, four of eight at the C locus, and four of twelve DR alleles (Black, Berman, and Gabbay 1980). Not only are the number of alleles in this race thus restricted, but they also are associated into relatively few of the many possible sets, called haplotypes (Black 1984). North American Indians have all the HLA antigens found in South America, plus a few more (Troup et al. 1982; Gorodezky, Castro-Escobar, and Escobar-Guiterez 1985). Other isolated populations, the Tuareg (Degos, Colombani, and Chavantre 1974), the Australian Aborigines (Bashir et al. 1973), the Papuans (Bhatia, Gorogo, and Koki 1984) and the Polynesians (Serjeantson, Ryand, and Thompson 1982) also have restricted gene pools, but it has been difficult to find populations with as little extraneous admixture as those of South America and hence their repertoires are less well defined.

Effects of Drift

The balance between the needs of defense and the economy in the South American forest gives rise to tribal units of between 100 and 1,000 persons. These small units provide the potential for very rapid genetic drift. As pointed out by Neel and Ward (1970), random drift in these tribes is greatly enhanced by the fact that a tribe commonly splits along kinship lines, thus maximizing the genetic differences between the two new units. Specific polymorphisms are often lost from individual successor groups, and tribes which came from a common group just a few generations earlier may differ dramatically in gene frequencies.

There are, however, balancing forces which prevent this trend toward diversification from maintaining its rapid pace. Genetic distances among apparently unrelated tribes are not much greater than among tribes of one cultural group. Some of this balancing effect is sociological. It is common practice to take women or children from other tribes as captives and give them full tribal membership. Also, for every tribe formed, another must disappear. This usually happens when a tribe falls to such low numbers that it cannot find marriage partners internally and voluntarily fuses with another group.

As well as the sociologic balancing factors, there are genetic pressures against the loss of diversity at some loci. Hedrick and Thomson (1983) note that the frequencies at which different HLA antigens are found are more uniform than in a fully random situation. Their study implies that any less common antigen has a selective advantage over any more common type, presumably because the rare type will seldom be homozygous. Most of the antigens which are available to the South American Indians are very widely and quite uniformly distributed, as would be predicted by Hedrick and Thomson's hypothesis. There are a few exceptions: B51, Cwl, and an unidentified C antigen have their highest incidence in the northern part of the continent, and B14 has been reported only from the Andean tribes. The genes coding for these antigens may have been brought to the continent by later migrants from North America, where they are widely distributed. A28 occurs in lower frequency than other A antigens, although it is widely distributed; it does not seem to share in the balancing selection.

Selective Effects Associated with Restricted Gene Pools

The impact of homozygosity at individual loci as observed by Hedrick and Thomson places no more than a small burden on any one generation. Neither they, nor we, working with the South American tribes, have demonstrated that the proportion of persons homozygous for any one antigenic type is lower than predicted by chance. What we (Black and Salzano 1981) and before us, Degos, Colombani, and Chavantre (1974), have shown is that there is a much greater deficit of persons homozygous over whole HLA haplotypes.

The HLA haplotypes are defined by genes linked along chromosome six. They are close enough together that crossovers with the A, B, C set occur only once in every 100 generations, but far enough apart that there is room for more than 1,000 other genes between them, genes which control much of the immune response. In the South American Indians, the antigens we have found could form 140 distinguishable sets, but only thirty-six different haplotypes have been found. This limitation stems largely from the fact that the haplotypes are sufficiently stable so that the small number of them, brought by the original migrants to the continent, has not been greatly augmented by crossover. Some of the thirty-six attain extremely high frequencies and wide distribution. For instance, A2, B39, and Cw7 and A31, B53, and Cw4, which have frequencies of 8.9 percent and 8.8 percent respectively in our Amazon population, are also present in higher than random frequency in the Mapuche of southern Chile-Argentina (Haas et al. 1985).

Because the number of different haplotypes in any one tribe is small, there is a substantial probability that a child will receive identical sets from its two parents. If, as seems often the case, these two haplotypes come from the same ancestor, the associated genes will also be identical. Thus, persons with homozygous haplotypes are homozygous for a large set of traits, and they may be much more sensitive to the selective force found by Hedrick and Thomson than persons homozygous at only one locus. In a small nonbellicose tribe the frequencies of a single haplotype may approach 0.5, and the proportion expected to be homozygous may exceed 0.25. On the average, these individuals experienced a 39 percent survival disadvantage.

Asurini of Trocará, the settled tribe mentioned with respect to hepatitis A, provide an example. Eighty percent of them carry the haplotype A24, B15, Cw3. We would expect 21 percent to be homozygous for this sequence, but fewer than 13 percent are. Eight percent of all conceptuses fail to survive because of the one coincidence that they received two copies of that particular haplotype. How serious a burden this places on the population depends on whether the loss occurs near the time of conception or after there has been substantial investment in the individual. A hypothesis for the reason for failure to survive comes easily to mind. The linked genes include many Ia genes which determine the ability to respond immunologically to specific

FIGURE 4.1

Proportion of Population Observed and Expected Homozygous for HLA Haplotypes, by Haplotype.[1]

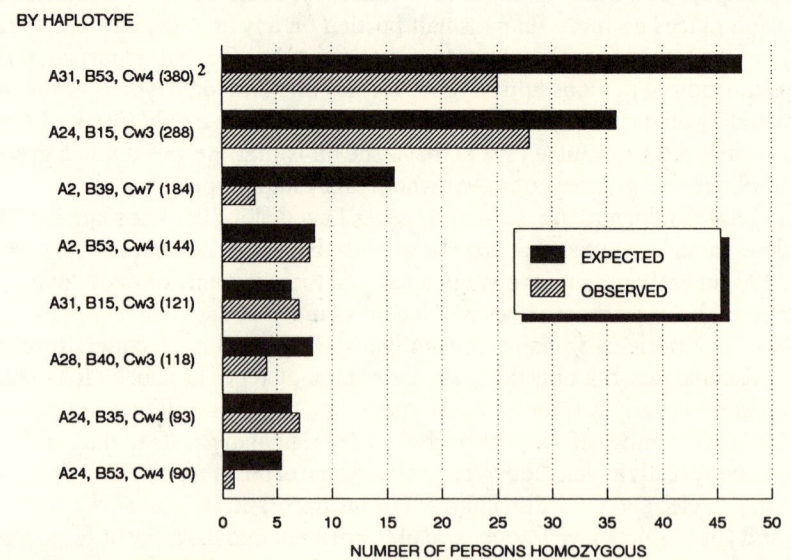

[1] Expected values determined from haplotype frequencies within each tribe separately and then summed, not the overall mean frequencies.

[2] Cases tested in parentheses.

FIGURE 4.2
Proportion of Population Observed and Expected Homozygous for HLA Haplotypes, by Tribe.[1]

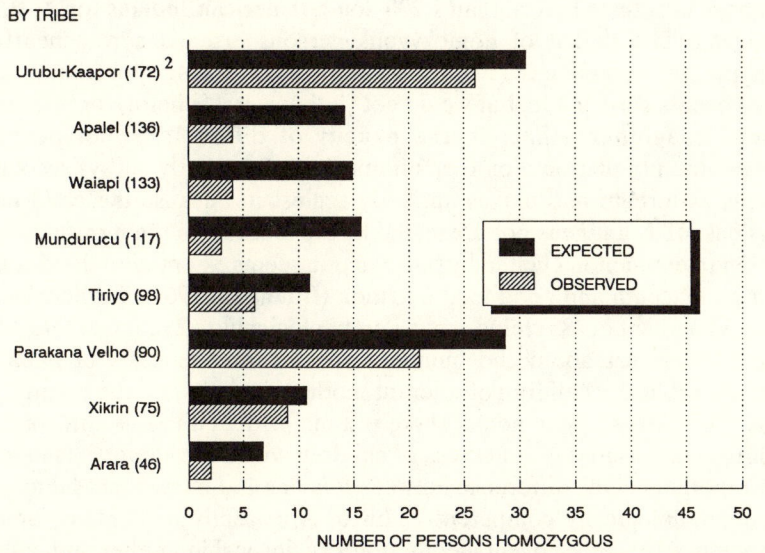

FIGURE 4.3
Proportion of Population Observed and Expected Homozygous for HLA Haplotypes, by Age.[1]

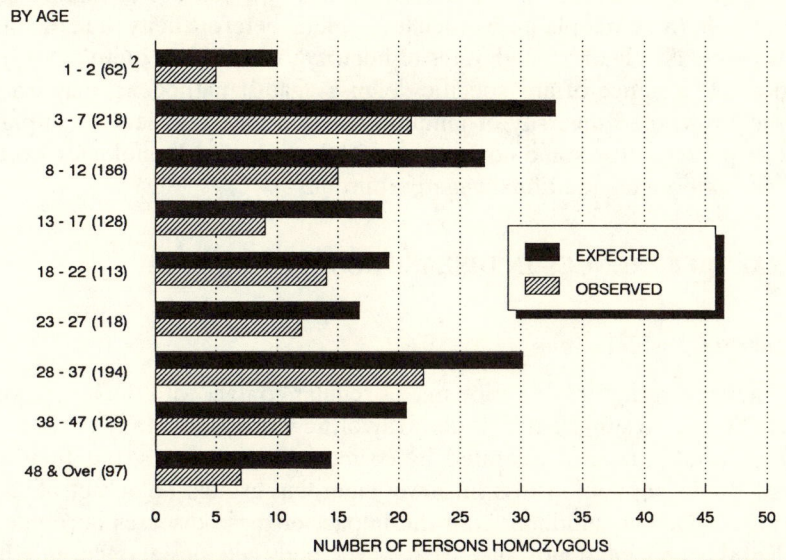

[1] Expected values determined from haplotype frequencies within each tribe separately and then summed, not the overall mean frequencies.
[2] Cases tested in parentheses.

antigens. These genes are codominant, and heterozygosity permits one to carry twice as many as the homozygous state.

We have now tested more than 1,200 South American Indians for A, B, and C antigens. The deficit of homozygous persons extends across nearly all haplotypes, tribes, and ages (Figures 4.1–4.3). The age data show that much of the loss occurs early in life, but we do not yet know it if is before or after birth.

There is another aspect to the paucity of different haplotypes. In a cosmopolitan population a mother's immune system nearly always recognizes the fetus as foreign and makes antibody against it, because the child nearly always has HLA antigens not possessed by the mother. In the mouse the graft rejection phenomenon elicited by this reaction seems essential to development of a large placenta and good fetal nutrition (Billington 1964). In the tribes we studied 34 percent of 285 children had immunologically tolerant mothers (Black 1985). This is just about the number expected on the basis of haplotype frequencies, but the children of tolerant mothers included all the homozygous children and, as has been noted, there is a major deficit in this category. The deficit is compensated by an excess of children with both haplotypes identical to their mothers'. One difference between humans and mice is that humans are more immunologically competent at birth. Apparently in humans, immune tolerance in fetal life is advantageous, if it is reciprocal in mother and child.

To summarize this section, those members of the Amerindian race who have remained largely uncontacted by Old World migrants have highly involuted ancestries, both in the far past and in recent times. Because of this history, because of their currently small breeding units, and because of high rates of neutral drift, these people have much less genetic heterogeneity than the other major races. This leads to high rates of homozygosity, which, quite apart from the possible absence of any specific defense against pathogens, may lead to relatively restricted diversity of immune reaction and does lead to impaired survival potential for some conceptuses. Maternal-child homologies do not, however, impose an additional negative burden.

RACIAL DIFFERENCES IN DISEASE SUSCEPTIBILITY

General Considerations

We have seen that when a tribe makes regular contact with the larger world society, it will be subject to a wide array of new diseases. Many of these are diseases which are well tolerated by cosmopolitan societies, but they have caused tragic population loss in newly emerging groups (Black et al. 1978; Barruzi 1977). The suddenness of the impact of these diseases accounts for much of the associated mortality. Nearly everybody gets sick at once, and there may be nobody strong enough to maintain basic services—carrying water, bringing food from the gardens, and collecting wood for fires (Neel et al. 1970). More than one disease may hit at the same time, exerting compounded effects.

The will to survive may be lost. Clearly these circumstantial factors play a major role in the associated mortality, but I am not satisfied that they provide the whole answer. Even where there has been good medical care, age-specific mortality rates from measles have been many times greater than in cosmopolitan populations (Livingstone 1958; Black et al. 1971; van Mazijk, Pinheiro, and Black 1982).

We have also seen that the forest tribes have very different genetic repertoires from the world's major groups. It is not that they have a unique set of genes, but that they have effectively fewer genes because they are so often duplicated. This phenomenon is particularly marked in those systems concerned with the immune response, systems which have been perfectly adequate to handle the endemic diseases but which face new challenges from the array of introduced diseases. The *possibility* that isolated populations are genetically less well prepared than others to fight diseases which are new to them is so obvious that it is often assumed to be true even though real evidence is very scarce. If such data are to be found, the Amazon tribes are an ideal place to look, and I have been looking there for several years. We have collected a lot of data, but still not enough to define specific genetic defects.

Measles

Our first positive finding was that the Amerindian tribes develop higher fever when infected with attenuated measles vaccine virus than other groups (Black, Woodhall, and Pinheiro 1969). The measles vaccine causes all the symptoms associated with the wild virus, but with greatly reduced severity and frequency. It therefore made a good model for the natural disease. The Indians had about twice as many high fevers as comparison groups, and their average fever was higher (Table 4.3). Note that the Icelandic temperatures were measured rectally, a method which gives higher values than axillary. The comparisons of elevation of temperature over that in controls eliminates this source of bias. The titers of antibody elicited by vaccination in the Indians were in the normal range, but titer is usually closely related to the intensity of infection, so these values were lower than expected.

TABLE 4.3
Febrile Reactions to Measles Vaccine in Amerinds and Cosmopolitan Groups.

Group	Number	Method	% > 39C	% > 40C	Mean Max. Temp. Elevation
Amerind Children	150	Axillial	25.3	3.3	0.97oC
Caboclo Children	142	Axillial	7.7	2.8	0.60
Amerind Adults	238	Axillial	13.0	2.9	0.91
Icelandic Adults	148	Rectal	7.4	1.4	0.60

These findings leave us still a long way from proving that the Indians are genetically more susceptible to measles. Two other possible explanations seemed particularly important to test, differences in nutrition and differences in prior experience with related viruses. Malnutrition is frequently associated with severe measles, and the studies of Holmberg (1949) and of Gross (1975) suggest that malnutrition might be a problem in our subjects. We took weight, height, arm circumference, and skin fold measurements on essentially all the tribes we have studied and never found evidence of protein-calorie deficiency. Vieira Filho has examined iodine and thyroxine levels in many of the same tribes and found that although the terrain is extremely poor in iodine, the Indian diet concentrates it adequately (Vieira Filho, Viero, and Russo 1979). When it comes to prior immune sensitization, the only viruses that cross-react with measles are canine distemper and rinderpest. They do not exist in the forest, but neither are they sufficiently prevalent in other parts of the world to play a regular role in modifying infection with measles virus. If prior sensitization were important in one area and not another, one would expect to find differences in timing of the events that follow infection. This we looked for but did not observe.

Any conclusive evidence of a genetic role in the different responses to measles vaccine requires association of the trait with specific genetic markers. It was for this reason that we started the HLA tests. Analysis of the variance of measles antibody titer revealed a strong association of titer with family and a weaker ($P = .015$) association with HLA haplotype. When we looked at individual haplotypes, we found that the haplotype A24, B53, Cw4 was associated with high titers (Black et al. 1982). A28, B40, Cw3 was associated with low titer in the Waiãpi but not the Parakanã. This intertribal variation suggested that the key gene was not one of those we were identifying directly but a gene linked to the HLA system. Different alleles of this gene might be associated with the same HLA sequence in different tribes.

Residual uncertainties in this study are twofold. First, we had no specific hypothesis to test beyond a general association of haplotype with variance in measles antibody titer; to be truly significant any association of antibody titer with an individual haplotype would have to have a P value lower than could be attained with the number of persons we could test. Second, immunity to measles is a very complex affair with sensitization of B-cells and various kinds of T-cells to a variety of epitopes on each of several proteins. Many different genes must have been involved in the reactions we measured. There are ways of tackling the latter problem, but now we can no longer use measles vaccine in field trials because the Brazilian Indian service has been sufficiently convinced of its value that they administer it as soon as possible — before we can get in to follow reactions.

Immunization Against Pneumococcal Polysaccharides

Recently we have concentrated on the pneumococcal vaccine as our test of immune response. Pneumonia is a major cause of death in the Indians. Although we do not know that the pneumococci are the chief cause of the Indians' disease, they are very important in New Guinea, where a similar situation pertained (Riley et al. 1977). The vaccine is composed of chemically defined polysaccharides from fourteen, or now twenty-three, different types of bacteria. Antibody to each type has been measured by Gerry Schiffman of Downstate Medical School. The immune reaction is largely B-cell dependent, and the various T-cell species play minor roles. We are dealing with immune reactions of one cell type to a set of distinct repeating sugar sequences.

The work is still in progress, but some noteworthy findings have been made. The reactions to the several polysaccharides are strongly correlated. A person who responds with a high titer to one polysaccharide always responds well to the others. Apparently, there is some common control over immune reactions to these polysaccharides as a class. Persons carrying the IgG allotype Kml and persons with the HLA haplotype A2, B51, C blank respond with more antibody than others. There are other positive associations between specific haplotypes and immune response but no negative association. It seems that the role of these genetic traits is to enhance the reaction over some basic level that is common to all members of our study population. The fact that the strongest of these enhancing effects is associated with the haplotype A2, B51, C blank is of some interest to us. This haplotype occurs in very high frequency in the Warao of the Orinoco delta, in moderate frequency in Brazil north of the Amazon River and only in low frequency south of the river. The components B51 and C blank are seldom found in combination with other antigens, suggesting that there has been little time for crossovers to accumulate. We have postulated that this haplotype was introduced relatively recently from the north; the fact that it has attained high frequencies suggests that it may confer some selective advantage.

CONCLUSIONS

The isolated South American Indian tribes are exposed to a long list of new diseases when they establish contact with the cosmopolitan world. These are diseases that would have been left behind on a migration through the Arctic, but many of them must have evolved in the Old World only after the populations of the two hemispheres had been separated. Most of the same diseases were new to the more populous parts of the New World when regularized contacts with the Old were established 500 years ago. It is likely that only a few introduced diseases, malaria being the most important, penetrated the isolation of the forest tribes and persisted among them before regular contacts were begun.

Information on the movement of disease in the reverse direction is more speculative. Among the forest tribes, endemic infectious diseases seem to be relatively benign, but these infections may not be so innocuous when they infect other communities where the ages attacked may be different and where cross-immunity from related infections may be lacking. It seems clear that the number of diseases that moved from the New World to the Old was much smaller than that moving the other way. This difference is at least partially explicable on the basis of the relative size and density of the two human populations.

Although 20,000 years of separation provided the time for evolution of quite different sets of diseases in the two hemispheres, the differences in defensive capability of the two human races has remained subtle. Much of the impact of the new diseases can be attributed to their social consequences, and part can be attributed to the inbreeding that is common in isolated New World populations. There is no evidence of any major gap in the immune defenses of the Amerindians, but some evidence of qualitative differences in the strength of responses to specific antigens. Inadequate defenses may not have been limited to one side of the exchange. If syphilis was in fact a New World disease, then its initial impact on the Old World peoples was as dramatically different from its effect among the forest people as was the impact of measles in the two hemispheres.

REFERENCES

Arnaud, E. 1961. Breve informacao sobre os indios Asurine e Parakanan; Rio Tocantins, Para. *Bos Museu E Goeldi* NS:1–22.

Barruzi, R. G. 1977. The Kreenakorore. In *Health and Disease in Tribal Societies*. Ciba Foundation Symposium No. 9. Amsterdam: Elsevier.

Bashir, H. V., J. M. MacQueen, D. N. Amos, et al. 1973. A study of the HLA system in an Australian Aboriginal population. In *Histocompatibility Testing*, J. Dausset and J. Colombani, eds. Copenhagen: Munksgaard.

Baur, M. P., and J. A. Danilovs. 1982. Reference table for two- and three-locus haplotype frequencies for HLA-A, B, C, DR, BF and GLO. In *Histocompatibility Testing*. Copenhagen: Munksgaard.

Bhatia, K., M. Gorogo, and G. Koki. 1984. HLA-A, B, C, and DR antigens in Asaro speakers of Papua, New Guinea. *Human Immunology* 9:189–200.

Billington, W. D. 1964. Influence of immunological dissimilarity of mother and fetus on placental size in mice. *Nature* 202:317–18.

Black, F. L. 1985. Mother-child HLA compatibility ratios in children of Amerindian parents who share common haplotypes. *American Journal of Human Genetics* 37:133–37.

————.1984. Interrelationships between Amerindian tribes of Lower Amazonia as manifest by HLA haplotype disequilibria. *American Journal of Human Genetics* 36:1318–1331.

————.1982. Geographic and sociological factors in the epidemiology of virus diseases. In *Virus Diseases of South-East Asia and the Western Pacific*. J. S. Mackenzie, ed. Sydney: Academic.

Black, F. L., L. L. Berman, and Y. Gabbay. 1980. HLA antigens in South American Indians. *Tissue Antigens* 16:368–76.

Black, F. L., W. H. Hierholzer, J. F. Lian-Chen, L. L. Berman, Y. Gabbay, and F. P. Pinheiro. 1982. Genetic correlates of enhanced measles susceptibility in Amazon Indians. *Medical Anthropology* 6:37–46.

Black, F. L., W. H. Hierholzer, F. P. Pinheiro, A. S. Evans, J. P. Woodall, E. M. Opton, J. E. Emmons, B. S. West, G. Edsall, W. G. Downs, and G. D. Wallace. 1974.

Evidence for persistence of infectious agents in isolated human populations. *American Journal of Epidemiology* 100:230–50.

Black, F. L., W. H. Hierholzer, J. P. Woodall, and F. P. Pinheiro. 1971. Intensified reactions to measles vaccine in unexposed populations of American Indians. *Journal of Infectious Disease* 124:306–17.

Black, F. L., F. P. Pinheiro, O. Oliva, W. H. Hierholzer, R. V. Lee, J. E. Briller, and V. A. Richards. 1978. Birth and survival patterns in numerically unstable proto-agricultural societies of the Brazilian Amazon. *Medical Anthropology* 2:95–127.

Black, F. L., and F. M. Salzano. 1981. Evidence for heterosis in the HLA system. *American Journal of Human Genetics* 33:894–99.

Black, F. L., J. P. Woodall, and F. P. Pinheiro. 1969. Measles vaccine reactions in a virgin population. *American Journal of Epidemiology* 89:168–75.

Crosby, A. W. 1972. *The Columbian Exchange: Biological and Cultural Consequences of 1492*. Westport, CT: Greenwood.

Degos, L., J. Colombani, and A. Chavantre. 1974. Selective pressure on HLA polymorphism. *Nature* 249:62–63.

Essex, M., M. F. McLane, P. Kanki, J. Allan, L. Kitchen, and T. H. Lee. 1985. Retroviruses associated with leukemia and ablative syndromes in animals and in human beings. *Cancer Research* 45:4534s–38s.

Fenner, F., and F. N. Ratcliffe. 1965. *Myxomatosis*. Cambridge, England: Cambridge University Press.

Gorodezky, C., C. E. Castro-Escobar, and A. Escobar-Guiterez. 1985. The HLA system in the prevalent Mexican Indian group: The Nahuas. *Tissue Antigens* 25:38–46.

Gross, D. R. 1975. Protein capture and cultural development in the Amazon Basin. *American Anthropologist* 77:526–49.

Haas, E. J. C., F. M. Salzano, H. A. Araujo, F. Grossman, A. Barbetti, T. A. Weimer, M.H.L.P. Franco, L. Verruno, O. Nasif, V. H. Morales, and R. Arienti. 1985. HLA antigens and other genetic markers in the Mapuche Indians of Argentina. *Human Heredity* 35:306–13.

Hedrick, P. W., and G. Thomson. 1983. Evidence for balancing selection at HLA. *Genetics* 104:449–56.

Holmberg, A. R. 1949. *Nomads of the Long Bow*. New York: Natural History Press.

Jacobson, D. L., and F. L. Black. 1986. Hepatitis A antibody in an isolated Amerindian tribe fifty years after exposure. *Journal of Medical Virology* 19: 19–20.

Kono, R., A. S. Sasagawa, S. Yamasaki, N. Nakazono, K. Minami, S. Otatsume, Y. Robin, J. Renaudet, M. Cornet, S. N. Afoakwa, A. A. Mingle, J. K. Obinin, and A. Huros. . 1981. Seroepidemiologic studies of acute hemorrhagic conjunctivitis virus (Enterovirus type 70) in West Africa. III. Studies with animal sera from Ghana and Senegal. *American Journal of Epidemiology* 114:362–68.

Lee, R. V., F. L. Black, W. J. Hierholzer, and B. S. West. 1978. Novel pattern of treponemal antibody distribution in isolated American Indian populations. *American Journal of Epidemiology* 107:46–53.

Levin, B. R., A. C. Allison, H. J. Bremermann, L. L. Cavalli-Sforza, S. A. Levin, R. M. May, and H. R. Thieme. 1982. Evolution of parasites and hosts. In *Population Biology of Infectious Diseases*. R. M. Anderson and R. M. May, eds. New York: Springer-Verlag.

Livingstone, F. 1958. Anthropological implications of sickle cell gene distribution in West Africa. *American Anthropology* 60:533–63.

Mourant, A. E., A. C. Kopec, and K. Domaniewska-Sobczak. 1976. *Distribution of Human Blood Groups and Other Polymorphisms.* Oxford: Blackwell.

Neel, J. V., W. R. Centerwall, N. A. Chagnon, and H. L. Casey. 1970. Notes on the effect of measles and measles vaccines in a virgin-soil population of South American Indians. *American Journal of Epidemiology* 91:418–29.

Neel, J. V., and R. H. Ward. 1970. Village and tribal genetic distances among American Indians and the possible implication for human evolution. *Proceedings of the National Academy of Sciences* 65:223–30.

Nihoul, E., L. Quersin-Thiery, and A. Weynants. 1957. ECHOvirus type 9 and the agent responsible for an important outbreak of aseptic meningitis in Belgium. *American Journal of Hygiene* 66:102–18.

Nutels, N. 1968. Medical problems of newly contacted Indian groups. *Pan American Health Organization, Scientific Publications* 165:68–76.

Riley, I. D., P. I. Tarr, M. Andrews, M. Pfeiffer, R. Howard, P. Challands, G. Jennison, and R. M. Douglas. 1977. Immunization with a polyvalent pneumococcal vaccine. *Lancet* i:1338–41.

Serjeantson, S. W., D. P. Ryand, and A. R. Thompson. 1982. The colonization of the Pacific: The story according to human leukocyte antigens. *American Journal of Human Genetics* 34:904–18.

Sibley, C. G. 1984. The phylogeny of the hominoid primatesas indicated by DNA-DNA hybridization. *Journal of Molecular Evolution* 20:2–15.

Troup, G. M., M. S. Schanfield, C. H. Singaraju, R. L. Harvey, J. Jameson, J. Capper, and B. Baker. 1982. Study of HLA alloantigens of the Navajo Indians of North America. *Tissue Antigens* 20:339–51.

van Loghem, E. 1984. The immunoglobulin genes: Genetics, biological and clinical significance. *Clinical Studies in Immunology and Allergy* 4:607–22.

van Mazijk, J., F. P. Pinheiro, and F. L. Black. 1982. Measles and measles vaccine in isolated Amerindian tribes. I. The 1971 Trio (Tiriyo) epidemic. *Tropical and Geographical Medicine* 34:3–6.

Vieira Filho, J. P. B., J. G. H. Viera, and E. M. K. Russo. 1979. Determiacao dos niveis sangineos de tiroxina, triiodtironina, testosterona e sulfato de deidroepiandrosterona dos silvicolas Xikrin e Surui. *Revista Associacao Medica Brasileira* 25:208–10.

5 DIABETES IN AMERINDIAN POPULATIONS: THE DOGRIB STUDIES

Emöke J. E. Szathmary

Among the diseases associated with "Westernization" (Zimmet 1979), non-insulin dependent diabetes mellitus (NIDDM) may be the most insidious. Its onset is unremarkable and asymptomatic, so that the disease can remain undiagnosed for years. Unfortunately diabetes, whether noninsulin dependent or insulin dependent (IDDM), is not a benign disease. In the United States it is one of the main causes of cardiovascular disease, kidney disease, blindness, and amputation, and it is ranked as the sixth most common cause of death (Bennett 1982).

PREVALENCE OF DIABETES IN NATIVE AMERICANS

There appears to be reasonably good evidence that two to three generations ago diabetes mellitus was very rare among Indian populations of North America. The evidence is based on records of Indian hospitals, testimonies of physicians who had Native patients, and interviews with knowledgeable elders (West 1974, 1978). Low prevalence was characteristic regardless of geographic origin, but by the late 1960s a different profile had emerged.

Niswander (1968) was among the first to note a new pattern in Indian diabetes: rates determined from hospital discharge records were on average twice as great in data obtained from Indian Health Hospitals as those from non-Indian hospitals. This observation is still a very important piece of evidence supporting the notion of an ongoing "epidemic" of diabetes among Native Americans. This is so because until 1979 there was no uniform set of diagnostic criteria and test procedures (see Table 5.1) applied by physicians and epidemiologists in their identification of diabetes mellitus (CSDA 1969; National Diabetes Data Group 1979). The majority of surveys, for example (see

Table 5.1.
Oral Glucose Tolerance Test Procedures and Criteria for the
Judgment of Diabetes Mellitus in Nonpregnant Adults.

Procedures:

Clinical examination
    Criteria: Symptoms of diabetes, for example, polyuria, polydipsia,
              ketonuria, rapid weight loss with gross hyperglycemia.
Fasting blood sample
    Criteria: Fasting glucose elevated on more than one occasion:
              venous plasma ≥ 140 mg / dl (7.8 mmol / l)
              venous whole blood ≥ 120 mg / dl (6.7 mmol / l)
              capillary whole blood ≥ 120 mg / dl (6.7 mmol / l)
Oral glucose tolerance test:
    a) on the 3 days preceding the test subjects should consume at least
    150 gm carbohydrate daily;
    b) test is administered in the morning after an overnight fast of 10-16
    hrs;
    c) fasting blood sample is obtained;
    d) within 5 minutes of the fasting sample the subject drinks a glucose
    load (or its carbohydrate equivalent) of 75 gm glucose (1.75 gm / kg
    body weight) in 250-350 ml water;
    e) a second blood sample is obtained within the fasting and hour 2
    samples; the last blood sample is obtained at hour 2.
    Criteria: 1. Fasting glucose is elevated as shown above on more than
             one occasion;
           2. Fasting glucose is normal, but on more than one occasion;
             the hour 2 specimen and some other sample drawn be-
             tween fasting and hour-2 are elevated as shown:
                venous plasma ≥ 200 mg / dl (11.1 mmol / l)
                venous whole blood ≥ 180 mg / dl (10.0 mmol / l)
                capillary whole blood ≥ 200 mg / dl (11.1 mmol / l)

Sources: National Diabetes Data Group (1979); WHO (1980).

Table 5.2), used methods and levels of abnormality that today would not be accepted as indicating diabetes. Estimates of the rate of clinical diabetes (see Table 5.3) also often relied on physicians' judgments based on responses to the oral glucose tolerance test in the absence of clinical complications (Prosnitz and Mandell 1967; Saiki and Rimoin 1968). Sometimes the rates of "diabetes" estimated from test responses were so discordant from the known rates of clinical diabetes (e.g., diagnosis based on "polyphagia, polydipsia, and polyuria, with the presence of reducing substances in the urine" [Bennett 1982: 38]) that the diagnostic utility of the oral glucose tolerance test for Native Americans was questioned (Schaefer, Crockford, and Romanowski 1972; Canadian Diabetic Association 1982). Table 5.2 provides an example of this problem: of the eighteen entries that give percentages of known diabetes, fifteen (or 83 percent) show that the percentage of hyperglycemia (called "diabetes" in the primary sources) is at least twice as great as the known amount of diabetes.

While "hidden" diabetes is a recognized problem in many countries (WHO 1980), this is unlikely to be the explanation for the elevated "abnormal" response rates shown in Table 5.2. It is more likely that the criterion of abnormality used in the studies was set too low. A second reason for not equating the rates of abnormal response with the incidence of diabetes is that in all cases but one (Alaskan Athabaskan, or Athapaskan, Indians) the rates were based on results obtained from a single test. Currently both the National Diabetes Data Group (NDDG) (1979) and the World Health Organization (WHO) (1980) recommend that, in the absence of clinical symptoms, diagnosis of diabetes mellitus be made only when abnormality of glucose level is detected on two separate occasions. For these reasons, and because test procedures in all cases but one (Kiowa-Comanche) deviate from current practice, it is clear that Table 5.2 does not provide good estimates of the prevalence of NIDDM in populations of Native Americans.

On the other hand, whatever the problems in determining whether the prevalence rates of reported diabetes are accurate, there seems to be no reason to doubt the veracity of the general statement that many Amerindian groups have higher rates of diabetes than non-Indians. Of the populations listed in Tables 5.2 and 5.3, very high frequencies of diabetes are known to be present in the Cherokee and Seneca (Iroquoian speakers) and in the Pima, Papago, and Cocopah (Uto-Aztecan speakers) (Bennett 1982). Regional prevalence data obtained since 1979 also show high rates of diabetes in several other populations (Table 5.3).

These findings should not be interpreted to mean that at the present time all Native Americans are equally at risk for diabetes. Notable among groups with low frequencies of disease are Athabaskan-speaking Indians of interior Alaska (Mouratoff, Carroll, and Scott 1969) and Canada's Northwest Territories (Szathmary and Holt 1983), as well as Eskimos in Alaska, Canada, and Greenland (Schaefer 1969). Nevertheless, even in these populations diabetes incidence is increasing (Mouratoff and Scott 1973; Schaefer, Crockford, and Romanowski 1972; Szathmary 1985). Although the increased number of cases is still absolutely small, the rise in frequency has prompted the question whether it is inevitable that these northern people will also experience the diabetes epidemic afflicting some of their southern brethren. The response to this depends upon our knowledge of the etiology of diabetes in Native Americans.

ETIOLOGY OF DIABETES IN NATIVE AMERICANS

NIDDM (also called "maturity-onset" diabetes or "Type II" diabetes) is considered to be the characteristic form of diabetes among Native Americans.

TABLE 5.2
Survey Results: Glucose Intolerance in Native Populations of North America.

Population[1] Location	Sample Size	Age	Dietary[2] State	Glucose or Glucose-Equivalent Load (gm)	Time(hr) After Ingestion	Abnormality[3] Criteria (mg/dl)	% Hyperglycemia	Known Clinical Diabetes (%)	Source[6]
Eskimo-Aleut Family									
Eskimo:									
40 mi radius of Bethel, Alaska	581	≥20	F	100	2	>140 wb	1.9	0.17	1
"	320	≥20	F	100	2	>150 wb	7.5	.30	2
Edmonton, Alberta[4]	20	<15	F	.8/lb body fat	see (d)	wb — see (d)	44.7	0.0	3
	112	>15	F	100					
Eastern and Central Arctic Canada	49	all ages	20NF 29F	100	see (d)	wb — see (d)	16.3	0.0	3
Aleut:									
Aleutian Islands	193	≥20	F	100	2	>150 wb	13.7[5]	2.10	4
Athabaskan Family									
Apache:									
White River, Arizona	268	>35	NF	75	2	≥160 p	11.0	not stated	5
San Carlos, Arizona	317	>35	NF	75	2	≥160 p	24.8	not stated	5
Navajo:									
Ft. Defiance, Arizona	55	>35	NF	75	2	≥160 p	12.8	not stated	5
Dogrib:									
Rae, LacLaMartre and Rae Lakes NWT, Canada	157	≥19	F	100	2	≥160 p	22.2	0.0	6
"	155	≥21	F	100	2	≥200 p	9.7	0.0	6

Slavey:									
Hay River and Ft. Providence NWT, Canada	70	≥15	F	100	2	≥160 p	4.3	not stated	7
"Athabascan"									
Alaska	360	≥20	F	100	2	≥150 wb	1.3	.33	8
Hokan Family									
Washo:									
Dresslerville, Nevada, and Woodfords, California	112	≥15	NF	75	2	>160 p	10.7	6.3	13
Iroquoian Fmaily:									
Cherokee:									
Qualla, North Carolina	448	>34	F and NF	1/kg body wt	2	≥150 wb	29.0	17.2	9
Seneca:									
Cattaraugus, New York	209	≥25	F	75	1	≥200 p	31.6	14.4	10
Muskogean Fmaily									
Alabama-Coushatta:									
Polk County, Texas	171	all ages	F	100 and .8/lb ideal body wt	2	≥120 wb	31.0	8.2	11
Seminole:									
Seminole County, Oklahoma	217	≥6	F	75	1–1 1/2	>160 p	38.7	13.0	12
Brighton, and Big Cypress Florida	254	≥6	F	75	1–1 1/2	>160 p	35.0	3.0	12
Uto-Aztecan Family									
Cocopah:									
Yuma County, Arizona	182	≥5	NF	75	2	≥160 p	17.0	5.5	17
Kiowa-Comanche:									
Oklahoma	200	≥19	F	75	2	>150 p	35.0	0.0	13

Table 5.2, continued

Population[1] Location	Sample Size	Age	Dietary[2] State	Glucose or Glucose-Equivalent Load (gm)	Time(hr) After Ingestion	Abnormality[3] Criteria (mg/dl)	% Hyperglycemia	Known Clinical Diabetes (%)	Source[6]
								Procedures and Diagnostic Criteria	
Paiute:									
Ft. McDermitt, Nevada	131	≥15	NF	75	2	>160 p	11.5	8.4	14
Papago:									
Sells & San Xavier, Arizona	627	≥9	NF	75	1	≥200 p	6.5	not stated	15
Pima:									
Gila River, Arizona	2917	≥5	NF	75	2	≥160 p	19.1	9.6	16
Upland Yuman (?Hualapai?)									
Peach Springs, Arizona	313	>35	NF	75	2	≥160 p	29.9	not stated	5
Zuni Language Isolate									
Zuni:									
West central New Mexico	652	≥20	NF	75	2	≥160 p	15.0	not stated	15

[1]Population classification is by language family as given in the Murdock, GP, O'Leary, TJ (1975) Ethnographic Bibliography of North America. New Haven: HRAF Press, and in Driver, HE (1961) Indians of North America. Chicago: University of Chicago Press, pp. 576.
[2]Fasting or Non-fasting at the start of the test.
[3]wb = whole blood, p = plasma. Whole blood values should be multiplied by 1.15 and a constant of 6 mg/100 ml added to convert whole blood glucose to plasma or serum glucose.
[4]Hospitalized patients from across the Canadian arctic. Moderately abnormal was defined as: any glucose value above 180 mg/dl, or two values above 170 mg/dl, or a two-hour value above 140 mg/dl.
[5]Percent given only for participants >39 years.
[6]Sources are numbered and are given in the following source notes.

1. Mouratoff, G.J., Carroll, N.V., and Scott, E.M. (1967) Diabetes mellitus in Eskimos. JAMA 199:107–112.
2. Mouratoff, G.J., and Scott, E.M. (1973) Diabetes mellitus in Eskimos after a decade. JAMA 226:1345–1346.
3. Schaefer, O. (1968) Glucose tolerance testing in Canadian Eskimos: A preliminary report and hypothesis. Can. Med. Assoc. J. 99:252–262.
4. Mouratoff, G.J., and Scott, E.M. (1976) Diabetes mellitus in the Aleutians of Alaska. Diabetes 25 (Suppl. 1):227.
5. Bennett, P.H., Rushforth, N.B., Miller, M., and LeCompte, P.M. (1976) Epidemiologic studies of diabetes in the Pima Indians. Rec. Prog. in Hormone Res. 32:333–375.
6. Szathmary, E.J.E., and Holt, N. (1983) Hyperglycemia in Dogrib Indians of the Northwest Territories, Canada: Association with age and a centripetal distribution of body fat. Human Biology 55:493–515.
7. Lathrop M., and Ward, R. (1979) Unpublished data.
8. Mouratoff, G.J., Carroll, N.V., and Scott, E.M. (1969) Diabetes mellitus in Athabaskan Indians in Alaska. Diabetes 18:29–32.
9. Stein, J.H., West, K.M., Robey, J.M. Tirador, D.F., and McDonald, G.W. (1965) The high prevalence of abnormal glucose tolerance in the Cherokee Indians of North Carolina. Arch. Intern. Med. 116:842–845.
10. Doeblin, T.D., Evans, K., Ingall, G.B., Dowling, K., Chilcote, M.E., Elsea, W., and Bannerman, R.M. (1969) Diabetes and hyperglycemia in Seneca Indians. Human Heredity 19:613–627.
11. Johnson, J.E. Jr., and McNutt, C.W. (1964) Diabetes mellitus in an American Indian population isolate. Texas Reports on Biology and Medicine 22:110–125.
12. Elston, R.C., Namboodiri, K.K., Nino, H.V., and Pollitzer, W.S. (1974) Studies on blood and urine glucose in Seminole Indians: Indications for segregation of a major gene. Am. J. Hum. Genet. 26:13–34.\
13. West, K.M., and Mako, M.E. (1976) Effect of prediabetes, preobesity and dietary sugar on insulin secretion. Diabetes 25 (Suppl. 1):389.
14. Bartha, G.W., Burch, T.A., and Bennett, P.H. (1973) Hyperglycemia in Washoe and northern Paiute Indians. Diabetes 22:58–62.
15. Workman, P.L. (1978) Genetic epidemiology and population structure. In: Genetic Epidemiology, N.E. Morton and C.S. Chung (eds.). New York: Academic Press, pp. 354–359.
16. Bennett, P.H., Burch, T.A., and Miller, M. (1971) Diabetes mellitus in American (Pima) Indians. Lancet 2:125–128.
17. Henry, R.E., Burch, T.A., Bennett, P.H., and Miller, M. (1969) Diabetes in the Cocopah Indians. Diabetes 18:33–37.
18. Young, T.K., McIntyre, L.L., Dooley, J., and Rodriguez, J. (1985) Epidemiologic features of diabetes mellitus among Indians in northwestern Ontario and northeastern Manitoba. Can. Med. Assoc. J. 132:793–797.
19. McNiven, M. (1978) Diabetes on the Wikwemikong Indian Reservation. Report to Health and Welfare Canada, Medical Services Branch.
20. Ede, M.C. (1966) Diabetes and the way of life on an Indian reservation. Guy's Hospital Reports 115:455–461.
21. Schaefer, O. (1968) Glycosuria and diabetes mellitus in Canadian Eskimos. Canad. Med. Assoc. J. 99:201–206.
22. Cohen, B.M. (1954) Diabetes mellitus among Indians of the American Southwest: Its prevalence and clinical characteristics in a hospitalized population. Ann. Intern. Med. 40:588–599.
23. Szathmary, E.J.E. (1985) The search for genetic factors controlling plasma glucose levels in Dogrib Indians. In: Diseases of Complex Etiology in Small Populations. R. Chakraborty and E.J.E. Szathmary (eds.). New York: Alan R. Liss. pp. 199–226.
24. Saiki, J.H., Rimoin, D.L. (1968) Diabetes mellitus among the Navajo. Arch. Intern. Med. 122:1–5.
25. White, W.D. (1966) Diabetes in the Oklahoma Indian. USPHS, 1st Proceedings, p. j21.
26. Brosseau, J.D., Elkema, R.C., Crawford, A.C., and Abe, T.A. (1979) Diabetes among the three affiliated tribes: Correlation with degree of Indian inheritance. Am. J. Pub. Health 69:1277–1278.
27. Montour, L.T., and Macauley, A.C. (1985) High prevalence rates of diabetes mellitus and hypertension on a North American Indian reservation. Can. Med. Assoc. J. 132:1112.
28. Drevets, C.C. (1965) Diabetes mellitus in Choctaw Indians. Oklahoma State Med. Assoc. 58:322–329.
29. Petersen, K. (1969) A profile of diabetes mellitus among the Indians of a Sioux/Assiniboine reservation. U.S. Public Health Service, 4th Proceedings, p. 35.
30. Long, T.P. (1978) The prevalence of clinically treated diabetes among Zuni reservation residents. Public Health Briefs 68:901–903.

TABLE 5.3
Clinical Records: Rates of Diabetes Mellitus in Native Populations of North America.

Population Location[1]	Group Size	Age	Type of Record and Duration of Assessment	Diagnostic Criteria[2]	% Diabetes	Comments	Source[3]
Eskimoan Family							
Eskimo: Greenland	32,000	All ages	Medical charts (1965)	Not stated	.03	All diabetics are of "racially mixed" parentage	21
Alaska	20,000	All ages	Medical charts (1967)	Not stated	.04	—	1
Canada	13,000	All ages	Hospital charts (1968)	Not stated	.02	—	21
Algonkian Family							
Cree and Ojibwa: NW Ontario and NE Manitoba	14,000	All ages	Hospital and Medical charts (1978–82)	Physician's diagnosis confirmed by NDDG criteria	2.75	three individuals under 15 years	18
Ottawa and Ojibwa: Wikwemikong, Ontario	3,000	All ages	Medical charts (1977–78)	Not stated	2.37	one "juvenile onset"	19
Passamaquody: Peter Dana Point, Maine	56	≥20	Hospital charts (1965)	Not stated	8.93	all noninsulin dependent	20
Athabaskan Family							
Apache: Ft. Apache, Arizona	2,103	All ages	Hospital admissions (July 1, 1950– June 30, 1952)	Not stated	.40	—	22
San Carlos, Arizona	2,266	All ages	Hospital admissions (July 1, 1950– June 30, 1952)	Not stated	.10	—	22
Dogrib: Rae, NWT	712	≥21	Hospital admissions diagnosis (1981)	FBS >140 mg/dl,p	.14	sole known diabetic in population	23
Navajo: Ft. Defiance, Arizona	11,412	≥20	Hospital discharge diagnosis (July 1958 –June 1963)	FBS >120 mg/dl wb or hr-2 >140 mg/dl,wb	.91	none developed diabetes before 20 years	24

Group	N	Age	Source	Criteria	Rate	Comments	Ref
Caddoan Family ?Pawnee?:							
Pawnee, Oklahoma	2,239	All ages	Health Service Clinic charts (1965)	FBS >140 mg/dl	11.70	predominantly adult-onset "ketosis-free"	25
Arikara:							
Ft. Berthold, N. Dakota	151	≥35	Health Service Clinic (active health records ?1978?)	Physician's diagnosis	39.00	full-blood Indians; diabetes uncommon in persons <35 yrs	26
Iroquoian Fmaily Mohawk:							
Kahnawake, Quebec	544	45–64	Hospital charts (1981)	Receiving treatment for diabetes by NDDG criteria OR preprandial >120 mg/dl, wb; postprandial at 2 hr >180 mg/dl, wb	12.00	—	27
Muskogean Family Choctaw:							
Talihina, Oklahoma	1,993	All ages	Hospital charts (Dec. 31, 1958)	FBS ≥130 mg/dl, wb 2 hr postprandial ≥150 mg/dl	5.30	all full-blood 1.83% diabetics in mixed blood	28
Siouan Family Assiniboine/Sioux:							
Poplar, Montana	3,500	All ages	Medical charts (1969?)	Not stated	2.90	markedly greater disease rate after 30; only 7% controlled by diet alone	29
Hidatsa:							
Ft. Berthold, N. Dakota	179	≥35	Health Service Clinic (active health records ?1978?)	Physician's diagnosis	21.20	full-blood 26	
Manda:							
Ft. Berthold, N. Dakota	59	≥35	Health Service Clinic (active health records ?1978?)	Physician's diagnosis	39.0	full-blood	26
Uto-Aztecan Family Mojave:							
Colorado River Agency, California & Arizona	1,427	All ages	Hospital admissions (July 1, 1950– June 30, 1952)	Not stated	2.2	—	22

Table 5.3, continued

Population Location[1]	Group Size	Age	Type of Record and Duration of Assessment	Diagnostic Criteria[2]	% Diabetes	Comments	Source[3]
Paiute & Shoshone: Walker River Agency, Nevada	1,685	All ages	Hospital admissions (July 1, 1950– June 30, 1952)	Not stated	1.0	—	22
Western Shoshone Agency, Nevada	751	All ages	Hospital admissions (July 1, 1950– June 30, 1952)	Not stated	.3	—	22
Papago: San Xavier Agency, Arizona	1,904	All ages	Hospital admissions (July 1, 1950– June 30, 1952)	Not stated	.4	—	22
Pima: Pima Agency, Arizona	2,898	All ages	Hospital admissions (July 1, 1950– June 30, 1952)	Not stated	3.2	—	22
Ute: Uintah & Ouray Agency, Utah	877	All ages	Hospital admissions (July 1, 1950– June 30, 1952)	Not stated	1.2	—	22
Yuma: Ft. Yuma Agency California	477	All ages	Hospital admissions (July 1, 1950– June 30, 1952)	Not stated	3.1	—	22
Zuni Language Isolate Zuni: Zuni, New Mexico	6,303	All ages	Hospital and Clinic charts (1975 and 1976)	Physician's diagnosis have diabetes	4.3	1/4 over 45 years	30

[1]Population classification by language as given in Murdock, GP, O'Leary, TJ (1975). Ethnographic Bibliography of North America. New Haven: HRAF Press, and Driver, HE (1961) Indians of North America. Chicago: The University of Chicago Press, pp. 576.
[2]NDDG = National Diabetes Data Group; FBS = Fasting blood sugar, p = plasma, wb = whole blood. See Table 1 for conversion of whole blood glucose to plasma glucose.
[3]Sources are numbered and are given in the source notes following Table 5.2.

Insulin dependent diabetes mellitus (IDDM) does occur, but it is very infrequent and contributes little to the Native American diabetes problem (West 1978).

Much of what we know about the epidemiologic and metabolic features of diabetes in Native Americans is based on detailed, longitudinal studies among the Pima people of Arizona. This group has the dubious distinction of having the world's highest frequency of NIDDM (Knowler et al. 1978). Many researchers assume that whatever etiological factors operate among the Pima will also apply to other Native Americans, including those who currently have very low rates of diabetes. While this assumption may be warranted, two observations suggest caution against overgeneralization: (1) genetic factors are thought to confer "susceptibility" to diabetes; and (2) environmental factors are also implicated.

Genetic Factors

That genes are involved in the onset of NIDDM is suggested by data obtained worldwide (Friedman and Fialkow 1980). However, the nature of the genetic mechanism that predisposes an individual to diabetes continues to be debated.

Among the Pima, until recently, the genetic basis of NIDDM was thought to be dependent on homozygosity for two autosomal recessive alleles (Steinberg et al. 1970). New analyses of accumulated data suggest the transmission pattern in autosomal dominant (Yamashita et al. 1984). These findings do not agree with results obtained from studies on other Amerindians. For example, segregation analysis of glucose levels of Seminole Indians from Oklahoma supported the recessive model the best (Elston et al. 1974), while analysis of Florida Seminole data supported neither model (Ibid.). Still different results were obtained from an Indian group currently undergoing cultural transition (Szathmary 1985) and will be detailed later in this chapter.

Focus on the contradictory results and on the problems associated with assumptions in the genetic models examined above (e.g., Neel 1976) distracts attention from one important point: if genetic factors are implicated, Native Americans should be expected to show variable frequencies of these genes. Considerable genetic heterogeneity characterizes Amerindian peoples (Spuhler 1972, 1979; Szathmary 1984), and in the absence of evidence for selection one may expect corresponding heterogeneity for the frequencies of the "susceptibility" alleles. It is very clear that selection has had little time to operate on the diabetic phenotype, given the short history of the disease in the Americas. Accordingly, "susceptibility genes" should not have decreased or increased in frequency in Native Americans, except as a consequence of random processes. The only way in which an increase could have occurred in all Native peoples is if these genes conferred a great advantage on the bearers in some other context.

The Thrifty Gene Hypothesis

As originally proposed by Neel (1962), the "thrifty gene" hypothesis stated that some individuals may be quicker than others in producing insulin when blood glucose levels are elevated. Such individuals would be able to take up glucose and store it as glycogen or fat more efficiently than those whose insulin response to carbohydrate is slower. The enhanced ability to store calories is an advantage under conditions of alternating food plenty and food shortage. Presumably those who had been able to store more glycogen or fat during the rich times had a greater chance of surviving the lean times. The survivors in turn would transmit to their offspring the thrifty gene(s) that coded for the "quick insulin trigger," allowing the increase of these genes in the next generation.

Neel (1962) also argues that the ability to respond quickly to carbohydrate stimulus has its costs when food availability is no longer episodic but continuous. Individuals who carry the thrifty gene(s) would overproduce insulin, become obese, and eventually exhaust the pancreatic B-cells that produce insulin. The net result would be diabetes.

Although the physiologic details of Neel's hypothesis have shifted considerably since it was first proposed (Neel 1982), the notion of a thrifty genotype more at risk for diabetes than other genotypes remains. Support for its plausibility is provided by studies on mice that are heterozygous for two genes that produce obesity and diabetes in these animals (ob/db); the heterozygotes are able to tolerate fasting for longer periods than the normal controls (Coleman 1979). The thrifty genotype model is also thought to apply to Pima Indians (Knowler et al. 1982).

The ancestors of the Pima were desert horticulturalists who were subjected to periodic bouts of feast and famine. Modern nondiabetic Pima have high concentrations of insulin in their blood and appear to be less efficient in reducing blood glucose levels than normal Caucasians (Nagulesparan et al. 1982). This evidence suggests some degree of resistance of cells to insulin action. However, fat cells of Pima individuals seem to have normal sensitivity to insulin. Knowler, Savage, et al. (1982) hypothesize that, in individuals with the thrifty genotype, cells differ in their responsiveness to insulin. Accordingly, insulin-mediated glucose transport is diminished in such people, but fat deposition in adipose tissue proceeds unhampered. Over time, the result of this process is obesity and NIDDM. This version of the thrifty genotype identifies a differential cellular response to insulin action rather than a "quick insulin trigger" as the basic mechanism that produces NIDDM.

Neel (1982) notes that the precise genetic basis of the thrifty genotype has never been elucidated, either in his original hypothesis or in its more recent versions. Nevertheless, if the hypothesis itself is correct, it has considerable ramifications for the expectation of NIDDM in Native Americans. For example, if it is assumed that Amerindians are the descendants of a single population that entered the Americas, then the existence of NIDDM in linguistically and culturally distinct groups suggests not just that thrifty genes are widely distributed among them but also that these genes are held by virtue of common ancestry. This would mean that all Amerindians should carry thrifty genes and that the latter were present in the founding population that entered North America. It is at this point in the argument that one has to question the thrifty gene concept by focusing specifically on the proposed mechanisms that selection is thought to have favored in the environment in which these ancient Americans lived.

Problems with the Thrifty Gene Model for Amerindians

Whether the basic mechanism favored by selection was the development of a quick insulin trigger or whether it was a difference in the sensitivity of specific cell types to insulin action, the thrifty gene hypothesis assumes a particular kind of nutritional environment in which selection took place. The dietary intake periodically had to include carbohydrate in amounts that exceeded the daily energy requirements. The liver converts and stores excess glucose as glycogen, and it also converts excess glucose into triglyceride and releases it for storage in fat cells as very low density lipoprotein (VLDL) (Tepperman 1980). Excess fat can also be stored, as can excess protein after suitable conversion of certain amino acids to triglyceride (Guyton 1971). However, such excesses occur only after all energy needs of the body have been met, and these needs place a priority on the availability of glucose for the brain, red cells, and kidney medulla. When the diet is severely restricted in carbohydrate, excess glucose will be unavailable, and the ingested protein and fat will have to provide the body's metabolic requirements. What might offer survival advantage when the diet provides for little or no carbohydrate is the enhancement of those mechanisms that allow for the endogenous derivation of glucose from noncarbohydrate sources.

We do not know much about the diets of the hunting bands that roamed across Beringia during the last glaciation, but we can make some educated guesses based on our knowledge of dietary intake components in Eskimos (Draper 1978) and subarctic Indians (Szathmary, Ritenbaugh, and Goodby 1987). In an arctic/subarctic climate year-round protein/fat intake is high, and carbohydrate intake is virtually nonexistent for much of the year. Even if one assumes that the peoples of Beringia had sufficient technological knowledge to store carbohydrate (e.g., berries) during the times such foods were available, it is doubtful that nomadic hunters could have carried sufficient quantities to last ten to eleven months of the year.

The difficulties a carbohydrate-deficient diet imposes on an individual are considerable. The American mixed diet, for example, in which approximately 46 percent of the calories are obtained from carbohydrate, 42 percent from fat, and 12 percent from protein, provides about 250 gm of glucose. Of this, the brain uses about 100 gm, and the remaining fuels the peripheral tissues (Draper 1978). Draper has estimated that the premodern, all-meat Eskimo diet supplied only about 10–20 gm of glucose per day. Year-round, approximately 98 percent of the calories consumed by Eskimos was obtained from meat and fat and only 2 percent from carbohydrate (Ibid.), the latter derived most commonly from rich animal tissues (Feldman, Ho, et al. 1972). When dietary carbohydrate is unavailable or is present in minimal amounts, glucose – the required fuel – can be obtained from available stores through the process of glycogenolysis. This supply, however, is limited. For this reason, continuous carbohydrate insufficiency means that the organism has to meet its needs through gluconeogenesis – the formation of glucose in the liver and kidneys (Kraus-Friedmann 1984). The substrates from which this new glucose forms are specific amino acids obtained primarily from the catabolism of skeletal muscle. A high protein diet permits gluconeogenesis without accompanying muscle wastage because the amino acids the diet supplies are used in the synthesis of new muscle (Tepperman 1980). When gluconeogenesis is taking place, triglyceride synthesis is greatly restricted (Ibid.) in spite of the fact that the circulation contains free fatty acids from mobilized lipid stores, as well as from the diet (Draper 1978). These free fatty acids are used to supply the energy requirements of peripheral tissues. The mechanism that permits this is the same as that which prevails during heavy exercise sustained over several hours (Hochachka and Somero 1984). The burning of fat as fuel saves endogenously produced glucose for the brain. Because this supply is still not enough, however, the brain and other tissues begin and progressively increase extracting energy from ketone bodies (Ibid.). The latter are produced in the liver from fatty acids whenever gluconeogenesis occurs (Tepperman 1980). During starvation, increased use of ketone bodies reduces the need of the brain for glucose to about 40 gm per day (Hochachka and Somero 1984).

Ordinarily, ketosis is considered to be an undesirable condition because accumulation of ketone bodies will lead to death. If ketones can be removed through use as fuel, however, an all-meat diet is not harmful. Vilhjalmur Steffanson and R. Anderson, for example, lived for one year on a diet consisting of 0.3 pounds of protein and 0.67 pounds of fat (plus occasional black coffee) without any apparent ill-effects (Folk 1984). Sinclair (1984) consumed a diet of seal, fish, mollusks, crustaceans, and water for a period of 100 days. He reported that even after a ten-mile walk he was unable to detect any ketone in his urine. Eskimos who were examined fifteen to twenty-six hours after a meal made up of their usual foods had levels of free fatty acids "seen only in prolonged starvation or diabetic ketoacidosis in US whites" (Feldman, Ho, et al. 1972: 50), yet no ketone bodies were detected in their sera. These observations suggest that a diet high in fat and protein does not necessarily lead to harmful levels of ketosis because the production of ketone bodies may be significantly less than under total starvation, such as for the ketones derived from branched chain amino acids (Schauder 1984), and the saturation point for ketone usage (Hall et al. 1984) is not attained. One additional advantage of ketone production may be that ketones can be used as substrates for formation of fat in adipose tissue (Ibid.).

Selective pressures under conditions of low to no carbohydrate intake should favor individuals in whom gluconeogenesis and free fatty acid release and utilization are enhanced. Gluconeogenesis is promoted by glucagon, epinephrine, and glucocorticoids, all of which are insulin antagonists (Kraus-Friedmann 1984). Plasma glucagon levels increase in normal individuals on low carbohydrate diets, and exercise triples glucagon levels (Ibid.). There is, in addition, experimental evidence from rats that shows that gluconeogenesis from amino acids increases in a cold environment (Nagai and Nakagawa 1973). Because glucose homeostasis is regulated through a complex interplay of counter-regulatory hormones and neural stimuli, it is worth emphasizing that metabolic responses of target tissues depend upon the relative amounts of the different hormones that are present. A protein meal, for example, stimulates the production of both glucagon and insulin, but triglyceride synthesis and fat deposition will be inhibited because the glucagon:insulin ratio favors gluconeogenesis and lipolysis (Tepperman 1980). A low carbohydrate, fat-rich meal significantly stimulates glucagon secretion but seems to have no enhancing effect on insulin production (Gutniak, Grill, and Efendic 1986).

Under arctic and subarctic conditions that favor a protein/fat food base, individuals whose metabolic systems inhibited gluconeogenesis would not have been likely to survive. Whether a low carbohydrate nutritional environment led to the selection of genes that enhanced gluconeogenesis is not known. If such selection occurred, and if the mechanism persists in at least some of the descendants of the groups that moved out of Beringia, then in the carbohydrate-rich environment of the "Westernized" diet, ingested glucose and endogenous glucose could lead to NIDDM. The primary defect would not have to be in the pancreas but could occur at the gastrointestinal level (Schaefer, Crockford, and Romanowski 1972; Hampton et al. 1986). For example, if adaptation to a high fat/protein, low carbohydrate diet led to an inability of gut hormones to respond appropriately to carbohydrate, that is, to release insulin and somatostatin (Tepperman 1980), and instead glucagon, insulin, and somatostatin were released, with the initial ratio in favor of glucagon (as in a low carbohydrate meal (Gutniak, Grill, and Efendic 1986)), hyperglycemia would be a consequence. To normalize plasma glucose, the glucagon:insulin ratio would have to shift in favor of insulin, with higher levels of insulin produced to deal with the higher levels of glucose. The rates of hyperglycemia in Table 5.2 suggest that Native Americans do have a propensity to respond abnormally to glucose challenge, yet these rates of hyperglycemia do not reflect known diabetes prevalence.

If Neel's thrifty gene model does apply to Native Americans, then one can predict that under modern conditions an overproduction of insulin should be demonstrable. Insulin excess, in particular, should be manifest in children (Neel 1982). To date, elevated serum insulin levels have been documented only in adult nondiabetic Pima (Aronoff et al. 1977) and Navajo Indians (Rimoin 1969), compared to Caucasians, but they have not been seen in Eskimos, either adults or adolescent boarding school pupils who consumed nontraditional diets (Feldman, Rubinstein, et al. 1978). Although adult diabetic Seneca displayed significantly higher insulin levels than normal Seneca, hyperinsulinemia in the normals was not reported (Frohman, Doeblin, and Emerling 1969). In relatively unacculturated adult South American Indians, insulin levels were indistinguishable from "white" Americans (Spielman et al. 1982). These data do not offer much support for the thrifty gene model, in part because they are based on few studies and because relevant age groups have not been tested. An alternative explanation may be that the thrifty gene mechanism is not present in Native Americans, and alternative explanations need to be sought for increase in NIDDM in these peoples.

Environmental Factors

The Pima studies show that, rather than diet, obesity (i.e., the body mass index [BMI] = [weight in kg] / [stature in m]^2) is a very important risk factor for the onset of diabetes (Knowler, Pettitt, et al. 1981). West (1978) has also argued that duration of obesity in Indians is diabetogenic. Increase in the mean weight of a population over time has been reported for Navajo (Niswander, 1968), but a weight increase paralleling an increase in diabetes in the same group has been reported only in Alaskan Eskimo (Mouratoff and Scott 1973). Within-population increases in mean weights of diabetics compared to normals have also been found in some (e.g., Seminole [Elston et al. 1974]) but not all Amerindians (Pima [Knowler, Pettitt, et al. 1981]; Seneca [Frohman, Doeblin, and Emerling 1969]). Other studies (e.g., Szathmary and Holt 1983) show no association between adiposity and hyperglycemia, whether the former is measured using principal components derived from fatfolds or with the BMI (Szathmary 1986). Instead, what is significantly associated is the development of truncal adiposity, a fat distribution pattern often called "centripetality." The latter has been shown to be diabetogenic (Kissebah et al. 1982) in non-Indian populations.

Although a great many studies have been done worldwide on the relationship between diet and NIDDM, only one published paper has focused on diet and diabetes in Native Americans. No association could be shown between any nutrient intake component and diabetes in the Pima (Reid et al. 1971). For this reason, some assume that dietary components have little to do with the onset of NIDDM in Indians. Rather, it is argued, excess caloric intake is the problem, for excess caloric intake when coupled with inactivity leads to obesity, and obesity is considered by many to be diabetogenic.

While this may be true, it is worth remembering that the Pima study is based on one population. The findings from one study do not warrant exclusion of the possibility that a shift in dietary intake components could have an effect on glucose metabolism independent of problems occasioned by obesity. The Pima diet, for example, did not differ significantly from that of white Americans in its daily proportions of fats, carbohydrates, and protein or in its ratio of polyunsaturated to saturated fats. Nevertheless, the diets of some other Native Americans do differ. Protein intake, for example, in both Nootka (Wakashan-speaking) and Chilcotin (Athabaskan-speaking) Indians of British Columbia exceeded Canadian standards in 1971 (Lee, Reyburn, and Carrow 1971), and caloric intake in adults of both groups as well as in Chilcotin children was less than in non-Indian Canadians. Such diversity is not seen when data are averaged for all Canadian Indians (e.g., Nutrition Canada 1975a). Nutritional intake patterns of Eskimos still tend to differ from those of non-Eskimos. Among Canadian Eskimos, for example, adult protein consumption exceeded the Canadian average in 1975, but total caloric intake and cholesterol levels were below median Canadian values. On the other hand, Eskimo children's caloric intake and protein consumption equalled that of other Canadian children, prompting Nutrition Canada (1975b) to suggest that Eskimo children were in the process of a dietary transition.

Anthropologists should not be surprised that dietary differences exist among Native Americans, given the variation in aboriginal subsistence patterns across the two continents. In pre-Columbian times, carbohydrates were far more readily available to corn-squash-pumpkin horticulturalists than to the fishing-gathering groups of the northwest coast or the hunter-fishers of the boreal forest. Whether the transition to a modern diet with its altered composition of proteins, fats, and carbohydrates is diabetogenic is unknown. Nevertheless, biological adaptation to an all-meat diet was postulated as the reason why the oral glucose tolerance test was incapable of identifying true diabetics among Eskimos and northern "bush" Indians and why change to a "white man's diet" might put native people at particular risk for diabetes (Schaefer, Crockford, and Romanowski 1972). A causal dietary shift was also postulated by Niswander (1968) who noted that the highest frequencies of diabetes were among those peoples who, aboriginally, practiced sedentary agriculture (e.g., maize, beans, pumpkins). In his scenario, such populations may have been acculturated more rapidly to the invaders' ways, and so showed the disease consequences of altered diets earlier than groups that aboriginally were hunters and gatherers.

THE DOGRIB STUDIES: A POPULATION IN CULTURAL TRANSITION

Research Design: Selection of the Population

One of the difficulties of determining cause in a disease such as NIDDM in Native Americans is that, by the time the disease becomes manifest, the changes that led to disease onset become obliterated and the altered "lifestyle" factors are fixed in the population. Recognizing this, the Diabetes Epidemiology Workgroup, National Conference on Diabetes (U.S.) recommended that populations that "are likely to undergo rapid cultural change be identified and studied for the prevalence of NIDDM and associated risk factors" (1981: 107). In similar fashion, but a few years earlier, Neel (1976) had argued that to understand the familial basis of Amerindian diabetes, studies needed to be conducted on populations before and after a major cultural transition. It is fact, however, that no Native American population in all of North America has remained untouched by the influence of surrounding non-Native cultures. Nevertheless, it is possible to approximate the recommendations above by identifying a population that because of historical accident is now undergoing the process loosely referred to as "Westernization."

The ideal study group would be a genetically identifiable, subdivided population. Among the subpopulations there should be clear-cut differences in European acculturation, and these should range from low to relatively high. I stress the term "relatively" because the whole group should be close to the transition line from aboriginal to modern, so that in the least acculturated subpopulation there is reasonable approximation of traditional lifeways, and the most acculturated is not yet experiencing complete cultural disruption. Because a genetic predisposition seems to exist for NIDDM, it is imperative that in this population non-Native and other-Native admixture be at a minimum. Lastly, because NIDDM is considered to be the end product of interaction between a genotype and cumulative environmental insult, such a population should not contain any clinical diabetics, at least at the time the study is launched.

Clearly, such populations do not exist in the southern parts of Canada or in the United States where the influence of the larger society is intensive, extensive, and of long duration and where Native patients present complications of diabetes mellitus. In the northern parts of Canada there are Indian groups that meet the "natural experiment" design requirements.

Population Description

Dogrib Indians are Athabaskan-speaking people who live between Great Slave and Great Bear Lakes in the Northwest Territories (NWT) of Canada. Their east-west distribution extends from the lowlands east of the Mackenzie River into the barrenlands. The Dogrib are the largest Indian group in the NWT (c. 1700 in 1970), and over 75 percent of the extant population are members of the Rae Band, that is, people who either reside in the hamlet of Rae or trade into that community (Helm 1981). The populations of the Lac La Martre, Rae Lakes, and Snare Lake settlements are also members of the Rae Band. This particular group of people was selected for investigation in 1979 and subsequently in 1985.

Helm, the principal ethnographer of the Dogrib, has noted that before 1950 "almost all Dogribs" pursued traditional subsistence and cultural activities and lived "in the bush" away from Euro-Canadian installations (1981:290). The major change in Dogrib lifestyles began during the 1950s when expansion in government-sponsored housing and schooling programs and health and welfare services encouraged sedentism at government's points-of-service, these being located within Dogrib regional band areas.

Aboriginally, the Dogribs were hunting-fishing nomads whose territory did not abut the Mackenzie River, the major trading waterway to the Arctic Ocean. Accordingly, they encountered non-Indians other than missionaries and some traders. Intensive European contact in their area did not begin until the discovery of gold in the mid 1930s led to the development of the present city of Yellowknife some 100 km from Rae. Unlike the Dogribs living in and around Yellowknife, members of the Rae Band were relatively untouched by these developments until after World War II (Helm 1981).

Although year-round sedentism now exists in all the Dogrib settlements, people in Lac La Martre, Rae Lakes, and Snare Lake live in their communities seasonally. Many still pursue traditional trapping, hunting, and fishing activities (Helm 1981). Personal experience attests (Szathmary and Holt 1983; Szathmary 1983a) that sometimes more than 55 percent of the "resident" adults may be absent from a community for such tasks as maintenance of winter trap lines.

Differences between Rae and the northern settlements can be highlighted both by what local people say about the communities and by detectable structural/socioeconomic differences. Dogrib opinion holds that people in the northern settlements live more like "real" Dogrib than the residents of Rae. Visible differences include the availability of road connections to the "outside," population size, the proportion of non-Indian residents, the number of available stores/cafes, and the fraction of men that earn at least some of their living by hunting and trapping. To date, only Rae is accessible overland by a permanent road, which ties the hamlet to the Mackenzie highway. The latter connects Yellowknife to Edmonton, Alberta. The highway was completed in 1967, and commercial bus service to Yellowknife became available around that time (Helm 1981). None of the northern settlements is connected to the outside or to Rae by permanent roads. Surface travel can be done by canoe in the summer, or by four-wheel drive vehicles over ice roads (i.e., frozen lakes) in the winter, or by snowmobile or dogsled through the bush. Weekly air service to Yellowknife now exists for those who can afford such trips.

Of the main Dogrib settlements, Rae is the largest, and Snare Lake is the smallest. In 1979 the population of Rae was approximately five times as great as that found in either Lac La Martre or Rae Lakes. Non-Dogribs represented about 8.7 percent of the population in Rae, while each of the northern settlements had two Euro-Canadian resident teachers (i.e., % non-Dogrib). Rae had two stores and one cafe, while each settlement had only one cooperative store. In the northern villages all men, with the exception of the aged and infirm, engage in hunting/fishing/trapping activity. However, in Rae, only around 60 percent of the adult males are involved in trapping (172 trappers in 1982-1983; Outcrop 1984). Other differences still manifest in 1985 included absence of flush toilets in Rae Lakes and Snare Lake, with the latter community also lacking (by community choice) electricity and piped running water. There is no doubt whatever that there are "acculturation" differences among the Dogrib communities.

With respect to other characteristics, the 1979 study showed that among the 157 adults who participated in the 1979 "blood sugar" survey (held in Rae, Lac La Martre, and Rae Lakes), the maximum amount of Caucasian admixture was less than 9 percent (Szathmary 1983a; Szathmary, Ferrell, and Gershowitz 1983). The mean amount of admixture is probably less than 5 percent. There was no evidence suggesting Black admixture. While inter-Indian gene flow is known to have occurred between the Dogrib and their neighbors, genetic distance analyses showed no detectable disruption of the Dogrib genome by such gene flow (Szathmary 1983b).

The last criterion that made the Dogrib suitable for investigation was the absence of known diabetics among them, this in spite of the fact that a mission hospital was established at Rae in the 1940s, and that a physician was attached in the 1950s (Helm 1981). The first case of clinically recognizable diabetes in conjunction with fasting plasma glucose 140 mg/dl was diagnosed in 1981 (Burke 1981) in an adult who had not participated in the 1979 survey.

Prevalence of Glucose Intolerance Among the Dogrib

Szathmary (1983a, 1985) and Szathmary and Holt (1983) summarize the methodology and results in the initial Dogrib survey. The 1979 investigation was held before any of the recommendations of the National Diabetes Data Group (1979) were published, hence there were some deviations from recommended procedures. Participation in the study was restricted to adults aged 21 years or older. The test challenge dose was 100 gm glucose to allow comparison with a study carried out on Alaskan Athabaskan-speaking Indians (Mouratoff, Carroll, and Scott 1969).

The 157 Dogrib participants represented 22 percent of the adults of the Dogrib Rae Band. Although participation was voluntary, the age structure of the sample did not deviate significantly from that of the target population, suggesting an absence of sampling bias, at least with respect to age and sex. Because the majority of adults had not even heard of diabetes at the time of survey, and because there were no such individuals among the Dogrib, it is very doubtful that there was any sampling bias toward participation (for or against) by relatives of possible diabetics.

In normal individuals, a glucose challenge dose of 100 gm does not produce a significant rise in plasma glucose level compared to that obtained with a 75 gm dose (Castro et al. 1970). Furthermore, reproducibility of response on test repetition is best accomplished with a 100 gm load (Toeller and Knussman 1973). However, in persons whose tolerance is impaired, the use of a test dose higher than 75 gm might make a difference in the outcome. Unfortunately, without a second screen it is not possible to tell who among those with abnormal response to glucose challenge is actually diabetic or merely showing "impaired glucose tolerance" (National Diabetes Data Group 1979).

Of the 157 participants, eight men and six women had either fasting blood sugar (FBS) ≥ 140 mg / dl or normal FBS but with both the hour 1 and hour 2 levels ≥ 200 mg / dl. At a minimum, these individuals suffer from impaired glucose tolerance. These numbers represent a prevalence rate of 13.3 percent and 6.3 percent by sex, respectively. The study definition of hyperglycemia required either that FBS was ≥ 140 mg / dl, or that hour 2 ≥ 200 mg/dl. Fifteen individuals (eight men, seven women) have such values representing prevalence of 13.3 percent and 7.4 percent by sex, respectively. Approximately four times as many Dogribs were abnormal on this initial screen as had been detected in Athabaskan Indians of Alaska by Mouratoff, Carroll, and Scott (1969).

In the 1985 follow-up of the Dogrib cohort surveyed in 1979, special effort was made to test again the fifteen hyperglycemic individuals detected earlier. Unfortunately not all survived the six years between screenings, and two were unwilling to undergo glucose challenge again. Of the eleven retested, only three had hour 2 plasma glucose equal to or greater than 200 mg / dl (11.1 mmol / l). Another four had now shifted to the impaired glucose tolerance (IGT) category (National Diabetes Data Group 1979), while the remaining four were now normal. Mouratoff, Carroll, and Scott (1969) had reported similar changes in the status of individuals they tested on two different occasions. The repeat tests allow an estimation of diabetes prevalence in the Dogrib: 3 / 153 = 1.96 percent, in comparison with a hyperglycemic prevalence of 9.6 percent. The difference in these figures underscores the need to distinguish between diabetes and the percentage of abnormal responses obtained from a single screen (Table 5.2). The two are not equivalent.

Genetic Effects

Distribution of hour 2 or hour 1 plasma glucose levels in most populations is unimodal but positively skewed. Exceptions to this include populations with high rates of diabetes, such as the Pima (Rushforth et al. 1971) and Micronesians from Nauru (Zimmet and Whitehouse 1978), among whom the distributions are clearly bimodal. The second mode in such distributions has been claimed to represent not just a diabetic phenotype but an underlying genotype (e.g., Elston et al. 1974). Dissenters (e.g., Neel 1976; Vogel 1985) point out that the second mode need not have such genetic underpinnings at all. If the bimodality is an artifact, a critical question is whether the bimodality would be lost were all clinical diabetics removed from the sample. This question can be tested in the Dogrib, for the sample included no clinical diabetics, although almost 10 percent displayed impaired glucose tolerance. In spite of this, the age-adjusted log plasma glucose (hour 2) was unimodal in this population (Szathmary 1985).

Covariance analysis of age-adjusted glucose levels and different categories of first degree relatives showed significant association among adult siblings (r =

+ .51, p < .01, df = 30), but not between parents and their adult offspring, nor husbands and their wives. Szathmary (1985) concludes that the model of glucose regulation that best fit these findings is complex and polygenic and includes genes with additive and dominant effects, as well as an intragenerational environmental effect. What this intragenerational effect may be is not known. However, fully 78 percent of the Dogrib sample were born prior to the major changes in lifestyle that occurred during the 1950s. Cohorts of sibs would have experienced this change together at a relatively young age. It is possible that the environmental effect involved in the onset of glucose intolerance has greatest impact on the young and so sets the path for emergence of disease in middle adulthood in those who are genetically susceptible.

As in other populations, glucose intolerance among the Dogrib appears to be familial; for example, 40 percent of the hyperglycemics are members of one pedigree. This and the covariance findings support the existence of a set of genetic factors in NIDDM in Indians, though not of a simple single gene variety.

Role of Obesity and Fat Patterning

Obesity is thought by many to be an important risk factor for NIDDM. The distribution of subcutaneous body fat is also thought to be important (e.g., Feldman, Sender, Siegelaub 1969; Kissebah et al. 1982). Szathmary and Holt (1983) address these issues by using skinfold data obtained on each participant. Principal components analysis allow the identification of components that are best interpreted as representing (1) "fatness," (2) increased upper trunk adiposity with a correspondingly decreased fat thickness in the distal limb appendages (i.e., "centripetality"), and (3) differences in the distribution of fat in the arms versus legs ("arm-leg vector"). Somewhat unexpectedly, they find that "fatness" does not differ significantly either among the villages or between hyperglycemics and normals. Centripetality, however, is different. This observation is made possible through the use of hierarchical analysis of variance, a procedure that controls for the effects of fatness before assessing the effects of glucose status ($\geq$ 200 mg / dl or 200 mg / dl) and village of location on the distribution of body fat. Not only is upper trunk adiposity greater among the hyperglycemics compared to normals, but it also differs significantly among the settlements, with the people of Rae having the highest scores (Szathmary 1983a). To date there are no conclusions concerning the hypotheses (e.g., Vague et al. 1979) presented to explain the conjoint occurrence of upper trunk obesity and NIDDM. However, Kissebah et al.'s (1982) longitudinal work certainly supports the notion that upper body obesity is diabetogenic. If so, one interpretation of the Dogrib findings is that some acculturation-associated factor in Rae is producing the higher rates of centripetality in that community and that this sort of fat patterning distinguishes normals from those with impaired glucose tolerance. Focussing on obesity alone, especially as measured by the body mass index (BMI), would not have allowed these findings to emerge.

That fatness as indicated by the first principal component was not significantly associated with hyperglycemia contravenes conventional wisdom that links obesity and NIDDM. Nevertheless, in the Dogrib not only is there no significant difference in the magnitude of the BMI between hyperglycemics and normals by sex, but the BMI is also unable to improve upon the variation in log glucose already explained by age (Szathmary 1986). In these people, adiposity does not have any demonstrable effects on glucose level. Because adiposity is influenced by the level of physical activity, one possible explanation is that the Dogrib remain active on average. This is certainly borne out by the men but may be less true for women, with the possible exception of the women of Rae Lakes.

The Role of Diet

Although acculturation-associated dietary changes are present in the Dogrib, there is also continuing reliance on the hunting-fishing food base. For example, Szathmary, Ritenbaugh, and Goodby (1987) found that protein intake is approximately twice the U.S. average and exceeds the ninety-fifth percentile for non-Native Canadians. Twenty-four-hour recall data obtained in the spring (i.e., June) showed that among men approximately 31 percent of the total calories were obtained from protein, 35 percent from fat, and 37 percent from carbohydrate. The intake pattern of women was nearly identical. Winter consumption patterns indicated a slight decrease in fat consumption balanced by a slightly greater increase in protein than in carbohydrate consumption.

Aboriginally, the Dogrib did not have access to carbohydrates beyond berries. Roots and tubers apparently were not consumed (Helm 1981), and berries were available only in August and early September. With the exception of berries, then, all carbohydrates and some protein and fat products that are eaten today are nontraditional foods. However, because flour, tea, sugar, lard, and baking powder have assumed the role of staples since the time they first became available (in 1852), the Dogrib consider these products and items prepared from them (e.g., bannock) to be traditional foods. As might be expected in a group that shows acculturation-associated differences across settlements, the Dogrib differ significantly in the percentages of calories, fats, and protein obtained from nontraditional foods. However, they do not differ in carbohydrate obtained from nontraditional foods, nor is there any difference in nutritional intake components derived from traditional foods. Age does have an effect on food consumption patterns: the oldest (i.e., 65 yrs.) consume little food in the nontraditional category, the middle aged consume more, and the youngest (> 25 yrs., < 45 yrs.) consume the most. Szathmary et al. (1987) conclude that dietary transition in the Dogrib appears to consist of addition of new foods to a stable traditional diet, rather than replacement of traditional foods. The net effect of this is increase in caloric content. The new food component that is consumed without difference across all the settlements is carbohydrate. Both of these observations fit expectations arising from mutually distinct hypotheses concerning the cause of NIDDM – for example, that increase of daily calories consumed may lead to the development of a diabetogenic obesity and that consumption of carbohydrate may be diabetogenic in Native Americans.

Of more importance than the separate observations is whether any of the nutritional intake components is associated with hyperglycemia in the Dogrib. Szathmary et al. (1987) could not identify any association with confidence, given the small size (seven persons) of the hyperglycemic subset in the total sample. Furthermore, settlement-associated differences in plasma glucose level were not discernible in 1986, even though differences were observable in dietary components, and differences in glucose levels were readily seen in the 1979 survey. What impact dietary change has on changing glucose levels in a transitional population, therefore, has still not been demonstrated.

CONCLUSION

The Dogrib studies show that traditional wisdom concerning the genetic and environmental factors involved in the onset of NIDDM in Indians may be challenged. Neither the genetic mechanisms nor the obesity expected from studies based on the Pima explained the occurrence of hyperglycemia in these subarctic Indians. Analysis of the 1985 data is continuing, the aim being to see what roles physical exercise, insulin, cholesterol, and triglyceride levels play in changing glucose levels in a Native American group currently undergoing cultural transition.

REFERENCES

Aronoff, S. L., P. H. Bennett, P. Gorden, N. Rushforth, and M. Miller. 1977. Unexplained hyperinsulinemia in normal and "prediabetic" Pima Indians compared with normal Caucasians. *Diabetes* 26:827–40.

Bartha, G. W., T. A. Burch, and P. H. Bennett. 1973. Hyperglycemia in Washoe and northern Paiute Indians. *Diabetes* 22:58–62.

Bennett, P. H. 1982. The epidemiology of diabetes mellitus. In *Diabetes Mellitus and Obesity*. B. N. Blodoff and S. I. Bleicher, eds. Baltimore: Williams and Wilkins.

Bennett, P. H., T. A. Burch, and M. Miller. 1971. Diabetes mellitus in American (Pima) Indians. *Lancet* 2:125–28.

Bennett, P. H., N. B. Rushforth, M. Miller, and P. M. LeCompte. 1976. Epidemiologic studies of diabetes in the Pima Indians. *Rec. Prog. in Hormone Res.* 32:333–375.

Brosseau, J. D., R. C. Elkema, A. C. Crawford, and T. A. Abe. 1979. Diabetes among the three affiliated tribes: Correlation with degree of Indian inheritance. *Am. J. Pub. Health* 69:1277–78.

Burke, E. 1981. Personal communication from the director of the Burke's Cottage Hospital, Edzo, NWT, Canada.

Canadian Diabetic Association (CDA). 1982. Acceptance of new criteria for diagnosis of diabetes mellitus and related conditions by the Canadian Diabetes Association. *Canadian Medical Association Journal* 126:473–76.

Castro, A., J. P. Scott, D. P. Grettie, D. Macfarlane, and R. E. Bailey. 1970. Plasma insulin and glucose responses of healthy subjects to varying glucose loads during three-hour oral glucose tolerance tests. *Diabetes* 19:842–51.

Cohen, B. M. 1954. Diabetes mellitus among Indians of the American Southwest: Its prevalence and clinical characteristics in a hospitalized population. *Ann. Intern. Med.* 40:588–99.

Coleman, D. 1979. Obesity genes: Beneficial effects in heterozygous mice. *Science* 203:663–65.

Committee on Statistics, American Diabetes Association. 1969. Standardization of the oral glucose tolerance test. *Diabetes* 18:299–307.

Diabetes Epidemiology Workgroup, National Conference on Diabetes. 1981. Research needs in the epidemiology of diabetes. *Journal of Epidemiology* 113:105–12.

Doeblin, T.D., K. Evans, G. B. Ingall, K. Dowling, M. E. Chilcote, W. Elsea, and R. M. Bannerman. 1969. Diabetes and hyperglycemia in Seneca Indians. *Human Heredity* 19:613–27.

Draper, H. H. 1978. Nutrition studies: The aboriginal Eskimo diet—A modern perspective. In *Eskimos of Northwestern Alaska*. P. L. Jamison, S. L. Zegura, F. A. Milan, eds. Stroudsburg, Penn.: Dowden, Hutchinson & Ross.

Drevets, C. C. 1965. Diabetes mellitus in Choctaw Indians. *Oklahoma State Med. Assoc.* 58:322–329.

Ede, M. C. 1966. Diabetes and the way of life on an Indian reservation. *Guy's Hospital Reports* 115:455–61.

Elston, R. C., K. K. Namboodiri, H. V. Nino, and W. S. Pollitzer. 1974. Studies on blood and urine glucose in Seminole Indians: Indications for segregation of a major gene. *American Journal of Human Genetics* 26:13–34.

Feldman, S. A., K. Ho, L. A. Lewis, B. Mikkelson, and C. B. Taylor. 1972. Lipid and cholesterol metabolism in Alaskan arctic Eskimos. *Archives of Pathology* 94:42–58.

Feldman, S. A., A. Rubenstein, C. B. Taylor, J. J. Ho, and L. Lewis. 1978. Metabolic parameters: Aspects of cholesterol, lipid, and carbohydrate metabolism. In *Eskimos of Northwestern Alaska*. P. L. Jamison, S. L. Zegura, F. A. Milan, eds. Stroudsburg, Penn.: Dowden, Hutchinson & Ross.

Feldman, R., A. J. Sender, and A. B. Siegelaub. 1969. Differences in diabetic and nondiabetic fat distribution patterns by skinfold measurements. *Diabetes* 18:478–86.

Folk, G. E., Jr. 1984. Stefansson and the discovery of essential fatty acids. In *Vilhjalmur Steffanson and the Development of Arctic Terrestrial Science*. G. E. Folk, Jr., and M. A. Folk, eds. Iowa City: University of Iowa Press.

Friedman, J. M., and P. J. Fialkow. 1980. The genetics of diabetes mellitus. *Progress in Medical Genetics* 4:199–232.

Frohman, L. A., T. D. Doeblin, and F. G. Emerling. 1969. Diabetes in the Seneca Indians. *Diabetes* 18:38–43.

Gutniak, M., M. D. Grill, and S. Efendic. 1986. Effect of composition of mixed meals—low- versus high-carbohydrate content—on insulin, glucagon, and somatostatin release in healthy humans and in patients with NIDDM. *Diabetes Care* 9:244–49.

Guyton, A. C. 1971. *Basic Human Physiology: Normal Function and Mechanisms of Disease.* New York: W. B. Saunders.

Hall, S. E., M. E. Wastney, T. M. Bolton, J .T. Braaten, and M. Berman. 1984. Ketone body kinetics in humans: The effects of insulin-dependent diabetes, obesity and starvation. *Journal of Lipid Research* 25:1184–94.

Hampton, S. M., L. M. Morgan, T. R. Cramb, and V. Marks. 1986. Insulin and C-peptide levels after oral and intravenous glucose. *Diabetes* 35:612–16.

Helm, J. 1981. Dogrib. In *Subarctic. Handbook of North American Indians.* vol. 6. J. Helm, ed. Washington: Smithsonian Institution.

Henry, R. E., T. A. Burch, P. H. Bennett, and M. Miller. 1969. Diabetes in the Cocopah Indians. *Diabetes* 18:33–37.

Hochachka, P. W., and G. N. Somero. 1984. *Biochemical Adaptation.* Princeton: Princeton University Press.

Johnson, J. E. Jr., and C.W. McNutt. 1964. Diabetes mellitus in an American Indian population isolate. *Texas Reports on Biology and Medicine* 22:110–25.

Kissebah, A. H., N. Vydelingum, R. Murray, D. J. Evans, A. J. Hartz, R. K. Kalkhoff, and P. W. Adams. 1982. Relation of body fat distribution to metabolic complications of obesity. *Journal of Clinical Endocrinology and Metabolism* 54:254–60.

Knowler, W. C., P. H. Bennett, R. F. Hamman, and M. Miller. 1978. Diabetes incidence and prevalence in Pima Indians: A 19-fold greater increase than in Rochester, Minnesota. *American Journal of Epidemiology.* 108:497–505.

Knowler, W. C., D. J. Pettitt, P. J. Savage, and P. H. Bennett. 1981. Diabetes incidence in Pima Indians: Contributions of obesity and parental diabetes. *American Journal of Epidemiology.* 113:144–56.

Knowler, W. C., P. J. Savage, M. Nagulesparan, B. V. Howard, D. J. Pettitt, J. R. Lisse, S. L. Aronoff, and P. H. Bennett. 1982. Obesity, insulin resistance, and diabetes mellitus in the Pima Indians. In *The Genetics of Diabetes Mellitus.* J. Kobberling and R. B. Tattersall, eds. New York: Academic.

Kraus-Friedmann, N. 1984. Hormonal regulation of hepatic gluconeogenesis. *Physiological Reviews.* 64:170–259.

Lathrop M., and R. Ward. 1979. Unpublished data.

Lee, M., R. Reyburn, and A. Carrow. 1971. Nutritional status of British Columbia Indians. *Canadian Journal of Public Health* 62:285–96.

Long, T. P. 1978 The prevalence of clinically treated diabetes among Zuni reservation residents. *Public Health Briefs* 68:901–3.

McNiven, M. 1978. Diabetes on the Wikwemikong Indian Reservation. *Report to Health and Welfare Canada*, Medical Services Branch.

Montour, L. T., and A. C. Macauley. 1985. High prevalence rates of diabetes mellitus and hypertension on a North American Indian reservation. *Can. Med. Assoc. J.* 132:1112.

Mouratoff, G. J., N. V. Carroll, and E. M. Scott. 1969. Diabetes mellitus in Athabaskan Indians of Alaska. *Diabetes* 18:29–32.

———. 1967. Diabetes mellitus in Eskimos. *Journal of the American Medical Association* 199:107–12.

Mouratoff, G. J., and E. M. Scott. 1973. Diabetes mellitus in Eskimos after a decade. *Journal of the American Medical Association* 226:1345–46.

Nagai, K., and H. Nakagawa. 1973. Cold adaptation III. Effects of catecholamines and thyroid hormone on induction of liver phosphoenolpyruvate carboxykinase on cold-exposure. *Journal of Biochemistry* 74:873–79.

Nagulesparan, M., P. J. Savage, W. C. Knowler, G. C. Johnson, and P. H. Bennett. 1982. Increased in vivo resistance in nondiabetic Pima Indians compared with Caucasians. *Diabetes* 31:952–56.

National Diabetes Data Group (NDDG). 1979. Classification and diagnosis of diabetes mellitus and other categories of glucose intolerance. *Diabetes* 28:1039–57.

Neel, J. V. 1982. The thrifty genotype revisited. In *The Genetics of Diabetes Mellitus*. J. Kobberling, and R. B. Tattersall, eds. New York: Academic.

———. 1976. Diabetes mellitus—a geneticist's nightmare. In *The Genetics of Diabetes Mellitus*. W. Creutzfeldt, J. Kobberling, and J. V. Neel, eds. New York: Springer-Verlag.

———. 1962. Diabetes mellitus: A "thrifty genotype" rendered detrimental by "progress?" *American Journal of Human Genetics* 14:353–62.

Niswander, J. D. 1968. Discussion. In *Biomedical Challenges Presented by the American Indian*. Scientific Publication No. 165, PAHO. Washington: WHO.

Nutrition Canada. 1975a. *The Indian Survey*. Ottawa: Bureau of Nutritional Sciences.

———. 1975b *The Eskimo Survey*. Ottawa: Bureau of Nutritional Sciences.

Outcrop, Ltd. 1984. *NWT Data Book 84/85*. Yellowknife, NWT: The Northern Publishers.

Petersen, K. 1969. A profile of diabetes mellitus among the Indians of a Sioux/Assiniboine reservation. *U.S. Public Health Service*, 4th Proceedings, p. 35.

Prosnitz, L. R., and G. L. Mandell. 1967. Diabetes mellitus among Navajo and Hopi Indians: The lack of vascular completion. *American Journal of Medical Science* 253:96/700–101/705.

Reid, J. M., S. D. Fullmer, K. P. Pettigrew, T. A. Burch, P. H. Bennett, M. Miller, and D. G. Whedon. 1971. Nutritional intake of Pima Indian women: Relationships to diabetes mellitus and gall bladder disease. *American Journal of Clinical Nutrition* 24:1281–89.

Rimoin, D. L. 1969. Ethnic variability in glucose tolerance and insulin secretion. *Archives of Internal Medicine* 124:695–700.

Rushforth, N. B., P. H. Bennett, A. G. Steinberg, T. A. Burch, and M. Miller. 1971. Diabetes in Pima Indians. Evidence of bimodality in glucose tolerance distributions. *Diabetes* 20:756–65.

Saiki, J. H., and D. C. Rimoin. 1968. Diabetes mellitus among the Navajo: Clinical features. *Archives of Internal Medicine* 122:1–5.

Schaefer, O. 1969. Carbohydrate metabolism in Eskimos. *Archives of Environmental Health* 18:144–47.

———. 1968. Glycosuria and diabetes mellitus in Canadian Eskimos. *Canad. Med. Assoc. J.* 99:201–6.

Schaefer, O., P. M. Crockford, and B. Romanowski. 1972. Normalization effect of preceding protein meals on "diabetic" oral glucose tolerance in Eskimos. *Canadian Medical Association Journal* 107:733–38.

Schauder, P. 1984. Effect of starvation, dietary protein, and pancreatic hormones on branched chain keto acid blood levels in man. In *Branched Chain Amino Acids and Keto Acids in Health and Disease*. S. A. Adibi, W. Fekl, U. Langenbeck, and P. Schauder, eds. Basel: Karger.

Sinclair, H. 1984. An Eskimo diet experiment in Greenland. In *Vilhjalmur Stefansson and the Development of Arctic Terrestrial Science*. G. E. Folk, Jr. and M. A. Folk, eds. Iowa City: The University of Iowa.

Spielman, R. S., S. S. Fajans, J. V. Neel, S. Pek, J. C. Floyd, and W. J. Oliver. 1982. Glucose tolerance in two unacculturated Indian tribes of Brazil. *Diabetologia* 23:90–93.

Spuhler, J. N. 1979. Genetic distances, trees, and maps of North American Indians. In *The First Americans: Origins, Affinities and Adaptations.* W. S. Laughlin, and A. B. Harper, eds. New York: Gustav Fischer.

———. 1972. Genetic, linguistic and geographical distances in native North America. In *The Assessment of Population Affinity in Man.* J. S. Weiner, and J. Huizinga, eds. London: Oxford University Press.

Stein, J. H., K. M. West, J. M. Robey, D. F. Tirador, and G. W. McDonald. 1965. The high prevalence of abnormal glucose tolerance in the Cherokee Indians of North Carolina. *Arch. Intern. Med.* 116:842–45.

Steinberg, A. G., N. B. Rushforth, P. H. Bennett, T. A. Burch, and M. Miller. 1970. On the genetics of diabetes mellitus. In *The Pathogenesis of Diabetes Mellitus.* E. Cerasi and R. Luft, eds. New York: John Wiley and Sons.

Szathmary, E. J. E. 1986. Diabetes in arctic and subarctic populations undergoing acculturation. *Collegium Anthropologicum* 10:145–58.

———. 1985. The search for genetic factors controlling plasma glucose levels in Dogrib Indians. In *Diseases of Complex Etiology in Small Populations.* R. Chakraborty and E. J. E. Szathmary, eds. New York: Alan R. Liss.

———. 1984. Peopling of northern North America: Clues from genetic studies. *Acta Anthropogenetica* 8:79–110.

———. 1983a. Athabaskan-speakers: Glucose intolerance, genes and obesity. *Final Report to the NHRDP,* Health and Welfare, Canada.

———. 1983b. Dogrib Indians of the Northwest Territories, Canada: Genetic diversity and genetic relationship among subarctic Indians. *Annals of Human Biology* 10:147–62.

Szathmary, E. J. E., R. E. Ferrell, and H. Gershowitz. 1983. Genetic differentiation in Dogrib Indians: Serum protein and erythrocyte enzyme variation. *American Journal of Physical Anthropology* 62:249–55.

Szathmary, E. J. E., and N. Holt. 1983. Hyperglycemia in Dogrib Indians of the Northwest Territories, Canada: Association with age and a centripetal distribution of body fat. *Human Biology* 55:493–515.

Szathmary, E. J. E., C. Ritenbaugh, and C. S. M. Goodby. 1987. Dietary change and plasma glucose levels in an Amerindian population undergoing cultural transition. *Social Science and Medicine.* 24:791–804.

Tepperman, J. 1980. *Metabolic and Endocrine Physiology.* Chicago: Yearbook Medical Publishers.

Toeller, M., and R. Knussman. 1973. Reproducibility of oral glucose tolerance tests with three different loads. *Diabetologia* 9:102–7.

Vague, J., R. Combes, M. Tramoni, J. S. Angeletti, P. Rubin, D. Hachem, M. F. Perey, C. Lansade, G. Ziras, G. Ramahandridona, R. Jouve, R. Sambuc, and J. Jubelin. 1979. Clinical features of diabetogenic obesity. In *Diabetes and Obesity.* J. Vague, P. Vague, and F. J. G. Eblin, eds. Amsterdam: Exerpta Medica.

Vogel, F. 1985. Epilogue and Summary. In *Diseases of Complex Etiology in Small Populations.* R. Chakraborty and E. J. E. Szathmary, eds. New York: Alan R. Liss.

West, K. M. 1978. Diabetes in American Indians. *Advances in Metabolic Disorders* 9:29–48.

———. 1974. Diabetes in American Indians and other native populations of the New World. *Diabetes* 23:841–55.

West, K. M., and M. E. Mako. 1976. Effect of prediabetes, preobesity and dietary sugar on insulin secretion. *Diabetes* 25 (Suppl. 1):389.

White, W. D. 1966. Diabetes in the Oklahoma Indian. *USPHS*, 1st Proceedings, p. 21.

Workman, P. L. 1978. Genetic epidemiology and population structure. In *Genetic Epidemiology*. N. E. Morton and C. S. Chung, eds. New York: Academic Press.

World Health Organization (WHO). 1980. WHO Expert Committee on Diabetes Mellitus. Second Report. Geneva: WHO Technical Report Series 646.

Yamashita, T., W. Mackay, N. Rushforth, P. J. Bennett, and H. Houser. 1984. Pedigree analyses of non-insulin dependent diabetes mellitus (NIDDM) in the Pima Indians. *American Journal of Human Genetics* 36:183S.

Young, T. K., L. L. McIntyre, J. Dooley, and J. Rodriguez. 1985. Epidemiologic features of diabetes mellitus among Indians in northwestern Ontario and northeastern Manitoba. *Canadian Medical Association Journal* 132:793–97.

Zimmet, P. 1979. Epidemiology of diabetes and its macrovascular manifestations in Pacific populations. The medical effects of social progress. *Diabetes Care* 2:144–53.

Zimmet, P., and S. Whitehouse. 1978. Bimodality of fasting and hour-2 glucose tolerance distributions in a Micronesian population. *Diabetes* 27:793–800.

6 TRANSITIONAL DIABETES AND GALLSTONES IN AMERINDIAN PEOPLES: GENES OR ENVIRONMENT?

Kenneth M. Weiss

Peoples with Amerindian genes are currently suffering high rates of adult-onset, noninsulin dependent diabetes mellitus (NIDDM) and of gallbladder disease (GBD) (Weiss, Ferrell, and Hanis 1984; Weiss et al. 1984; Weiss and Ferrell 1985; Diehl, in press; Bennett, in press; West 1974, 1978a, 1978b; Devor 1982; Knowler, Carraher, and Pettitt 1984; Knowler et al. 1984; Szathmary, this volume; Sievers and Fisher 1981). These diseases are associated with a tendency to become obese early in adult life. Together, this constitutes a major epidemic among Amerindian groups at least from Mexico northward.

The evidence is that this epidemic has arisen in the last forty to fifty years. Therefore, environmental changes must be involved. Because of an association between risk level and Amerindian admixture, however, it is also likely that genetic susceptibility plays a role. We have hypothesized (Weiss, Ferrell, and Hanis 1984; Weiss, Ferrell, Hanis, and Styne 1984; Weiss and Ferrell 1985) that the collection of diseases may constitute a syndrome, which we have referred to as the "New World syndrome" (NWS) (Weiss, Ferrell, and Hanis 1984). The term denotes the hypothesis that the collection of disorders is related to a common underlying genetic cause, interacting with some environmental factor(s). Individuals may be affected to a variable extent, both in the severity of disease and in the specific components of the syndrome which they manifest.

There is currently no consensus concerning the cause of this epidemic, nor that it constitutes a syndrome. Selected aspects of this problem are discussed in this chapter, in an attempt to outline the hypothesis for a syndrome in clear terms, to identify areas where research is currently inconclusive or may suggest alternative explanations, and to outline ways by which the problem may be addressed in future research.

The term "New World peoples" denotes Amerindians, in particular those of North and Central America. This includes peoples with Amerindian genetic ancestry, though some (such as Mexican-Americans) are not typically thought of as Amerindians. Eskimos and Aleuts are not included and will be considered only briefly in this chapter.

An understanding of this pattern of disease may reveal much about gene-environment interaction and can possibly inform us about the settlement history of the New World. Evolutionary, ecological, historical, and other anthropological considerations may be brought to bear, making the problem an interesting one for anthropology, beyond its considerable epidemiological and public health importance (Weiss 1985; Weiss, Ferrell, and Hanis 1984; Weiss and Ferrell 1985).

BASIC NATURE OF THE EPIDEMIC

Emöke Szathmary, in Chapter 5, has compiled the most careful and detailed tables of Amerindian diabetes rates yet assembled. The tables show that Amerindians from widespread parts of North America have manifest high rates of adult-onset diabetes (NIDDM). These are much higher than generally observed in Caucasians, Blacks, or most Asians. For example, prevalence of NIDDM in Caucasian adults over the age of 25 is about 2–5 percent (Stern et al. 1983; Brousseau et al. 1979; Palumbo et al. 1976; Barrett-Conner 1980). Mexican-Americans have values of about 7–10 percent (Hanis et al. 1983; Stern et al. 1983).

In a study in progress, Weiss, Georges, and Levy, have measured serum glucose and glycosylated hemoglobin levels on Mayan Mexican Indians from the Yucatan peninsula. The results are summarized in Table 6.1. While diabetes rarely presents frank, late-stage pathology in this area as in many Amerindian populations, it is clear that it is either a latent problem or an incipient one, because the prevalence of diabetes or of elevated glucose is as high there as in Mexican-Americans and many North American Amerindians. One village, Village C, which is isolated and least modernized, has no diabetes. Small modernization effects apparently can trigger evidence of susceptibility.

Amerindian peoples have traditionally been divided into "paleo-Indians" and "Athabaskans," based on various cultural and linguistic criteria and supported to some extent by biometrical ones. The prevalence of glucose intolerance in at least some Athabaskans is high, comparable to that in Amerindians, but the percent of diagnosed diabetics is relatively smaller. In general, the survey results (glucose tolerance) are probably a better indicator of real biological differences at the times studies were carried out; hospital studies suffer from a diversity of problems, not the least of which are the many factors which can lead individuals to, or not to, show up ill at a hospital. The Athabaskan data are important because it has been suggested that they may have settled the New World subsequent to the initial movement of "paleo-Indians" here and may be genetically different from the latter. Similarly, Eskimos and Aleuts are thought

Table 6.1
Prevalence of Confirmed and Suspected Diabetes in Several Mayan Villages and Comparison Populations.

Population	Confirmed Diabetes[1]		Suspected Diabetes[2]		Total
	Number	%	Number	%	%
Village C	0	0.0	0	0.0	0.0
Village B	3	12.5	1	4.2	16.7
Village H	4	22.3	2	11.2	33.5
Village P	2	13.3	2	13.3	26.6
Village T	7	17.9	8	20.5	38.4
Starr County[3]		6.9		not available	
San Antonio[4]		9.5		not available	
Pima Indians[5]		24.3		not available	
US Caucasians[6]		2.0–5.0			

[1] Confirmed diabetes is diabetes diagnosed by physician, or shown by glycosylated hemoglobin value above 8% or casual blood glucose level over 120 mg / dl.

[2] Criteria for suspected diabetes (which may be pre-diabetes) are either: glycosylated hemoglobin value above 7.5%; serum glucose over 100; or those reporting symptoms suggestive of diabetes (frequent thirst, sugar in urine, easily fatigued, frequent urination; at least two positive responses were needed to classify). Values for last four lines are prevalances among adults over age 25 based on random population samples. Mean age in Maya was 35–45 in the different village samples, which were mostly females.

[3] Starr County Mexican-American values from Hanis et al. (1983).

[4] San Antonio Mexican-American values from Stern et al. (1981).

[5] Pima Indian values from Knowler et al. (1983).

[6] Caucasian values are typical (e.g., Palumbo et al. 1976; Barrett-Conner 1980).

by many to be later arrivals, and the evidence is still unclear as to the extent to which they suffer from these problems – or, indeed, the extent to which they may actually differ genetically from other native American peoples (Szathmary and Holt 1983).

Fewer data are available concerning Amerindian obesity. Amerindians were typically reported to be of healthy appearance in travelers' and explorers' reports before the days of research or photography. (However, the classic Mayans, including those in the area of Yucatan referred to above, apparently had a fat god (Coe 1984), of unknown function). Subsequently, obesity has become a major problem in many, if not most, Amerindian populations (see West 1974, 1978a, 1978b; Joos et al. 1984; Szathmary and Holt 1983; Stern et al. 1983; Weiss et al. 1984; Weiss and Ferrell 1985). There are data showing that obesity and/or a history of upper-body fatness and weight gain are associated with disease in the Pima (Knowler et al. 1981), in Mexican-Americans (Mueller et al. 1984), in Oklahoma Amerindians (Lee et al. 1985; West 1978a), and in the Dogrib of northern Canada (Szathmary, this volume; Szathmary and Holt 1983). In San Antonio Mexican-Americans, diabetes is associated with socioeconomic status in both sexes, as is the degree of genetic admixture, but an obesity gradient is found only in males (Malina et al. 1984). In Minnesota, obesity and diabetes are more prevalent among urban Amerindians than corresponding Whites, and both conditions are comparable to those in Mexican-Americans (Gillum, Gillum, and Smith 1984).

Because of the variable results regarding obesity, it is likely that obesity reflects pathogenic processes, rather than being a primary cause. In the Pima there is a bimodal distribution of glucose tolerance. Individuals move from the lower to the upper group during their lives; obesity appears to trigger this shift (Bennett et al. 1982). Hence, there may be a kind of threshold mechanism either in obesity or in glucose tolerance which could obscure correlations between them, especially in a population in which both prevalences are very high.

An elevated prevalence of GBD in Amerindians has been as widely reported as that for NIDDM, and from a wide variety of types of data and types of study. Positive reports of high prevalence have been reported along the west coast of North America from Alaska to British Columbia to Arizona to Mexico, along the East Coast from Nova Scotia to New York to Alabama, and throughout the center from the Northwest Territories and northern Ontario through the Great Lakes and Rockies to Texas. Risk levels which appear to be correlated with levels of Amerindian admixture also occur in New Mexico, Mexico, Bolivia, and Chile (Medina, Fascual, and Medina 1983). By age 70, in Caucasian populations, the prevalence of clinical GBD diagnosed by a physician reaches 10–18 percent in females and 8 percent in males, but 30–34 percent in Mexican-American and Amerindian females and 14 percent in males. The prevalence of either clinical or asymptomatic gallstones can reach nearly 90 percent by the end of life, as found in the Pima (Sampliner et al. 1970). For details and supporting references, see Bennett, in press; Diehl, in press; Samet, in press; Sievers and Fisher 1981; Weiss, Ferrell, and Hanis 1984; Weiss et al. 1984; Weiss and Ferrell 1985).

Most New World populations have not been studied in regard to gallstones, which requires either the existence of good hospital records or a cholecystographic survey, but gallbladder cancer (GBCA), for which persistent gallstones are a well-known risk factor (DeVor 1982), is an indicator disease for GBD because there are more data on GBCA. It is elevated in New World

Figure 6.1
Standardized Mortality or Morbidity Ratios for Gallbladder Cancer in Selected New World and Comparison Populations.

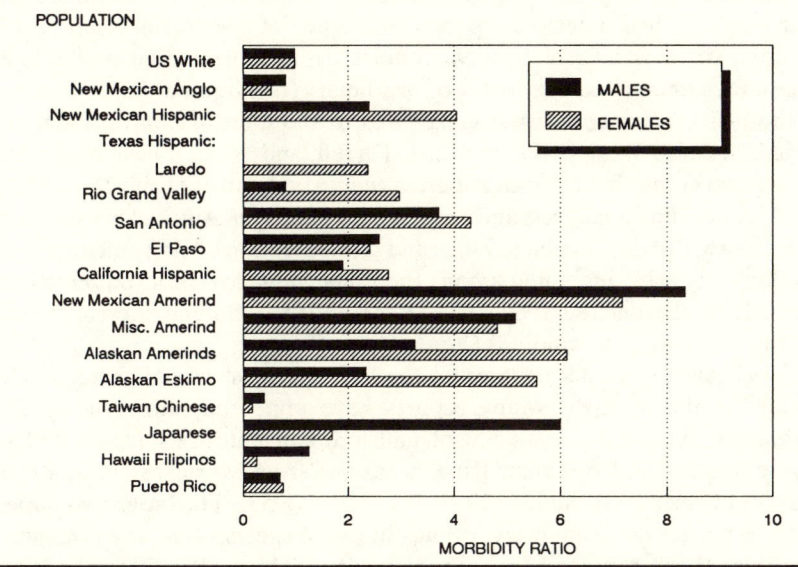

Source: Weiss, Ferrell, Hanis, and Styne, (1984). See original for source details.

peoples, especially in North America including Mexico (Devor 1982; Samet 1985; Weiss, Ferrell, and Hanis 1984), and Bolivia (Henson 1983; Rios-Dalenz et al. 1983). This is shown in Figure 6.1.

While in many ways the recency of this epidemic is clear, there is still skepticism. The supporting evidence comes from direct and indirect reports, mainly from after 1945, of elevated disease and from a few reports from before that time showing little disease. The controversy lies in the fact that diagnostic efficacy has improved greatly since World War II, for both NIDDM and GBD. It is possible that physicians failed to diagnose disease which was present or that changing attitudes toward medicine have led to a greater tendency for patients to complain of symptoms and for physicians to look for, and diagnose, these diseases. For example, before X-ray based cholecystography, which began in the 1930s, it was difficult to diagnose gallstones definitively. Once such a tool becomes available, it may be that incidence would rise simply because diagnosis was possible.

The best evidence for recency pertains to NIDDM. Before the war, many reports specifically looked for or tested for diabetes. The tests may not have been up to current standards, but they were up to contemporary standards as applied to Caucasians and Europeans, and the reports stressed the relative rarity of the disease in Amerindians (West 1978a; Geare 1915; Hoffman 1928;

Hamlin 1933; Salsbury 1937, 1947; Urquhart 1935; Sievers and Fisher 1981). These studies include physicians' reports, hospital admissions, glucose tests, and, indirectly, the absence of data suggesting high rates of diabetes-related conditions, such as amputations, blindness, kidney disease (e.g., Hoffman 1928; Salsbury 1937). These negative reports cover much of North America.

By contrast, a wealth of positive reports, from Amerindian and related populations, summarized effectively by Szathmary (this volume) have appeared since the 1940s, which encompass most of North and some of Central and South America (see also West 1978a, b; Weiss, Ferrell, and Hanis 1984). Suggestive evidence also comes from South America (e.g., Spielman et al. 1982).

The secular trend is clearest and explicitly proven in the American Southwest, where Geare (1915), Joslin (1940), and others reported low incidence of "pathologic" obesity, including among the Pima, who have suffered increasing risk as late as the decade 1967–1977 (Bennett 1985). Similar increases were noted in Oklahoma Amerindians (West 1978a).

In the absence of cholecystography, the best and most reliable evidence for gallstones is the autopsy. Many reports have appeared, most since 1940, documenting the high prevalence of gallstones in autopsies performed on Amerindian peoples from many tribal areas and from Mexicans (West 1978b; Sievers and Fisher 1981; Steiner 1954; Tragerman 1953). The latter two papers refer to autopsies covering prewar times in Los Angeles; while the rates were higher than those reported in hospital surveys (Geare 1915; Hamlin 1933; Hancock 1933), they show an excess in Mexican-Americans. In Laredo, Texas, where we have reviewed all hospital inpatient records for this entire century, only twenty cholecystectomies were performed up to 1945, but about 270 have been performed annually since then. We do not think that this is due only to better and safer surgical methods.

Hospital reports suggest that gallstones became a major problem in Amerindian peoples roughly after the war. In the Navajo, they represented only a modest fraction of hospital admissions in the period 1931–1935 (Salsbury 1937) but had increased by 1.5–3.0 times by 1947 to represent 1–1.5 percent of all admissions (Salsbury 1947) and are now one of the leading conditions for admission among the Navajo (Brown and Christensen 1967). This is true for most studied tribal groups (Weiss et al. 1984).

In regard to GBCA, an autopsy survey found, from 1918 to 1948, a pattern suggesting excess risk in Mexican-Americans (Steiner 1954; Tragerman 1953). GBCA was unseen in Laredo before 1940 and has increased since then such that there have been about seven cases annually. In the state of Texas, a registry existed between 1944 and 1966 (MacDonald and Heinze 1978). This was an imperfect registry, but the data clearly show that in Blacks and Caucasians there was a slight increase in GBCA rates through this period. Mexican-American males experienced a greater, and females a much greater, increase. In the Navajo, GBCA did not occur between 1931 and 1935, and only three times from 1940 to 1942, in females aged 50, 52, and 60. In general, the rate of GBCA in the

Navajo is known to have increased substantially in later years, to become one of their more common tumors (Rudolf, Cohen, and Gascoigne 1970), as it has in other native Americans (e.g., Weiss, Ferrell, and Hanis 1984; Weiss et al. 1984).

ENVIRONMENTAL FACTORS

Many have argued that these diseases are environmental (e.g., West 1978a). However, it has been difficult to identify specific factors. The suggestion that either local foods or generalized excess consumption may be related (e.g., Mayberry and Lindeman 1963; West, 1978a, 1978b) has not been supported by most existing studies, in which little in the way of useful associations was found (e.g., Johnston, Williams, and Weldon 1977; Reid et al. 1971). In a prospective study in the Pima, however, Bennett et al. (1984) found an association, in women, with consumption of an increased proportion of total, and of complex, carbohydrate in the diet. These were correlated with total calorie and fat intake. Many potential confounding factors make these results difficult to interpret (Bennett et al. 1984).

RELEVANT GENETIC OBSERVATIONS

The geographic pattern suggests that environmental factors are not all that is responsible for this epidemic. Otherwise, one would expect, for example, to find similar disease patterns in American-Hispanic populations with high Black, but low Amerindian, admixture, but this has not been the case (e.g., Weiss, Ferrell, and Hanis 1984).

On the other hand, a correlation within populations between putative Amerindian ancestry and diabetes prevalence would not be expected, but such has been found in Oklahoma Choctaw (Drevets 1965; Brosseau et al. 1979) and in the Pima based on putative ancestry (Bennett 1985). There is a similar association across populations, including subpopulations of Mexican-Americans, and this is quantitatively consistent with genetic causation (polygenic or recessive monogenic). Such a pattern is unlikely to have arisen by chance, because it would require a finely tuned correlation between environment and admixture.

There are some more direct genetic data. In the Pima, an association between the presence of the HLA-A2 allele and diabetes has been found (Williams et al. 1981). The overall disease pattern there has been interpreted as being consistent with a single dominant Mendelian allele (Bennett 1985; Knowler et al. 1981; Knowler et al. 1983; Yamashita et al. 1984). In the Seminoles, segregation analysis of family data on serum glucose levels showed evidence for a single Mendelian locus in Oklahoma but not in Florida, though the results were equivocal in the latter (Elston et al. 1974). Szathmary (herein) has found evidence for genetic etiology but not for a single locus pattern. Also in the Pima, obesity was found not to be a risk factor for NIDDM unless there is a parental history of the disease, suggesting a genetic component (Knowler et al. 1981). This has also been found in Oklahoma Amerindians of diverse tribes (Lee et al. 1985).

Data in support of a genetic etiology for GBD are of a similar nature. The population data suggest that the prevalence of GBD is correlated with admixture. This includes results from Starr County and Laredo, Texas (Hanis et al. 1985; Weiss et al. 1984), and similar gradients of risk in tricultural New Mexico (Morris et al. 1978), in Bolivia (Rios-Dalenz et al. 1983), and in Los Angeles (Mack and Menck 1982). The Los Angeles data show a greater elevation in risk for those born in Central America, which might suggest a higher average Amerindian fraction than in other Los Angeles Hispanics. An association with subjects' known amount of Amerindian ancestry and GBD prevalence was found by Thistle et al. (1971) in the Chippewa. Similar findings have been made in the Pima (Knowler et al. 1984). There are incidental reports of multiple occurrence of GBCA in three Amerindian families (Sperling 1964; Devor and Buechley 1979) and an excess of gallbladder disease in family members of Mexican-Americans in Starr County, Texas (Hanis, Schull, and Ferrell 1985).

CONTRASTING POPULATIONS

One way to isolate genetic risk factors would be to find populations of relevant genetic relationship to the Amerindians and to ascertain their risk patterns. The most potentially informative group of this nature would be the East Asian ancestors of all Amerindians. If they share the susceptibility, then any relevant genes must have been present for a considerable time period. If they are not susceptible, there may be genetic risk variants which have arisen since the separation of American from Asian peoples.

Separating environmental from genetic susceptibility is not easy. There are a few reports to suggest that Asians in general may be susceptible to these diseases. The data come mainly from Indians in South Africa (e.g., Walker 1981) and Fiji (Zimmet, Taylor, and King 1982), and from Polynesians (e.g., Bennett, Harris, and Murphy 1983; Prior and Tasman-Jones 1981; Zimmet, Taylor, and King 1982). Excepting the Polynesians, the reports are isolated and may not be of general relevance; there are, for example, some differences in age of onset and other characteristics in the South African sample (Walker 1981). While NIDDM is elevated in some more westernized Chinese or Japanese, the evidence for extremely high rates of diabetes is equivocal (e.g., Bennett, Harris, and Murphy 1983; Cheah and Yeo 1983; Glober and Stemmermann 1981). Susceptibility has not been as high in Melanesians (Sinnett and Whyte 1981; Zimmet, Taylor, and King 1981) or in Australian aborigines (Moodie 1981), both derived from or related to Mongoloid ancestors. Obesity may be more a risk factor in Pacific females than in Amerindians (King et al. 1983).

The data in regard to GBD generally suggest that Asians are less susceptible than Amerindians to GBD. Although gallstones are increasing in prevalence, the rates of GBCA in most Japanese and Chinese populations living in the West are substantially lower than found in Amerindians (e.g., Henderson, Kolonel, and Foster 1982; Locke and King 1980; King and Locke 1980; Kolonel 1980; Menck and Henderson 1982), although the rates in Japanese in British Columbia may be nearly comparable (Gallagher and Ellwood 1979). Gallstone prevalence is elevated in some New Zealand Polynesians (Prior and Tasman-Jones 1981), but (based on the pattern of GBCA rates) this does not seem to be generally true in the Pacific basin (Henderson, Kolonel, and Foster 1982; Menck and Henderson 1982).

SOME THOUGHTS ON POSSIBLE MECHANISMS

There are no definitive leads as yet as to the nature of the kinds of primary defect which could underlie the NWS. However, several observations suggest plausible directions for research. Studies in diverse populations have shown associations between HLA types (or glyoxylase, which is closely linked to HLA) and diabetes (e.g., Williams et al. 1981; Serjeantson et al. 1983). The associations are not consistent or strong, nor do the diseases appear to segregate in a Mendelian way with HLA. Gm allotypes have also been found to be associated with NIDDM; this has been reported in two non-Amerindian populations (Berg et al. 1967; Scholz, Knussman, and Daweke 1975) and suggestive indications may have been found in the Pima (Bennett, personal communication) and the Dogrib (Szathmary, personal communication), though the latter two remain unpublished at present. These may reflect an immunological aspect to the diseases, or they may be linked to other nonimmunological risk loci. However, these are highly variable loci, and the associations may simply reflect the admixture between susceptible and nonsusceptible types in hybrid populations with different haplotypes at these loci.

It is clear from the worldwide literature that there are statistical associations among obesity, diabetes, and gallstones, in the sense that they are risk factors for each other or share common risk factors. For example, having at least one child is a risk factor for diabetes and for gallstones. The obese are found to be at higher risk for NIDDM and GBD almost everywhere in the world. In this sense, these conditions must constitute a clinical syndrome of sorts, though in Amerindians the associations are much stronger.

There are some suggestions of mechanisms which may increase the plausibility that the three conditions could be related to some relatively simple underlying physiological differences. Elevated insulin is associated with NIDDM; there may be a similar association with gallstones (Scragg, Calvert, and Oliver 1984). In this study (of non-Amerindians) increased triglycerides were also associated with GBD, and there was a negative correlation between high-density lipoprotein (HDL) levels and gallstones. These were unrelated to obesity or diet.

Similar findings have been made in New World peoples. Typically, insulin levels are high. Triglyceride levels have been reported to be high and HDL levels to be low in Mexican-Americans (Stern et al., in press), the Pima (Howard et al. 1984). Triglycerides are higher in Minneapolis Amerindians than in San Antonio Caucasians and roughly comparable to the Mexican-Americans there (Gillum, Gillum, and Smith 1984). Trigylcerides were even slightly elevated in healthy, non-Westernized Tarahumara Amerindians of Mexico (Connor et al. 1978). The relationships are complex and do not suggest an easy or simple explanation. However, high levels of insulin may trigger the synthesis and/or release of triglycerides into the bloodstream, and high insulin also may trigger the synthesis of trigylcerides and cholesterol by the liver, much of which is excreted into the bile. Hence, the underlying defect may simply lead to high levels of insulin, with the other conditions following as consequences (Weiss and Ferrell 1985).

THE NEW WORLD SYNDROME HYPOTHESIS

It is consistent with the facts that NIDDM and GBD are, independently, the result of modernization, specifically an increase in the intake of calories and a decrease in physical exercise (e.g., West 1978a; Trowell and Burkitt 1981). There has in fact been a worldwide increase of both NIDDM and GBD in modernizing populations. Racial differences in prevalence would simply reflect differences in the risk factors rather than genetic differences.

One kind of environmental explanation for the widespread and dramatic increase in NWS diseases could be that modernization affected Amerindian tribes so rapidly that today's adults are metabolically incapable of responding. For example, they could have adopted a damaging set point in regard to fat storage and insulin levels, in response to rapid environmental changes taking place within their own lives. If this is true, the children, who have been exposed to these conditions from birth, would be expected to manifest less, or less severe, disease, by virtue of being better adapted or habituated. This, however, cannot explain the NWS: the second and third postwar generations of Mexican-Americans and Pima have been manifesting more, and more serious, disease than their parents and grandparents (Bennett 1985).

Though the component diseases of the NWS all typically increase with modernization (Trowell and Burkitt 1981), they do not seem to arise with the co-occurrence pattern found in the Amerindians. For example, modernization has not yet produced the degree of elevated risk in Japanese, Chinese, Melanesians, and other Asians, and, even in the Polynesians, GBD does not appear to be markedly elevated. This suggests a different etiology in Amerindians.

More specific hypotheses have been advanced, in particular that diabetes is the evolutionary product of efficient nutrient-storage metabolism in humans generally (Neel 1962, 1982) or in certain populations, like the Polynesians (Baker 1984; Prior 1971) or the Pima, specifically (Knowler et al. 1983). In the latter case, local factors, like unpredictable water supply for agriculture, have been offered to explain the advantage in Darwinian fitness a bearer of an efficient genotype might have. Such a genotype may only have become pathogenic in the modern world. The widespread nature of Amerindian susceptibility surely shows, however, that factors local to the Pima are not a sufficient explanation.

Our hypothesis takes the general logic, but not the details, of Neel's hypothesis, applied specifically to Amerindian peoples and their particular settlement history (Weiss 1985; Weiss, Ferrell, and Hanis 1984; Weiss and Ferrell 1985). It is that a gene or genes arose or existed early in the settlement of the New World which, under the conditions of arctic food supplies, was more efficient at storing nutrients than other available genotypes. Some new genotypes conferred an advantage on both sexes for survival or on females for fertility and were selected for in the small ancestral hunting-gathering bands that were the forebears of Amerindians (the data will eventually determine whether of all Amerindians plus Eskimo-Aleuts or of a smaller subset). These genes became virtually fixed in the small ancestral populations. In subsequent times, they continued to confer a beneficial effect or at least were not harmful. Now, with exposure to some aspects of modernization, they are deleterious.

In this author's opinion, a single gene locus (or, perhaps, several such loci segregating in different families) may be responsible for the NWS. The degree of interpopulation variance in susceptibility seems to be less than would be expected if the problem were polygenic; the variation observed is consistent with non-Amerindian admixture and variable environmental exposures. One would expect that many other gene loci would also contribute to the nature and expression of pathology in this complex gene-environment situation, and in that sense a single locus is not likely to explain the whole pattern.

Ward (1985) has shown that it might be difficult to maintain a selective balance between helpful and harmful genotypes across widely variant environments over 12,000 to 20,000 years, from the original arctic, to all of those inhabited by Amerindians precontact, to current modernized conditions. For that kind of reason, it seems likely that the gene(s) were fixed in the ancestral population; the genetic details remain to be proven, however.

If the same genes are responsible for the NWS components, those components must eventually be proven to be associatied intraindividually. This has been difficult to document, partly due to the high prevalence of all conditions in those Amerindian populations where a joint assessment has been attempted, and partly to the difficulty in classifying individuals (e.g., a diabetic with subclinical gallstones scored as "unaffected" by GBD). In the Pima, there is evidence for an association between NIDDM and clinical GBD (Knowler et al. 1984), and there is similar suggestive evidence in Texas Mexican-Americans (Hanis, Schull, and Ferrell 1985).

It is possible that all Asians will eventually prove to be susceptible, as mentioned earlier. This would necessitate fundamental changes in the origins aspect of the NWS hypothesis. But it is also possible that the high susceptibility in some Pacific populations is due to the independent evolution of the same or similar mutants. This is certainly precedented in the instance of many disorders, most noteworthy, perhaps, being the malaria-associated hemoglobinopathies. There have seemed to be a gradient of disease risk with admixture in the Pacific (Serjeantson et al. 1983) and a relationship between disease and settlement history (e.g., Baker 1984).

COMPLICATING FACTORS AND RESEARCH DESIGNS

To date, no studies have undertaken to test the hypothesis that the NWS components in fact constitute a genetic syndrome. There are several criteria which must be met in order to do this. They include:

1. Phenotypes must vary in the study population. It is obviously difficult to obtain individual or family associations among conditions and genes if they are so prevalent in a population that virtually everyone is affected. This probably has been a problem in the Pima. If the susceptibilty genotypes have been fixed, or nearly so, it may be necessary to study these problems in populations, like Mexican-Americans, which are admixed with lower-risk populations. Similarly, it is important to work in populations in which exposures to dietary and other environmental components vary among individuals or are easiest to assess. For example, we think that dietary risk factors will be understandable in a population such as the Maya, where diets are simpler and quantifiable and where dietary changes are recent and datable. Differentiating among models of causation will obviously be easier when there are more contrasts, genetic and environmental.

2. Correct specification of the phenotype. In the absence of a knowledge of genotypes of family members, it is important to specify the phenotypes in a way which is most highly correlated with the unknown genotypes, that is, with the highest penetrance. Because the NWS diseases are common and have gradual, late-age onset, there is a danger that subjects not affected at study time will falsely be classified as "unaffected"; many of them may become affected later in their lives and may even manifest some subclinical precursor phenotypes.

   Older adults will be the most informative. However, because the processes are known to be cumulative (e.g., glucose tolerance or fasting glucose levels and subclinical gallstones), susceptible genotypes, if they exist, are probably phenotypically expressed by a gradually increasing degree of pathology, eventually leading to clinical disease. I have called this process "phenotype amplification" (Weiss 1985). Family studies should classify individuals in terms of the most primary phenotypic measure possible. If good precursor measures can be found, and if they are genetic in origin, they might be identifiable even from birth.

3. Correct definition of the proband. Every study to date has been based on classifications of individuals' disease status in terms of only one NWS component. Study subjects, probands, family members have all been classified in the same way. Clearly such an approach cannot address the existence of a syndrome in which susceptible individuals may manifest only one, or some, of the components.

To test the syndrome hypothesis, probands and others in the study must be classified as "affected" if they manifest any of the components (measured by the most primary phenotype, as discussed above). It is not clear that reconstruction of a correct study population can be done with data collected on the basis of a single trait as the defining condition for probands or controls.

4. Ascertainment and sampling by unbiased and efficient strategy. Because of the difficulty of distinguishing between affected and unaffected individuals, proband-based (case-control or family) studies should be designed so as to maximize the probability of correct classification. One way to do this with degenerative conditions is to sample only from the older generation in the population where, as noted above, the unaffected probably will remain unaffected (especially if precursor states are measured). Proband ascertainment from among such adults should be possible without serious problems of ascertainment bias.

Perhaps an even better approach, given the uncertainties of disease classification, is randomly to sample a fraction of the entire population of advanced age, rather than selecting probands. In high-risk populations, enough affecteds (with each syndrome component) would be found to address the risk factors for the components as well as the syndrome or to divide the probands into unaffected and affected groups.

5. Linkage and genetic markers should be sought. Clearly the NWS will remain an unproven hypothesis unless a linked marker or variant gene product can be found. If the problem is essentially a polygenic one, of course, this will not occur. Because of the potential for understanding, therapy, and prevention, however, it is important to look for identifiable genes.

CONCLUSIONS

New World Syndrome is a major health problem for Native American peoples, and it is one which seems to involve a complex interaction between some aspect of a recently changed environment and the genotype of the host. While we cannot assert that a genetic syndrome hypothesis has been proven, the evidence clearly merits an energetic search for genetic factors. This series of disease produces more morbidity in Amerindian populations than any other diseases. Yet, it is clearly preventable. Genetic susceptibility, if it exists, cannot be prevented, but the environment can be modified in some way which would reduce the risk. A better understanding of current environmental risk factors and of the mechanism of the disease pathogenesis will be needed to determine the most feasible strategy for prevention.

Regardless of the cause, this syndrome of diseases is a clear and very important instance of transitional disease. It is a problem on which anthropologists can work with a level of understanding which may not be found in traditional epidemiological research. One hopes the problem will be solved and will contribute toward a methodology for solving other, similar problems elsewhere in the world.

NOTE

I wish to thank Dr. Emöke J.E. Szathmary specifically for her critical comments on an earlier draft of this chapter. Also, many points were raised at the Wenner-Gren Conference, and I hope these have been addressed herein. I wish to thank the Wenner-Gren Foundation for providing this forum. A considerable literature has accumulated since the 1985 conference at which this paper was presented, but the essence of the argument has not changed.

REFERENCES

Baker, P. T. 1984. Migrations, genetics, and the degenerative diseases of South Pacific Islanders. In *Migration and Mobility*. A. J. Boyce, ed. London: Taylor & Francis.

Barrett-Conner, E. 1980. The prevalence of diabetes mellitus in an adult community as determined by history of fasting hyperglycemia. *American Journal of Epidemiology* 111: 705–12.

Bennett, P. H. 1985. Chronic diseases in American Indians. In *Proceedings of a Conference on Chronic Diseases Among Mexican-Americans: A Public Health Issue*. C.L. Hanis and W. J. Schull, eds. Unpublished.

Bennett, P. H., M. Harris, and R. S. Murphy. 1983. Geographic and ethnic differences in diabetes frequency in the Americas. In *Diabetes 1982*. E. N. Mngola, ed. Proc., 11th Cong. Intl. Diab. Fed., Nairobi, Nov., 1982. Amsterdam: Excerpta Medica.

Bennett, P. H., W. C. Knowler, H. R. Baird, W. J. Butler, D. J. Pettitt, and J. M. Reid. 1984. Diet and development of noninsulin-dependent diabetes mellitus: an epidemiological perspective. In *Diet, Diabetes and Atherosclerosis*. G. Pozza, P. Micossi, A. Catapano, and R. Paoletti, eds. New York: Raven.

Bennett, P. H., W. C. Knowler, D. J. Pettitt, M. J. Carraher, and B. Vasquez. 1982. Longitudinal studies of the development of diabetes in the Pima Indians. In *Advances in Diabetes Epidemiology*. E. Eschwege, ed. INSERM Symposium, No. 22. Amsterdam: Elsevier.

Berg, K., S. Aarseth, J. Lundevall, and L. Reinskou. 1967. Blood groups and genetic serum types in diabetes mellitus. *Diabetologia* 3:30–34.

Brosseau, J. D., R. C. Eelkema, A. C. Crawford, and T. A. Abe. 1979. Diabetes among the three affiliated tribes: Correlation with degree of Indian inheritance. *American Journal of Public Health* 69:1277–78.

Brown, J., and C. Christensen. 1967. Biliary tract disease among the Navajos. *Journal of American Medical Association* 202:1050–52.

Cheah, J. S., and P. P. B. Yeo. 1983. Prevalence of diabetes in the developing countries of Asia and Africa with special reference to the Chinese and Indians. In *Diabetes 1982.* E. N. Mngola, ed., Proc. 11th Cong. Intl. Diab. Fed., Nairobi, Nov. 1982. Amsterdam: Excerpta Medica.

Coe, M.D. 1984. *The Maya.* 3d ed. New York: Thames & Hudson.

Connor W. E., M. T. Cerqueira, M. S. Rodney, R. W. Connor, R. B. Wallace, M. R. Malinow, and H. R. Casdorph. 1978. The plasma lipids, lipoproteins, and diet of the Tarahumara Indians of Mexico. *American Journal of Clinical Nutrition* 31:1131–42.

Devor, E. 1982. Ethnographic patterns of gallbladder cancer. In *Epidemiology of Cancer of the Digestive Tract.* P. Correa and W. Haenszel, eds. The Hague: Nijhoff.

Devor, E., and R. Buechley. 1979. Gallbladder cancer in hispanic New Mexicans. II. Familial occurrence in two northern New Mexico kindreds. *Cancer Genetics and Cytogenetics* 1:139–45.

Diehl, A. K. 1985. Gallbladder disease in Mexican-Americans. In *Proceedings of a Conference on Chronic Disease in Mexican-Americans: A Public Health Issue.* C. L. Hanis and W. J. Schull, eds. Unpublished.

Drevets, C. C. 1965. Diabetes mellitus in Choctaw Indians. *Journal of the Oklahoma Medical Association* 58:322–29.

Elston, R., K. Namboodiri, H. Nino, and W. Pollitzer. 1974. Studies on blood and urine glucose in Seminole Indians: Indications for segregation of a major gene. *American Journal of Human Genetics* 26:13–34.

Gallagher, R. P., and J. M. Elwood. 1979. Cancer mortality among Chinese, Japanese, and Indians in British Columbia, 1964–73. National Cancer Institute. Monographs. 53:89–93.

Geare, R. 1915. Some diseases prevalent among Indians of the Southwest and their treatment. *Medical World News* 33:305–10.

Gillum, R. F., B. S. Gillum, and N. Smith. 1984. Cardiovascular risk factors among urban American Indians: Blood pressue, serum lipids, smoking, diabetes, health knowledge, and behavior. *American Heart Journal* 107:765–76.

Glober, G., and G. Stemmermann. 1981. Hawaii ethnic groups. In *Western Diseases: Their Emergence and Prevention.* H. C. Trowell, and D. P. Burkitt, eds. Cambridge: Harvard University Press.

Hamlin, H. 1933. A health survey of the Seminole Indians. *Yale Journal of Biology and Medicine* 33:155–77.

Hancock, J. 1933. Diseases among the Indians. *Southwestern Medicine* 17: 126–29.

Hanis, C. L., R. E. Ferrell, S. A. Barton, L. Aguilar, A. Garza-Ibarra, B. R. Tulloch, C. A. Garcia, and W. J. Schull. 1983. Diabetes among Mexican-Americans in Starr County, Texas. *American Journal of Epidemiology* 118:659–72.

Hanis, C. L., W. J. Schull, and R. E. Ferrell. 1985. Gallbladder disease among Mexican-Americans in Starr County, Texas. *American Journal of Epidemiology* 122:120–29.

Henderson, B. E., L. N. Kolonel, and F. Foster. 1982. Cancer in Polynesians. National Cancer Institute. Monograph. 62:73–78.

Henson, D. 1983. Conference and workshop on cancer epidemiology in Latin America. *Journal. National Cancer Institute* 70:979–85.

Hoffman, F. L. 1928. The health progress of the North American Indian. Boston: Prudential Life Ins.

Howard, B. V., W. C. Knowler, B. Vasquez, A. L. Kennedy, D. J. Pettitt, and P. H. Bennett. 1984. Plasma and lipoprotein cholesterol and triglyceride in the Pima Indian population: comparison of diabetics and nondiabetics. *Arterio-sclerosis* 4:462–71.

Johnston, J. L., C. N. Williams, and K. L. M. Weldon. 1977. Nutrient intake and meal patterns of Micmac Indian and Caucasian women in Shubenacadie, NS. *Journal of the Canadian Medical Association* 116:1356–59.

Joos, S. K., W. H. Mueller, C. L. Hanis, and W. J.Schull. 1984. Diabetes Alert Study: Weight history and upper body obesity in diabetic and non-diabetic Mexican American adults. *Annals of Human Biology* 11:167–71.

Joslin, E. P. 1940. The universality of diabetes. A survey of diabetic morbidity in Arizona. *Journal of the American Medical Association* 115:2033–38.

King, H., and F. B. Locke. 1980. Cancer mortality among Chinese in the United States. *Journal. National Cancer Institute* 65:1141–48.

King, H., P. Zimmet, L. R. Raper, and B. Balkau. 1983. Risk factors for diabetes in three Pacific populations. *American Journal of Epidemiology* 119:396–409.

Knowler, W. C., M. J. Carraher, and D. J. Pettitt. 1984. Diabetes mellitus, obesity, and cholelithiasis. In *Epidemiology and Prevention of Gallstone Disease*. L. Capocaccia, G. Ricci, F. Angelico, M. Angelico, and A. F. Attili, eds. Lancaster, Penn.: MTP Press.

Knowler, W. C., M. J. Carraher, D. J. Pettitt, and P. H. Bennett. 1984. Epidemiology of cholelithiasis in the Pima Indians. In *Epidemiology and Prevention of Gallstone Disease*. L. Capocaccia, G. Ricci, F. Angelico, M. Angelico, and A. F. Attili, eds. Lancaster, Penn.: MTP Press.

Knowler, W. C., D. J. Pettitt, P. H. Bennett, and R. C. Williams. 1983. Diabetes mellitus in the Pima Indians: Genetic and evolutionary considerations. *American Journal of Physical Anthropology* 62:107–14.

Knowler, W. C., D. J. Pettitt, P. J. Savage, and P. H. Bennett. 1981. Diabetes incidence in Pima Indians: Contributions of obesity and parental diabetes. *American Journal of Epidemiology* 113:144–56.

Kolonel, L. N. 1980. Cancer patterns of four ethnic groups in Hawaii. *Journal. National Cancer Institute* 65:1127–39.

Lee, E. T., P. S. Anderson, J. Bryan, C. Bahr, T. Coniglione, and M. Cleves. 1985. Diabetes, parental diabetes, and obesity in Oklahoma Indians. *Diabetes Care* 8:107–13.

Locke, F. B., and H. King. 1980. Cancer mortality risk among Japanese in the United States. *Journal. National Cancer Institute* 65:1149–56.

Macdonald, E., and E. Heinze. 1978. *Epidemiology of Cancer in Texas*. New York: Raven.

Mack, T., and H. Menck. 1982. Epidemiology of cancer of the gallbladder and extra-hepatic biliary passages. In *Epidemiology of Cancer of the Digestive Tract*. P. Correa and W. Haenszel, eds. The Hague: Nijhoff.

Malina, R. B., B. B. Little, M. P. Stern, S. P. Gaskill, and H. P. Hazuda. 1984. Ethnic and social class differences in selected anthropometric characteristics of Mexican-American and Anglo adults: The San Antonio heart study. *Human Biology* 55:867–83.

Mayberry, R., and R. Lindeman. 1963. A survey of chronic disease and diet in Seminole Indians in Oklahoma. *American Journal of Clinical Nutrition* 13:127–34.

Medina, E., J. P. Pascual, and R. Medina. 1983. Frecuencia de la litiasis biliar en Chile. *Revista Medica de Chile* 111:668–75.

Menck, H. R., and B. E. Henderson. 1982. Cancer incidence patterns in the Pacific Basin. National Cancer Institute. Monograph. 62:101–09.

Moodie, P. M. 1981. Australian aborigines. In *Western Diseases: Their Emergence and Prevention.* H. C. Trowell, and D. P. Burkitt, eds. Cambridge: Harvard University Press.

Morris, D., R. Buechley, C. Key, and M. Morgan. 1978. Gallbladder disease and gallbladder cancer among American Indians in tricultural New Mexico. *Cancer* 42:2472–77.

Mueller, W. H., S. K. Joos, C. L. Hanis, A. N. Zavaleta, J. Eichner, and W. J. Schull. 1984. The diabetes alert study: growth, fatness and fat patterning, adolescence through adulthood in Mexican Americans. *American Journal of Physical Anthropology* 64:389–99.

Neel, J. V. 1982. The "thrifty genotype" revisited. In *The Genetics of Diabetes Mellitus.* J. Kobberling and J. Tattersall eds. New York: Academic.

———. 1962. Diabetes mellitus: a "thrifty" genotype rendered detrimental by "progress"? *American Journal of Human Genetics* 14:353–62.

Palumbo, P. J., L. R. Elveback, C-P. Chu, D. C. Connolly, and L. T. Kurland. 1976. Diabetes mellitus: Incidence, prevalence, survivorship, and causes of death in Rochester, Minnesota, 1945–1970. *Diabetes* 25:566–73.

Prior, I. 1971. The price of civilization. *Nutrition Today* 6:2–11.

Prior, I., and C. Tasman-Jones. 1981. New Zealand Maori and Pacific Polynesians. In *Western Diseases: Their Emergence and Prevention.* H. C. Trowell, and D. P. Burkitt, eds. Cambridge: Harvard University Press.

Reid, J. M., S. D. Fullmer, K. D. Pettigrew, T. A. Burch, P. H. Bennett, M. Miller, and G. D. Whedon. 1971. Nutrient intake of Pima Indian women: Relationships to diabetes mellitus and gallbladder disease. *American Journal of Clinical Nutrition* 24:1281–89.

Rios-Dalenz, J., A. Takabayashi, D. Henson, B. Strom, and R. Soloway. 1983. The epidemiology of cancer of the extra-hepatic biliary tract in Bolivia. *International Journal of Epidemiology* 12:156–60.

Rudolf, R., J. Cohen, and R. Gascoigne. 1970. Biliary cancer among Southwestern American Indians. *Arizona Medicine* 27:1–4.

Salsbury, C. 1947. Incidence of certain diseases among Navajos. *Arizona Medicine* 4:29–31.

———. 1937. Disease incidence among the Navajos. *Southwestern Medicine* 21:230–33.

Samet, J. 1985. Cancer epidemiology in Hispanics of the West and Southwest. In *Proceedings of a Conference on Chronic Diseases Among Mexican-Americans: A Public Health Issue.* C. L. Hanis, and W. J. Schull, eds. Unpublished.

Sampliner, R., P. H. Bennett, L. Comess, F. Rose, and T. Burch. 1970. Gallbladder disease in Pima Indians: Demonstration of high prevalence and early onset by cholecystography. *New England Journal of Medicine* 283:1358–64.

Scholz, W., R. Knussmann, and H. Daweke. 1975. Distribution of blood and serum protein group characteristics in patients with diabetes. *Diabetologia* 11:77–82.

Scragg, R. K. R., G. D. Calvert, and J. R. Oliver. 1984. Plasma lipid and insulin in gallstone disease: A case-control study. *British Medical Journal* 289:521–25.

Serjeantson, S. W., D. Owerbach, P. Zimmet, J. Nerup, and K. Thoma. 1983. Genetics of diabetes in Nauru: Effects of foreign admixture, HLA antigens, and the insulin-gene-linked polymorphism. *Diabetologia* 25:13–17.

Sievers, M., and J. Fisher. 1981. Diseases of North American Indians. In *Biocultural Aspects of Disease.* H. Rothschild, ed. New York: Academic.

Sinnett, P., and M. Whyte. 1981. Papua New Guinea. In *Western Diseases: Their Emergence and Prevention*. H. C. Trowell, and D. P. Burkitt, eds. Cambridge: Harvard University Press.

Sperling, M. 1964. Familial biliary tract carcinoma. *Journal of the American Medical Association* 190:944–45.

Spielman, R. S., S. S. Fajans, J. V. Neel, S. Pek, J. C. Floyd, and W. J. Oliver. 1982. Glucose tolerance in two unacculturated Indian tribes of Brazil. *Diabetologia* 23:90–93.

Steiner, P. E. 1954. *Cancer, Race and Geography*. Baltimore: Williams and Wilkins.

Stern, M. P., S. P. Gaskill, C. R. Allen, V. Garza, J. L. Gonzalez, R. Waldropo. 1981. Cardiovascular risk factors in Mexican Americans in Laredo, Texas. I. Prevalence of overweight and diabetes and distribution of serum lipids. *American Journal of Epidemiology* 113:546–55.

Stern, M. P., S. P. Gaskill, H. P. Hazuda, L. I. Gardner, and S. M. Haffner. 1983. Does obesity explain excess prevalence of diabetes among Mexican-Americans? *Diabetologia* 24:272–77.

Stern, M. P., S. M. Haffner, H. P. Hazuda, and M. Rosenthal. 1985. Cardiovascular disease in Mexican-Americans. In *Proceedings of a Conference on Chronic Diseases Among Mexican-Americans: A Public Health Issue*. C. L. Hanis, and W. J. Schull, eds. Unpublished.

Szathmary, E. J. E. 1987. Genetic and environmental risk factors. In *Diabetes in the Canadian Native Population: Biocultural Perspectives*. T. K. Young, ed. Toronto: Canadian Diabetes Association.

———. 1983. Peopling of northern North America: Clues from genetic studies. *Acta Anthropogeneica* 8:79–110.

Szathmary, E. J. E., and N. Holt. 1983. Hyperglycemia in Dogrib Indians of the Northwest Territories, Canada: Association with age and a centripetal distribution of body fat. *Human Biology* 55:493–516.

Thistle, J., K. Eckhart, R. Neusel, F. Nobrega, G. Poehling, M. Reimer, and L. Schoenfield. 1971. Prevalence of gallbladder disease among Chippewa Indians. Mayo Clinic. Proceedings. 46:603–08.

Tragerman, L. J. 1953. Primary carcinoma of the gallbladder: Review of 173 cases. *California Medicine* 78:431–37.

Trowell, H., and D. Burkitt, eds. 1981. *Western Diseases: Their Emergence and Prevention*. Cambridge: Harvard University Press.

Urquhart, J. A. 1935. The most northerly practice in Canada. *Canadian Medical Association. Journal* 33:193–96.

Walker, A. 1981. South African black, Indian and coloured populations. In *Western Diseases: Their Emergence and Prevention*. H. C. Trowell, and D. P. Burkitt, eds. Cambridge: Harvard University Press.

Ward, R. H. 1985. Isolates in transition: A research paradigm for genetic epidemiology. In *Diseases of Complex Etiology in Small Populations: Ethnic Differences and Research Approaches*. R. Chakraborty, and E. J. E. Szathmary, eds. New York: Liss.

Weiss, K. M. 1985. Phenotype amplification, as illustrated by cancer of the gallbladder in New World native peoples. In *Etiology of Complex Diseases in Small Populations*. R. Chakraborty and E. J. E. Szathmary, eds. New York: Raven.

Weiss, K. M., and R. E. Ferrell. 1985. The New World "syndrome" of disease: Evidence for gene-environment interaction. In *Proceedings of a Conference on Chronic*

Diseases Among Mexican-Americans: A Public Health Issue. C. L. Hanis, and W. J. Schull, eds. Unpublished.

Weiss, K. M., R. E. Ferrell, and C. L. Hanis. 1984. A New World syndrome of metabolic diseases with a genetic and evolutionary basis. *Yearbook of Physical Anthropology* 27:153–78.

Weiss, K. M., R. E. Ferrell, C. L. Hanis, and P. N. Styne. 1984. Genetics and epidemiology of gallbladder disease in New World native peoples. *American Journal of Human Genetics* 36:1259–78.

West, K. M. 1978a. Diabetes in American Indians. R. Levine and R. Luft, eds. *Advances in Metabolic Disorders* 9:29–48.

———. 1978b. *Epidemiology of Diabetes and Its Vascular Lesions.* New York: Elsevier.

———. 1974. Diabetes in American Indians and other native populations of the new world. *Diabetes* 23:841–55.

Williams, R. C., W. C. Knowler, W. J. Butler, D. J. Pettitt, J. R. Lisse, P. H. Bennett, D. L. Mann, A. H. Johnson, and P. I. Terasaki. 1981. HLA-A2 and type 2 (insulin independent) diabetes mellitus in Pima Indians: An association of allele frequency with age. *Diabetologia* 21:460–63.

Yamashita, T., W. Mackay, N. Rushforth, P. Bennett, and H. Houser. 1984. Pedigree analyses of non-insulin dependent diabetes mellitus (NIDDM) in the Pima Indians. *American Journal of Human Genetics* 36:183S.

Zimmet, P., R. Taylor, and H. King. 1981. In *Advances in Diabetes Epidemiology.* E. Eschwege, ed. INSERM Symp. No. 22. Amsterdam: Elsevier.

II INFECTIOUS DISEASE AND NUTRITION IN TEMPORAL PERSPECTIVE

7 HEALTH AND DISEASE IN PREHISTORIC POPULATIONS IN TRANSITION

George J. Armelagos

The study of disease in prehistory offers a unique opportunity for the anthropologist. Paleopathologists have contributed significantly to our knowledge about the history and geography of numerous pathological conditions. While there is still a vigorous debate concerning the chronology and geographic distribution of diseases such as syphilis, tuberculosis, and rheumatoid arthritis, we know a great deal about their occurrence in many regions. However, paleopathology can potentially provide a broader understanding of the relationship between disease and human populations. For example, the interaction between human populations and the disease process provides information about biocultural adaptation. The cultural system can dramatically influence the disease process, and disease can significantly alter the cultural adaptation.

Populations in transition often experience change in ecological relationships that alter their disease patterns. The paleopathology of prehistoric populations provides a means for examining these changes from an evolutionary perspective. While early human populations subsisted primarily as gatherer-hunters, there was a dramatic shift to primary food production about 10,000 years ago. I will discuss the impact of this shift and subsequent changes on the disease profile of populations undergoing these major transitions.

During the last four million years human disease ecology has changed significantly as a function of changes in the environment, evolution of the species, and cultural adaptation. These processes created different environments for the pathogens and altered their interaction with human populations. There is a substantial literature that describes the evolutionary impact of disease on human populations. These studies (Armelagos 1967; Armelagos and Dewey 1970; Armelagos and McArdle 1975; Cockburn 1971;

Boyden 1970; Fenner 1970; Polgar 1964) agree that there has been dramatic change in the pattern of disease and the human response, especially within the last 10,000 years. When gathering and hunting were the sole means of human subsistence (a period lasting from 4,000,000 years ago to the beginning of the Neolithic), population size was small, and density was quite low.

Human population size and density presumably remained quite low throughout the Paleolithic. It is assumed that fertility and mortality rates in these small gathering-hunting populations were balanced and that population growth was low and stable. Controversy continues as to the demographic factors which created this stability. Some demographers argue that gatherer-hunters were at their maximum natural fertility and this was balanced by high mortality. Other demographers argue that gatherer-hunters maintained a stable population with controlled moderate fertility balanced by moderate mortality.

A critical key to resolving this controversy is to understand the demographic changes that occurred during the Neolithic period. The Neolithic not only heralded a major shift in subsistence, it also resulted in a dramatic increase in population size and density. The reasons for this increase are complex. There are those who have argued that the Neolithic economy generated food surpluses which provided the key to population growth. The abundance of food would have led to a better nourished and healthier population with a reduced rate of mortality. Since populations were at their natural maximum fertility, there would have been a rapid increase in population.

While this scenario is appealing in its simplicity, the empirical evidence paints a different picture. The biological consequence of the shift from gathering and hunting to agriculture presents a much bleaker picture of health and disease. Instead of experiencing improved health, there is evidence of an increase in infectious and nutritional disease.

DISEASE IN GATHERER-HUNTERS

A consideration of the disease ecology of contemporary gatherer-hunters provides insights into the types of disease that would have affected our gatherer-hunter ancestors. Polgar (1964) suggests that gatherer-hunters would have two types of disease to contend with in their adaptation to their environment. One class of disease would be those organisms that had adapted to prehominid ancestors and persisted with them as they evolved into hominids. Head and body lice (*Pediculus humanus*), pinworms, yaws, and possibly malaria would be included in this group. Cockburn (1967b) adds to this list most of the internal protozoa found in modern humans and such bacteria as salmonella, typhi and staphylococci.

Livingstone (1958) dismisses the potential of malaria in early hominids because of the small population size and an adaptation to the savannah, which would not have been within the range of the mosquitos that carry the malaria plasmodium. The second class of diseases is the zoonotics, which have nonhuman animals as their primary host and only incidentally infect humans. Humans can be infected by zoonoses through insect bites, by preparing and eating contaminated flesh, and from wounds inflicted by animals. Sleeping sickness, tetanus, scrub typhus, relapsing fever, trichinosis, tularemia, leptospirosis, and schistosomiasis are among the zoonotic diseases which could have afflicted earlier gatherers and hunters.

The range of the earliest hominids was probably restricted to the tropical savannah. This would have limited the pathogens that were potential disease agents. During the course of human evolution there was eventually an expansion of habitat into the temperate and eventually the tundra zones. As Lambrecht (1964, 1985) points out, the hominids would have avoided large areas of the African landscape because of tsetse flies and thus avoided the trypanosomes they carried. The evolution of the human species and its expansion into new ecological niches would have led to a change in the pattern of trypanosome infection. While this list of diseases that plagued our gathering-hunting ancestors is informative, those diseases that would have been absent are also of interest. The contagious community diseases such as influenza, measles, mumps, and smallpox would have been missing. Burnet (1962) states that there would have been few viruses infecting these early hominids. On the other hand, Cockburn (1967b), in a well-reasoned argument, suggests that the viral diseases found in nonhuman primates would have been easily transmitted to humans.

DISEASE IN AGRICULTURAL POPULATIONS IN TRANSITION

Given the limited list of diseases found in gatherer-hunters, it should not have been surprising that a shift to primary food production (agriculture) would increase the number and the impact of disease in sedentary populations. Sedentism would undoubtedly increase parasitic disease spread by contact with human waste. In gathering-hunting groups, the frequent movement of the base camp and frequent forays away from base camp by men and women would decrease their contact with human wastes. In sedentary populations the proximity of habitation area and their waste deposit sites to the water supply would be a source of contamination. While sedentism could and did occur prior to the Neolithic period in those areas with abundant resources (acorns in California and marine resources in the Northwest Coast), the shift to agriculture would necessitate sedentary living.

The herding of animals would also increase the frequency of contact with zoonotic diseases. The domestication of animals in the Neolithic would have provided a steady supply of disease vectors. The zoonotic infections would likely increase because of domesticated animals, such as goats, sheep, cattle, pigs, and fowl. Products of domesticated animals such as milk, hair, and skin, as well as the dust raised by the animals, could transmit anthrax, Q fever, brucellosis, and tuberculosis (Polgar 1964). Breaking the sod during cultivation exposes workers to insect bites and diseases such as scrub typhus (Audy 1961).

Livingstone (1958) showed that slash-and-burn agriculture in west Africa exposed populations to *Anopheles gambiae*, a mosquito which is the vector for *Plasmodium falciparum*, which causes malaria.

The development of urban centers is a recent event in human history. In the Near East, cities as large as 50,000 people were established by 3000 B.C. In the New World, urban settlements of half a million were in existence by 5000 B. C. Settlements of this size increase the already difficult problem of removing human wastes and delivering uncontaminated water to the people. Cholera, which is transmitted by contaminated water, was a potential problem. Diseases such as typhus (carried by lice) and the plague bacillus (transmitted by fleas or by the respiratory route), could be spread from person to person. Viral diseases such as measles, mumps, chicken pox, and smallpox could be spread in a similar fashion. We had, for the first time, populations which were large enough to maintain disease in an endemic form. Cockburn (1967b) estimates that populations of one million would be necessary to maintain measles as an endemic disease.

There were also social changes and social upheavals, which resulted in a different mode of disease transmission; for example, the crowding of urban centers, changes in sexual practices, such as prostitution, and an increase in sexual promiscuity may have been factors in the venereal transmission of the treponema, the pathogen which causes syphilis (Hudson 1965). The period of urban development can also be characterized by the exploration and expansion into new areas which would result in the introduction of novel diseases to populations that had little resistance to them (McNeill 1976).

The evolutionary picture of infectious disease suggests that agriculturalists faced considerable difficulties. However, there exists a possible paradox that deserves further consideration. Zoonotic diseases in gatherer-hunters would likely have the greatest impact on the segment of the society that contains the producers (those between age 20 and 40). This segment, in its daily rounds, is more likely to come into contact with the animals that are the vector of disease. As Lambrecht (1985: 642) points out, exposure to fly bites is unavoidable in tsetse fly country. The degree of exposure to fly bites is influenced by the choice of habitat and the behavior of the potential host. He writes, "In many areas, Rhodesian sleeping sickness is significantly higher in men than women. This is related to men's activity such as hunting and honey collecting which brings them in close contact with *morsitans* savanna flies, major vector of *T. b. rhodesiense*." The infection is called "honey collector's disease" by the native groups.

The occurrence of endemic diseases in larger urban agriculturalist areas would most likely kill the very young infants, young children, and the very old adults. In this situation, the predictability of mortality allows them to reduce birth spacing to meet the increase in mortality. Sedentary societies can wean infants earlier, allowing the women to become pregnant again. The social costs of disruption from this pattern of endemic disease mortality may not be as great as the impact of zoonotic diseases on the gatherer-hunters. Even the energetic costs of endemic diseases that are fatal would not be as great. Infants require relatively little energetic investment when compared to older children and young adults. Those who do survive (because of acquired immunity) will be protected from these pathogens. The protected producers segment would be able to reproduce and continue to extract the resources essential for survival.

The process of industrialization, which began a little over 200 years ago, would lead to an even greater environmental and social transformation. City dwellers would have to contend with industrial wastes and polluted water and air. Slums that rise in industrial cities become the focal point for poverty and the spread of disease. Epidemics of smallpox, typhus, typhoid, diptheria, measles, and yellow fever in urban settings are well documented (Polgar 1964). Tuberculosis and respiratory diseases such as pneumonia and bronchitis are even more serious problems with harsh working situations and crowded living conditions.

In the modern era, there are organized public health and medical practices to control infectious diseases in many western societies. Yet, in many of the developing nations, infectious diseases still extract a great toll of human life. Even with public health and medical advances, nations such as the United States experience new outbreaks of infectious disease which they find very threatening. The current AIDS epidemic generates great fear among the public.

The above discussion has focused our concerns on the ecology of disease in these populations in transition. The issue of the biological response of the host and pathogen remains. It has been assumed that the pathogen-host interaction would result in a decrease in the virulence of the pathogen and an increase in the resistance of the host. The short generation time of the pathogens makes it possible for them to evolve mechanisms which decrease their pathogenicity. This evolutionary strategy would be effective if the virulence of the pathogen threatened the extinction of the host. A dead host is of little value in maintaining the reproductive potential of the pathogen.

The potential response of the human host is still an open question. It is often assumed that human populations have developed genetic resistance to disease. For example, generalized host factors and highly specific genetically determined resistance factors (r) would have evolved (Motulsky 1963). The development of resistance factors (r) is assumed but difficult to demonstrate. Since the interaction of the endemic pathogen and the human host is quite recent in evolutionary terms, there is a question of the potential for a human genetic response to have evolved. The 5,000 years since the development of large urban centers may not have been an adequate time for evolution to occur. However, according to Lederberg (1963), it is possible that the human host-pathogen contact may have preceded the Neolithic period. He suggests that during the Paleolithic period, animals may have acted as a reservoir for diseases. If there had been intense and continuing contact between the human population and the animals, then a potential for humans to develop a genetic response to diseases would have existed.

NUTRITIONAL DEFICIENCY AND THE ORIGIN OF AGRICULTURE

The evidence suggesting that nutritional problems plagued Neolithic groups is more surprising. It would seem that agriculturalists could control their food supply by generating surpluses. Even though there is the potential of periodic famines and blight, the surpluses should be theoretically able to buffer the society through these critical periods.

The nutritional difficulties of agriculturalists may be more problematical. Periodic famines have been and remain a problem. Hollingsworth (1973) has documented thousands of famines that occurred during the historical period. Presently, vast areas of Africa are experiencing famines that are extracting a toll on the populations. It is estimated that a million people will die during a single year.

Even without the occurrence of famine or blight nutritional deficiencies can result from the intensification of agricultural production. The intensification of agriculture through irrigation often leads to a reliance on cereal grains. Diets which rely on cereal grains can be deficient in essential nutrients. Maize, for example, is deficient in the essential amino acid lysine. Other cereal grains contain phytates which combine with important minerals decreasing their bioavailablility.

The development of social classes within Neolithic societies also has nutritional implications. Since class, by definition, reflects differences in the access to resources, there is the probability that there will be individuals within the society who are not receiving adequate nutrition.

THE EVIDENCE FROM SKELETAL REMAINS: DEAD MEN (AND WOMEN) DO TELL TALES

The response of the human skeleton to normal and abnormal growth is deceptively simple. Bone is limited to a process by which osteons (the building unit of bone) can be deposited or they can be resorbed — or they can combine these processes in response to a stimulus.

An individual who weighs 160 pounds will have a skeleton comprised of 206 bones the sum weighing about thirty pounds. These thirty pounds of bones, which are composed of about fifteen pounds of calcium, seven pounds of water and a few ounces of major, minor, and trace minerals, are responsible for supporting our muscle structure, protecting vital organs such as the brain and the eyes, producing red blood cells, and maintaining chemical balance in the body.

Many diseases leave their mark on bone, and these marks can be used to diagnose disease occurrence. Tuberculosis, syphilis, and leprosy have skeletal "signatures" which aid in their diagnosis. In severe cases of tuberculosis, for example, there is often a collapse of the vertebral body and frequently resorptive lesions in other parts of the skeleton which are diagnostic.

Many pathogens leave only generalized changes in the skeleton. For example, we often find a periosteal reaction that reflects a pathogenic change to a number of organisms. These nonspecific lesions (periosteal reactions) are confined to the outer layer of bone and show a roughened appearance caused by the inflammatory process. The periosteal reaction occurs when the fibrous outer layer is stretched and subperiosteal hemorrhages occur. Micro-organisms such as staphylococcus and streptococcus and other pathogens can cause these changes. Unfortunately, there are many pathogens (viruses) that leave no evidence on bone. These viruses can cause an illness and even death without any skeletal response.

Nutritional deficiencies can also leave specific lesions which are easily diagnosed from bone. Deficiencies of vitamin D (rickets) result in a constellation of characteristics that are very distinct. Similarly, vitamin C deficiency (scurvy) leaves unique changes but these are more difficult to diagnose in prehistoric remains.

A major breakthrough in analyzing nutritional disease resulted from a movement away from using single indicators of stress to an approach that considers multiple indicators which are systematically analyzed to provide an understanding of nutritional disease stress. For example, there are a number of lesions such as porotic hyperostosis, defects in enamel development, and premature bone loss that, when coupled with evidence of growth retardation, can provide clues to a pattern of nutritional deficiency.

Porotic hyperostosis, which potentially occurs on the cranium and the roof of the eye orbits, can be used to diagnose iron deficiency anemia. The lesion, as the name implies, has a very porous, coral like appearance, which develops when diploe (the trabecular portion of the cranial bone that separates the inner and outer surfaces) expands. Then the outer layer of bone becomes thinner and may eventually disappear, exposing the trabecular bone (diploe) which is quite porous. The expansion of the diploe can be caused by any anemia that stimulates red blood cell production. While there are a number of anemias (sickle cell anemia, thalassemia, iron deficiency) that can cause these changes, the relatively minor manifestation of the lesion on the cranial surface and roof of the orbits and its high frequency in children between ages one and three and in young adult females would suggest iron deficiency anemia as the most likely cause.

In conjunction with the analysis of porotic hyperostosis, other stress indicators such as a decrease in long bone growth may provide information about the individual's physiological state. Since we are by necessity using cross-sectional data, comparison with longitudinal growth studies are very difficult. Growth patterns are determined by averaging long bone lengths of individuals whose developmental age is determined by tooth eruption patterns. These lengths are then compared to standards that exist for living populations. There are few growth standards from peasant agriculturalists, and it is often necessary to use growth standards developed from well-nourished children from the United States. Even with these difficulties, we can often see indications of growth retardation. However, internal comparison of populations experiencing shifts in subsistence may be the most useful method for understanding the impact of these changes on growth.

Recently, histological techniques have provided additional tools for analyzing the impact of nutritional deficiencies on bone growth and maintenance. Microscopic analysis of cross-sections of femora reveal that some children have very thin cortical bone. By examining the percentage of cortical bone for each individual and comparing it with an age-matched sample, we can determine those individuals experiencing nutritional difficulties. It is even possible to ascertain if the bone loss is the result of a lack of osteonal deposition or an increase in bone resorption.

Finally, two additional methods can be used to determine disruption of normal growth and development. Harris lines (lines of increased radiopaque density) found by radiographic analysis have been used as an indicator of growth arresting and recovery. Recent research suggests that Harris lines are more likely to be evidence of recovery and therefore can be used to assess the ability of the individual to respond to stress.

The Harris lines can also be used to assess the age at which an individual experienced growth disruption and subsequent recovery. Since growth occurs at both ends of a long bone, the Harris lines will maintain their relative position to the midshaft. If a researcher knows the relative growth rates of the proximal and distal portion of the long bone, then the age at which a line developed can be estimated.

The analysis of defects in dental enamel is another measure of growth disruption. Dental enamel hypoplasia is a deficiency in enamel thickness that results from a disruption in the formation of the matrix. Enamel defects can result from systemic disruption, hereditary conditions, or localized trauma. Since systemic disruption is likely to affect more than one tooth, we use the occurrence on multiple teeth as the criteria for assessing a systemic cause. Unlike bone, once enamel matures it can not be remodeled. Enamel is secreted in a regular ringlike pattern, and the crown development provides a permanent chronological record of any physiological disruption. An understanding of rates of enamel formation allows one to define the time in development at which the metabolic disruption occurred.

There are two ways in which the chronological distribution can be used. First, we can examine the chronological pattern of hypoplasia in adults to see the age at which they were exposed to physiological disruption. Second, we can evaluate the impact of this disruption on other aspects of their morbidity and mortality. Do adults who were stressed as children suffer from other insults, and do they live as long as those who were not stressed?

Trauma is another insult that provides information on the adaptation of the group. The location of the callus formation which results from the healing of the fracture provides clues to their cause. For example, fractures of the bones of the forearm (the radius and ulna) at the midshaft usually result from raising the arm

Table 7.1
Frequency of Infectious Lesions (Periostitis and Osteomyelitis) and Porotic Hyperostosis.

Dickson Population		Postcranial Infectious Lesions		Porotic Hyperostosis		Porotic Hyperostosis and Infectious Lesions	
	N	N	%	N	%	N	%
Late Woodland	44	9	20.5	6	13.6	3	6.5
Mississippian Acculturated Late Woodland	93	45	48.4	29	31.2	20	21.5
Middle Mississippian	101	74	73.3	52	51.5	41	40.6
Total	238	128	53.8	87	36.5	64	26.9

Source: Huss-Ashmore, Goodman, and Armelagos (1982).

to parry or ward off a blow. These fractures, called "parry fractures," are a good index of strife in a population. When individuals extend an arm to break a fall, however, they frequently fracture the bones of the forearm at the wrist. These fractures, "Colles and Potts" fractures, are indices of klutziness.

DICKSON MOUNDS: A PREHISTORIC POPULATION IN TRANSITION

The change in subsistence from ?900 to 1250 A.D. at the Dickson Mounds, Illinois, was profound. In the period from ?900 A.D. to 1175 A.D., there was a shift from a late woodland adaptation, which can be characterized as a general gathering-hunting strategy, to one which emphasized agriculture. The latter phase of this development (Mississippian Acculturated Late Woodland) was a period in which maize agriculture became established at Dickson Mounds.

From 1175 to 1250 A.D. there was an intensification of agriculture in what has been called the Middle Mississippian period. When these earlier groups from Dickson Mounds are compared to the Middle Mississippian people, there is evidence of a remarkable deterioration of health. In this short period there was a fourfold increase in iron deficiency anemia (porotic hyperostosis) and a threefold increase in infectious disease (periosteal reaction) (see Table 7.1). The frequency of individuals with both iron deficiency and infectious lesions increases from 6 percent in the Late Woodland period to 40 percent in the Middle Mississippian period. Furthermore, individuals with both conditions display a synergistic disease interaction (Lallo et al. 1977; Lallo et al. 1978), that is, they experience more severe manifestation of each condition.

Figure 7.1
Life Expectancy for the Dickson Mounds Population for Those Dying Within the First Ten Years.

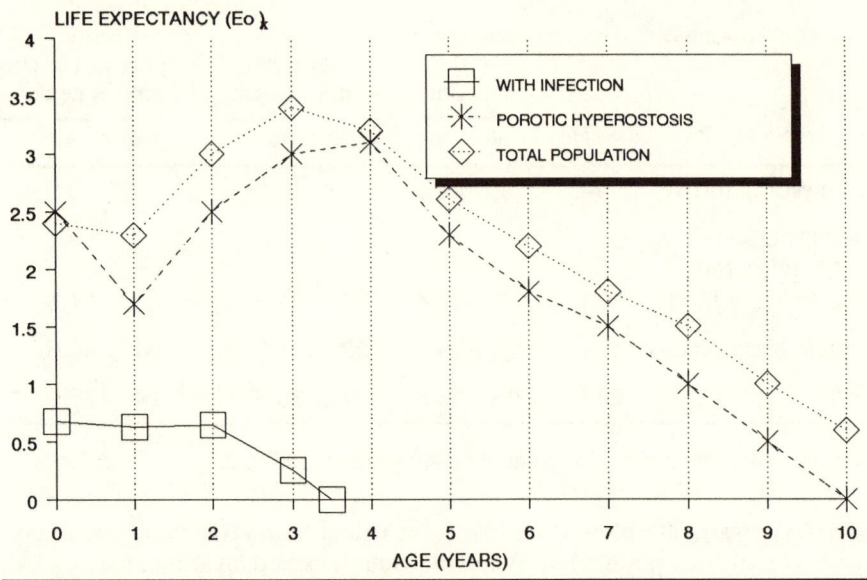

Source: Huss-Ashmore, Goodman, and Armelagos (1982). Reprinted by permission from Academic Press.

The relationship of infection and anemia in children can be ascertained by examining the age of onset and distribution of the lesions by age. The infectious lesion in children under ten years of age peaks during the first year while the anemia shows its highest frequency during the second and third year. This pattern suggests that individuals who do survive the infectious pathogen may have problems in maintaining adequate iron reserves. The exposure to the pathogens that are the consumers of iron and iron deficiencies due to nutritional intake are the most likely explanation of this pattern. The biological cost of infection and anemia can be determined from an analysis of a life expectancy constructed for individuals who died before their tenth year (Figure 7.1). It is apparent that individuals with infections show a dramatic decrease in life expectancy. Those chidren in the group with periosteal lesions at birth can be expected to live less than a year. Even those suffering from iron deficiency display a decrease in life expectancy of up to six months at each age group.

The impact of the shift to agriculture at Dickson Mounds can be seen in other aspects of growth and development. There is evidence of delayed growth in the long bone length and circumference of Mississippian children from their fifth through fifteenth year (Goodman et al. 1984).

The frequency and the chronology of hypoplastic defects in the dental enamel of the Dickson Mounds population supports the argument that the shift to agriculture had deleterious effects on the health of the group. There is an increase in hypoplasia from 0.90 defects per individual (Late Woodland) to 1.61 per individual in the Middle Mississippian period. The proportion of individuals with one or more hypoplasias increases from 45 percent to 80 percent during the same period (Goodman et al. 1984). Since the chronological development of the enamel is well understood, it is possible to determine the age at which the hypoplasias occurred during the life of the individual. The hypoplastic lines in adults provide "metabolic memory" of events which occurred during their childhood.

The chronology of enamel hypoplasia shows that the Dickson Mounds population experienced peak stress between the ages of two and four, which corresponds to the period of weaning. The pattern of porotic hyperostosis in this population occurs at about the same phase of development. The comparison of the chronology between the earlier groups and the intensive agriculturalists

Figure 7.2
The Cumulative Frequency of Enamel Hypoplasias in Two Dickson Mounds Populations.

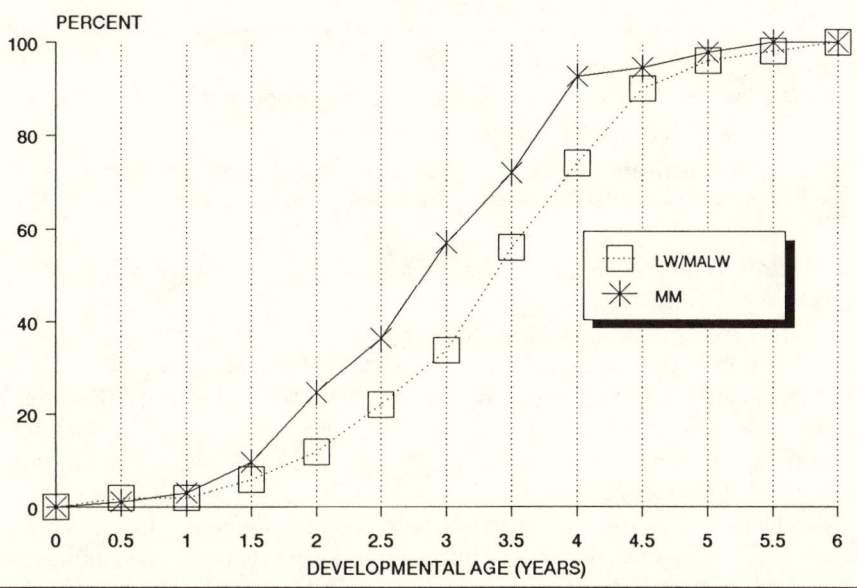

Key: LW   =   Late Woodland
MALW =   Mississippian Acculturated Late Woodland
MM   =   Middle Mississippian

Source: Goodman, Armelagos, and Rose (1984). Reprinted by permission.

Figure 7.3
Mean Ages at Death of Dickson Mounds Adolescents/Adults by
Number of Hypoplasias-Stress Periods Between 3.5–7.0 Years
Developmental Age.

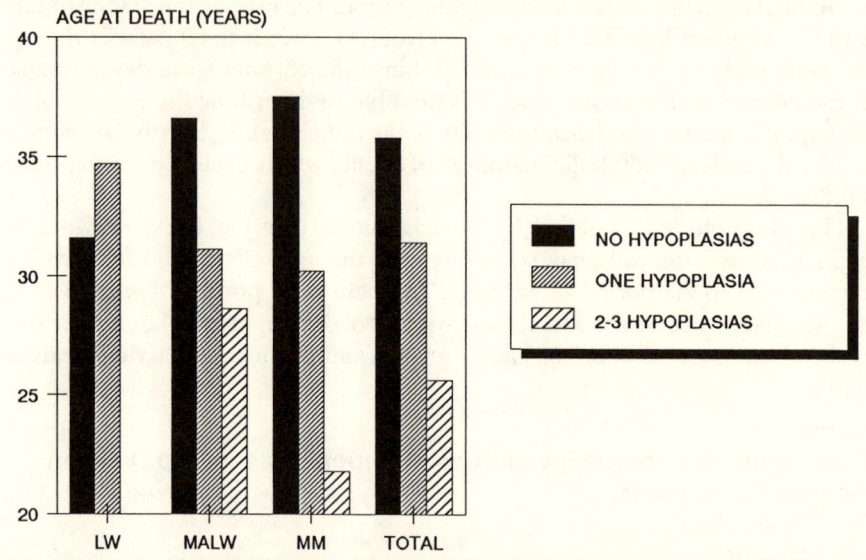

Key: LW   =   Late Woodland
      MALW   =   Mississippian Acculturated Late Woodland
      MM   =   Middle Mississippian

Source: Goodman and Armelagos (1988). Reproduced by permission of the American Anthropological Association from *American Anthropologist* 90:4, 1988.

at Dickson Mounds (Figure 7.2) shows an earlier age of onset of hypoplasia, suggesting an earlier age of weaning.

Enamel hypoplasia is considered a relatively benign pathology. However, Goodman and Armelagos (1988) have calculated the mean age at death for those with and without hypoplasias and find significant differences. Individuals with no lesions have a mean age at death five years greater than individuals with one hypoplasia and nine years greater than individuals with two or more hypoplastic episodes (Figure 7.3).

Two hypotheses have been proposed to explain the difference in mean age at death. The first suggests that those with hypoplasia represent a group of individuals who were challenged by the insult early in their lifetime and continued to be subjected to insults during the rest of their lives. This increased "wear-and-tear" throughout their lives leads to an earlier death. Another hypothesis suggests that major insults occur at a critical period of immunological development. Individuals experiencing severe stress during the development of their immunological system

Figure 7.4
Comparison of Life Expectancies for Two Dickson Mounds Populations.

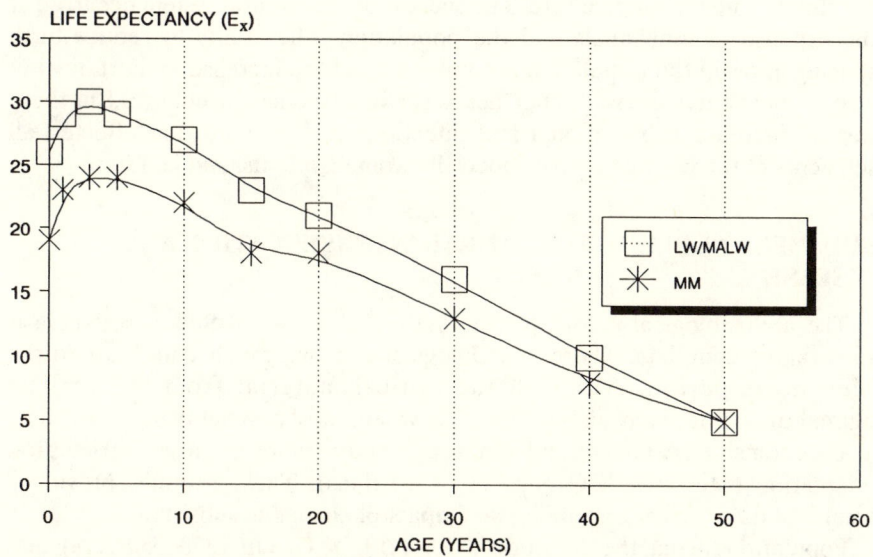

Key: LW   =   Late Woodland
     MALW =   Mississippian Acculturated Late Woodland
     MM   =   Middle Mississippian

Source: Goodman et. al. (1984). Reprinted by permission.

may irreparably damage their ability to fight infection throughout their lifetime. The "damaged goods" hypothesis suggests that significant thymolymphatic growth, which is essential for developing effective immunological competence, occurs prenatally, in infancy and early childhood.

Clark (1985) and co-workers (Clark et al. 1986) use the growth of the vertebral column to offer support to the "damaged goods" hypothesis. The size of the vertebral neural canal (VNC) is a good measure of childhood growth. The VNC is completed in childhood and is not subjected to catch-up growth. Since the VNC is growing during the phase of the neurological (of which it is a part) and the thymolymphatic development, it may reflect disruptions that occur during this period which affect immunological development. Multivariate, bivariate, and nonparemetric analyses show that small VCN are associated with greater vertebral wedging (a measure of morbidity) and decreased mean age at death (Clark et al. 1986).

The impact of multiple stressors affected the mortality pattern of the Dickson Mounds population. Change in the mortality profile is the final measure of the biological cost of the shift to agriculture at Dickson Mounds. A comparison of life expectancy (Figure 7.4) shows a decrease in life expectancy at all ages for the intensive agriculturalists.

In summary, the population at Dickson Mounds suffered biologically from the shift to intensive agriculture. The success of the cultural system occurred at the expense of individuals and the population. The ability to reduce birth spacing allowed the population not only to meet the increase in mortality but also to meet the increased labor needs for intensifying agriculture. But there was an increase in nutritional and infectious disease load that affected all segments of the population but especially women, infants, and children.

SUDANESE NUBIA: AGRICULTURAL INTENSIFICATION AND DISEASE

The archaeological record for the Wadi Halfa area of Sudanese Nubia is remarkably complete. There are biological remains which date back to the Mesolithic period. Although the critical material from the earliest agriculturalists is not available, there are two series of populations which reflect a less intensive (A-Group and G-Group) and a more intensive agricultural adaptation (Meroitic, X-Group, and Christians). These samples provide a wealth of data for understanding the impact of change in subsistence.

Populations from the Meriotic (350 A.D.), X-Group (350–550 A.D.) and Christian (550–1300 A.D.) periods show a pattern of pathology similar to that at the Dickson Mounds. There is, for example, similarity in the distribution of porotic hyperostosis (iron deficiency anemia) in which the children between two and six years of age and young adult females are affected. A significant difference did exist in frequency of infectious disease in the Nubian population. The frequency of periosteal reaction was much lower. This surprising finding can be explained by the consumption of a broad spectrum antibiotic. The Nubians ingested tetracycline (Basset et al. 1981) produced by mold-like bacteria (*Streptomycetes*) which contaminated the grain. The contaminated grain may have been brewed into beer that provided them with therapeutic doses of the antibiotic, a serendipitous factor in controlling infectious diseases which affect bones.

Growth retardation in the Nubians is extremely difficult to demonstrate from the cross-sectional data (Armelagos et al. 1972). Since we are not able to follow the growth of individuals during the various phases of their lifetime, we rely on averaging the long bone lengths for the various developmental ages and infer growth pattern from these data. Long bone length and widths fail to show any definitive evidence of growth retardation. The comparison with standards developed from United States data shows that the Nubians are smaller but are experiencing similar patterns of growth. However, when the long bone lengths and widths are compared with the thickness of cortical bone, problems in growth become evident. The cortices are very thin and are equivalent to the thicknesses found in two-year-old children. Microscopic analysis confirms this observation. Huss-Ashmore (1981) finds that the premature osteoporosis results from an increase in intercortical resorption. Martin and Armelagos (1979) show that young adult women (ages 19–25) from this same population also have problems maintaining cortical bone. There is a significant increase in rates of endosteal resorption (when compared to males of the same age). While these women are able to form osteons on their periosteal surface, there is no indication that these osteons are being mineralized. Instead, the resorption of osteons from the endosteal surface is the source for calcium for the lactating women.

THE TEST: PREHISTORIC POPULATIONS IN TRANSITION

These two cases studies do not prove that a shift to agriculture will always result in a deterioration of health. There is other evidence that provides information to further test this hypothesis. In *Paleopathlogy at the Origins of Agriculture* (Cohen and Armelagos 1984a), there are seventeen case studies (in addition to the Nubian and Dickson Mounds examples) that examine the impact of subsistence change on the health of both New World and Old World populations. In general, the shift to a sedentary habitation pattern (with or without agriculture) may have triggered the most significant changes in disease profile. As expected, the sedentary populations show a dramatic shift in infectious diseases. The increased contact between individuals and close contact with human wastes which contaminate the environment are undoubtedly the major causes of this change in disease pattern.

Twelve of the case studies published in *Paleopathology at the Origins of Agriculture* (Cohen and Armelagos 1984a), for which observations on the pattern of infectious disease were available, show an increase in infections in the agricultural groups when compared with the gatherer-hunters. This increase is due to the increase in sedentism, the increase in population size, and the synergism between malnutrition and infection (Cohen and Armelagos 1984b). One study records a decrease in infections from the gathering-hunting to the early farming period, with an increase as agriculture became intensified (Norr 1984).

The same sample demonstrates that the intensification of agriculture consistently led to poorer nutrition as evidenced by the occurrence of porotic hyperostosis (an indicator of iron deficiency anemia). In sixteen groups where data are available, twelve show an increase with the intensification of agriculture.

CONCLUSIONS

1. The small population size of paleolithic gatherer-hunters made con-tagious or infectious disease a relatively minor problem for these earlier groups.
2. The impact of zoonotic diseases may have presented more of a problem to gatherer-hunters because of the greater impact of disease on the

producer segment of the population. In small populations an increase in mortality among the producers would be potentially more socially and economically disruptive.

3. The transition to sedentism among gatherer-hunters with a stable and abundant food supply and among early agriculturalists potentially represents a new ecological setting. Population and pathogens are placed in new relationships that can result in an increase in parasitic and infectious diseases.

4. Beyond the problems associated with sedentism, the transition to agriculture increases the potential problems with infectious diseases. The increase in population size and density will increase the possibility of infectious disease transmission.

5. Although primary food production can generate surpluses, there is a potential for nutritional deficiencies from blight, drought, and the reliance on single crops which may be deficient in essential nutrients.

6. Agricultural populations which experienced an increase in nutritional and infectious disease were able to increase their population size. The predictability of mortality in these sedentary populations (deaths of the very young and very old) and a producer segment of the population with acquired immunity to disease may have been able to respond to the increase in mortality. The population size can be maintained or increased by decreasing the birth spacing. Furthermore, the acquired immunity of those who survive these childhood diseases may act to protect the producer segment of the population and thus make infectious disease socially less disruptive.

7. The rise of population in urban centers was relatively late in human history. In the Old World, preindustrial urban centers developed only 5,000 years ago and 2,400 years ago in the New World. This suggests that human populations have been exposed to endemic diseases for a relatively short time in evolutionary terms. For this reason, specific genetic adaptation to specific pathogens is unlikely. The development of a generalized physiological response is more likely than the evolution of a specific genetic response.

8. Lederberg (1963) argues that a genetic response may have occurred earlier than the post-Neolithic period. He claims that a specific genetic response may have evolved in situations in which humans and animals develop an intense and long-term interaction. In that situation the animals could act as reservoirs for pathogens and repeatedly infect humans.

9. In the last 10,000 years, *Homo sapiens* has experienced a number of periods of rapid transition that have had a dramatic impact on health and disease patterns. The shift to a neolithic economy that relied on primary food production, the development of urban centers, the In-

dustrial Revolution, and the development of rapid long distance travel changed the pattern of disease in human population. The interaction of pathogens and people has been influential in shaping our biology and culture.

REFERENCES

Armelagos, G. J. 1967. Man's changing environment. In *Infectious Diseases: Their Evolution and Eradication*. T. A. Cockburn, ed. Springfield, Ill.: Charles C. Thomas.

Armelagos, G. J., and J. Dewey. 1970. Evolutionary response to human infectious disease. *Bioscience* 20(5):271–75.

Armelagos G. J., and A. McArdle. 1975. Population, disease, and evolution. In *Population Studies in Archaeology and Biological Anthropology: A Symposium*. A. C. Swedlund, ed. *Memoir of the Society of American Archaeology*, No. 30.

Armelagos, G. J., J. H. Mielke, K. H. Owen, D. P. Van Gerven, J. R. Dewey, and P. E. Mahler. 1972. Bone growth and development in prehistoric populations from Sudanese Nubia. *Journal of Human Evolution* 1:89–119.

Audy, J. R. 1961. The ecology of scrub typhus. In *Studies in Disease Ecology*. J. M. May, ed. New York: Hafner.

Basset, E., Margaret Keith, George J. Armelagos, Debra L. Martin, and A. Villanueva. 1981. Tetracycline-labeled human bone from prehistoric Sudanese Nubia (A.D. 350). *Science* 209:1532–34.

Boyden, S. V. 1970. *The Impact of Civilization on the Biology of Man*. Toronto: University of Toronto Press.

Burnet, F. M. 1962. *Natural History of Infectious Disease*. Cambridge: Cambridge University Press.

Clark, G. A. 1985. Hetrochrony, allometry and canalization in the human vertebral column: Examples from prehistoric American populations. Ph.D diss., University of Massachusetts, Amherst.

Clark, G. A., N. R. Hall, G. J. Armelagos, G. A. Borkan, M. M. Panjabi, and G. T. Wetzel. 1986. Poor growth prior to early childhood: Decreased health and life-span in the adult. *American Journal of Physical Anthropology* 70:145–60.

Cockburn, T. A. 1971. Infectious disease in ancient populations. *Current Anthropology* 12(1):45–62.

———. 1967a. Infections of the order primates. In *Infectious Diseases: Their Evolution and Eradication* T. A. Cockburn, ed. Springfield, Ill.: Charles C. Thomas.

———. 1967b. The evolution of human infectious diseases. In *Infectious Diseases: Their Evolution and Eradication*. T. A. Cockburn, ed. Springfield, Ill.: Charles C. Thomas.

Cohen, M. N., and G. J. Armelagos, eds. 1984a. *Paleopathology at the Origins of Agriculture*. Orlando: Academic Press.

———. 1984b. Paleopathology at the origins of agriculture: Editors' summation. In *Paleopathology at the Origins of Agriculture*. M. N. Cohen and G. J. Armelagos, eds. Orlando: Academic Press.

Fenner, F. 1970. The effects of changing social organization on the infectious diseases of man. In *The Impact of Civilization on the Biology of Man*. S. V. Boyden, ed. Canberra: Australia National University Press.

Goodman, A. H., and G. J. Armelagos. 1988. Childhood stress, cultural buffering, and decreased longevity in a prehistoric population. *American Anthropologist* 90:936–44.

Goodman, A. H., G. J. Armelagos, and J. C. Rose. 1984. The chronological distribution of enamel hypoplasia from prehistoric Dickson Mounds. *American Journal of Physical Anthropology* 65:259–266.

Goodman, A. H., J. Lallo, G. J. Armelagos, and J. Rose. 1984. Health changes at Dickson Mounds, Illinois (A.D. 950–1300). In *Paleopathology at the Origins of Agriculture*. M. N. Cohen and G. J. Armelagos, eds. Orlando: Academic Press.

Goodman, A. H., D. L. Martin, and G. J. Armelagos. 1984. Indications of stress from bone and teeth. In *Paleopathology at the Origins of Agriculture*. M. N. Cohen and G. J. Armelagos, eds. Orlando: Academic Press.

Haldane, J. B. S. 1949. Disease and evolution. Supplement to *La Ricerca Scientifica* 19:68–76.

Hollingsworth, T. H. 1973. Population crises in the past. In *Resources and Population*. B. Cox and J. Peel, eds. New York: Academic.

Hudson, E. H. 1965. Treponematosis and man's social evolution. *American Anthropologist* 67:885–901.

Huss-Ashmore, R. 1981. Bone growth and remodeling as a measure of nutritional stress. In *Biocultural Adaptation Comprehensive Approaches to Skeletal Analysis*. University of Massachusetts, Department of Anthropology, Research Reports No. 20, pp. 84–95.

Huss-Ashmore, R., A. H. Goodman, and G. J. Armelagos. 1982. *Advances in Archaeological Method and Theory*, vol. 5. Orlando, Fla.: Academic Press.

Lallo, J., G. J. Armelagos, and R. P. Mensforth. 1977. The role of diet, disease and physiology in the origin of porotic hyperostosis. *Human Biology* 40:471–83.

Lallo, J., G. J. Armelagos, and J. C. Rose. 1978. Paleoepidemiology of infectious disease in the Dickson Mounds population. *Medical College of Virginia Quarterly* 14:17–23.

Lambrecht, F. L. 1985. Trypanosomes and hominid evolution. *Bioscience* 35(10):640–46.

———. 1964. Aspects of evolution and ecology of tsetse flies and trypanosomiasis in prehistoric African environments. *Journal of African History* 5:1–24.

Lederberg, J. 1963. Comments on A. Motulsky's "Genetic systems in disease susceptibility in mammals." In *Genetic Selection in Man*. W. J. Schull, ed. Ann Arbor: University of Michigan Press (Comments are interspersed with the Motulsky text).

Livingstone, F. B. 1958. Anthropological implications of sickle-cell gene distribution in West Africa. *American Anthropologist* 60:533–62.

McNeill, W. H. 1976. *Plagues and People*. Garden City: Anchor/Doubleday.

Martin, D. L., and G. J. Armelagos. 1979. Morphometrics of compact bone: An example from Sudanese Nubia. *American Journal of Physical Anthropology* 51:571–578.

Motulsky, A.G. 1963. Genetic systems involved in disease susceptibility in mammals. In *Genetic Selection in Man*. W. J. Schull, ed. Ann Arbor: University of Michigan Press.

Norr, L. 1984. Prehistoric subsistence and health status of the Coastal peoples from the Panamanian Isthmus of Lower Central America. In *Paleopathology at the Origins of Agriculture*. M. N. Cohen and G. J. Armelagos, eds. Orlando: Academic Press.

Polgar, S. 1964. Evolution and the ills of mankind. In *Horizons of Anthropology*. S. Tax, ed. Chicago: Aldine.

8 OLD AND NEW TRANSITIONS AND NUTRITION IN MEXICO

Luis A.Vargas

The purpose of this volume is to delineate specific research questions that bear on the health and disease of populations in transition. In this chapter I will try to bring out these questions in relation to three phases in Mexican history.

TRANSITIONS AND DISEASE IN MEXICAN HISTORY

Mexican history is fairly well documented from a distant past. Archaeological excavations have provided data from the beginning of the populating of America to the eve of the arrival of Europeans on Mexican territory. The writings, sculpture, architecture, and other cultural productions of the varied pre-Hispanic groups that inhabited Mexico provide insights on how they lived and on the main changes that occurred over time. The initial period of the Conquest is exceptionally well documented through the writings of the Spaniard soldiers and priests, including such well-known figures as Hernan Cortes, Bernal Diaz del Castillo, and Bernardino de Sahagun.

Three Moments in Mexican History

Despite the numerous wars and turmoils that have occurred in Mexico since the beginning of the Conquest, the country can claim an adequate continuity of its historical sources, with continuous awareness of the importance of maintaining archives and historical sources for future studies. A good example is the role that the Archivo General de la Nacion has played in keeping, classifying, and making available Mexico's historical record.

It is easy to identify the moments in Mexican history when important transitions have occurred. The first is the passage from hunting and gathering to intensive agriculture, but, without doubt, the most important moment in Mexican history was the Conquest, when two different and isolated worlds met. Although both transitions are now past history, there are still lessons to be learned from them. The third period that I have chosen is contemporary Mexico, starting in 1910, which has witnessed spectacular social and economic transformations that have had an important impact on health and disease. I will focus on health problems related to nutrition, since they have particularly good documentation in physical anthropology, archaeology, and history, and they are of relevance for Mexico's future.

Illness and Disease

In the discussion that follows I will attempt to examine issues of health problems from two perspectives: from the perspective of illness and, to the extent that the data permit, from the perspective of disease.

By the term illness, I refer to the classification of human illnesses that can be found in pathology textbooks, where they are presented in terms of a series of causes, such as trauma, infection, immunity, deficit or excess of nutrients, heredity, and the like. Each illness or nosological entity has its own etiology, pathology, and clinical picture. Thus physicians can identify, for example, a fracture of the neck of the femur, salmonellosis, a bronchogenic carcinoma, or schizophrenia. But human reaction to illness is not limited to a biological deviation from normality. Physicians constantly encounter persons who feel sick, even though a complete medical examination, with laboratory tests, X-rays, and all the modern paraphernalia, cannot find any illness. They do have a disease, which may relate to their social or psychological adaptation, but that leaves no biological lesion on their bodies. On the other hand, a specific illness, such as a fracture of a finger, will have a very different impact on diverse individuals, as in the case of a pianist, a person who is on vacation, or one who needs an excuse not to do an important task. This is to say that one illness can mean different diseases in different persons.

Humans react to illness in relation to their age, sex, physiological condition, culture, knowledge, and, in general, their personal biography and their biopsychosocial integrity. The term "disease" (*padecer* in Spanish) encompasses the way that each individual personally reacts to his illness (*enfermeded* in Spanish) from the biological, psychological, and social perspective.

Illness and Disease in the Past

Studies done on past populations can deal with illness, but they yield little insight into disease. The types of illness that can be studied are those that leave morphological changes in bone and teeth, and, in exceptional circumstances, this can be expanded to other tissues when mummies or remains of soft tissues or body products are found. But disease is elusive and can seldom be reconstructed. Fortunately, careful studies of historical sources may allow research of this type to be undertaken (Aguirre Beltran 1963; Ladurie 1982). Disease, of course, is what we are interested in. It is important to know how societies and individuals reacted to their illnesses. For example, how did hunger and malnutrition, and the morbidity and mortality that it brought, affect ways of life, political decisions, and social survival?

With these ideas in mind, we can focus on the three phases of Mexican history that we have chosen to exemplify transitions that affect nutrition and thus human health and illness.

THE TRANSITION TO INTENSIVE AGRICULTURE

Mexico's pre-Hispanic history has been studied in the context of numerous chronological and/or developmental sequences; for example, Pina Chan (1967) divided Mexican pre-Hispanic history into several horizons, which are accepted by most archaeologists: (1) *Primitive*, with four stages: Lithic, Protoagricultural, Early Agricultural, and Protopreclassic; (2) *Formative*, which has three stages: Lower Preclassic, Middle Preclassic, and Upper Preclassic; and (3) Evolutionary, which includes: Protoclassic, Early Classic, Late Classic, Protopostclassic, Early Postclassic, and Late Postclassic. Most of the archaeological frameworks employed in Mexico utilize this terminology, although many variations occur as well in the literature.

Agriculture appears at about 5000 B.C., in the Early Agricultural period. In the three Preclassic periods, from about 2000 B.C. until about 200 B.C., agriculture becomes more and more complex, incorporating new plants and new techniques. However, there is little advance in the domestication of dogs and turkeys that had started earlier. The Classic period, from about 200 to 700 A.D., includes the establishment of intensive agriculture and the appearance of large cities and a clear social stratification. The Postclassic period, from 900 to 1500 A.D., includes the formation of military states and an agriculture supported by intensive irrigation, with special types of cultivation, such as *chinampas* (floating garden plots).

The Skeletal Evidence of Nutritional Status

There are good human skeletal samples for most of these periods from several parts of the country which have been the subject of extensive study; several researchers have examined changes in height over the centuries. Haviland (1967) found differences in stature among fifty-five skeletons from several historical periods of Tikal. A marked reduction in stature appeared among males in the late Classic while considerable sexual dimorphism in height remained constant in this site.

Nickens (1976) studied four Mesoamerican skeletal series from Zaculeu, Tikal, Altar de Sacrificios, and Tehuacan. The series covered approximately

3,500 years, from the Preclassic to the Postclassic. In males, he found a trend toward smaller stature over time. The decrease in stature seems to be correlated with the appearance of more skeletal lesions, which, in this instance, can apparently be attributed to inadequate nutrition.

One of the few studies in the northern part of Mexico is from Casas Grandes, Chihuahua (Weaver 1980), in which skeletal remains were compared from two cultural phases: Viejo (700–1060 A.D.) and Medio (1060–1340 A.D.). Some of the outstanding trends during this transition include the development of a broader trade network, the introduction of a greater variety of maize, and the creation of more nucleated communities, together with an increase in population. Vargas (1978) compared skeletal pathology related to nutritional deficiencies and infections: porotic hyperostosis and periosteal reactions. His data show an increase in periotic reactions, which he interprets as evidence of a change in sanitary risks and infectious disease. Coruccini (1982) questions this conclusion, suggesting that these data do not provide skeletal evidence of changes in health during this particular period.

The only study by a Mexican published so far on this subject is on the Maya (Marquez Morfin 1984b). Other articles dealing with nutrition are of a descriptive character and offer no basis for analyzing changes due to social or economic transitions. Marquez Morfin studied fifteen pre-Hispanic series of her own and five from other authors, in addition to materials from a contemporary cemetery in Merida. The pre-Hispanic series covers a long period, from the Preclassic to the Postclassic. Unfortunately, only male skeletons are available for the Preclassic. She finds a definite trend for males to become shorter in the transition from the Preclassic to the Classic but no changes of importance from the Postclassic to modern times. This can be attributed to a series of causes, but Marquez Morfin considers the most probable explanation to be that the transition from the Preclassic to the Classic was a transition to a more densely populated society, with a higher workload and fewer people engaged in food-producing activities, all of which increased nutrient requirements and reduced the food supply.

Another technique for investigating nutritional change was employed by Schoeninger (1979) in her study of diet in Chalcatzingo, a Formative period village in the highlands of Central Mexico. She studied strontium contents of bones in ninety-one skeletons from this site, which could be assigned to specific social strata. Her findings show that strontium levels correspond to differences of socioeconomic group that, in turn, may indicate differences in the availability of meat in the diet. It would be very useful to do a similar study in series that date from different cultural stages.

A more general reconstruction of the influence of diet and nutrition on population dynamics in the Basin of Mexico has been attempted by Santley and Rose (1979). They reconstructed food availability at different periods and correlated it with estimates of population growth. The stage that corresponds to Pina Chan's Lower and Middle Preclassic is one of slow but sustained population growth. The Protoclassic and the Classic were found to be times of a reduction in population growth, probably due to nutritional stress. The situation seemed to reverse in the Post-classic, when population growth rose again, due to an intensification of commerce and the inclusion of new foods in the diet. Within the necessary limitation that estimates of this type must necessarily have, the results agree with the conclusions previously discussed.

Methodological Problems in the Study of the Hunting-Gathering to Agricultural Transition

The studies of food habits and nutrition of ancient Mexicans have tended to be somewhat ethnocentric, placing emphasis on foods that are familiar in the West. The finding that the large meat- or milk-yielding animals, such as cattle, pigs, sheep, or goats, did not exist in America has perpetuated the idea of low protein diets in Mesoamerican and the New World in general. Several authors (Casillas and Vargas 1984; Hunn 1982; Ortiz de Montellano 1978; Vargas 1984) have stressed the importance of less obvious sources of plant and animal protein, which in Western categories are considered "exotic" or "nonconventional." Some authors have already shown the important role that amaranth, spirulina, and other algae of the lakes could have played in the past. Little attention has been given to migrant waterfowl, insects, and small mammals and reptiles which are still eaten in some parts of Mexico. Thus, previous conceptions about protein and other food resources need to be revised.

Probably the most serious limitation on assessing the impact of nutrition on the health of pre-Hispanic Mexicans has been the lack of information from archaeological sources, which has only recently improved. Although there is considerable knowledge about the evolution of the domestication of some plants, others are practically unknown. This is the case for amaranth in Central Mexico and ramon or chava in the Maya area. There is more archaeological evidence for the domestication of chenopodium than amaranthus. On the other hand, there are new publications or current research projects that have identified remains of edible plants in archaeological contexts (McClung de Tapia, 1977, 1980, in press; McClung De Tapia, Serra, and Limon de Dyer, 1986).

Data on the history of food processing techniques, such as *tortilla* making or the use of fermented products, are still not complete. There should be ceramic evidence for the preparation of maize in the form of *nixtamal* (the process of soaking maize in hot water containing lime, previous to grinding it into meal), since this cooking technique leaves calcium deposits in the vessels that are used in its preparation. The cooking of *tamales* or *tortillas* also needs special ware, such as *comales*, pottery in which steam can be generated. Techniques can be found to identify calcium or the type of pottery used in certain forms of food preparation.

Also lacking are more thorough analyses of pollen, seeds, and phytoliths in archaeological sites and a careful examination of human remains *in situ*. Most archaeologists and physical anthropologists have a sense of urgency to clean their sherds and bones with running water and forget to take soil samples, which leaves important clues to the past in the earth or in the drain. Fortunately, this situation is rapidly changing and some very adequate archaeological excavations are done now in Mexico.

It is also important to note that the great majority of Mexican physical anthropological studies are descriptive in nature. Most of them are very well done, but so far only a few have attempted comparisons in time and space. Again, this is a rapidly changing situation.

Golden opportunities are lost each day in Mexico, where studies of children could give a better insight into the evolution of those skeletal lesions that we associate with malnutrition. It is also relatively easy to gather contemporary skeletal material of known age, sex, and cause of death, since by Mexican law, unless a fee is paid, human remains are dug from their tombs at the end of seven years after burial. Autopsy material is also abundant.

Finally, very few planned excavations designed to look for answers to specific questions have been carried out. More often, physical anthropologists remove the human remains from sites where archaeologists needed to dig. For instance, the number of skeletons from the Classic period is very scarce, but sites that could yield them are well known. Mexican scholars, so far, have not had the problems that other countries are having concerning the possibility of obtaining human remains from archaeological sites for scientific study. Work is progressing and some excavations of human skeletal remains have now been done with modern techniques.

Nutrition and Health Impact of the First Transition

So far, it has been possible to draw a rough sketch of some of the illnesses that affected ancient Mexicans in the long transition from hunting and gathering to advanced agriculture. Disease is still far from our reach. It may be possible to get more information about it from good osteological and paleopathological studies of individuals and communities. Some help may be gained from the analysis of representations of human beings in stone, clay, or other forms. Still, for this period in history, the information that can be gained is necessarily scanty, due to the subjective nature of disease.

The present evidence suggests that the slow transition of Mexican societies from hunting-gathering to intensive agriculturalist did have an impact on their nutrition and their health. The main mechanisms that have been postulated to explain this impact are an increasing dependence on plant protein, a shift to living in larger human groups, which enhances the possibilities for the transmission of infectious diseases, and the appearance of specialists in activities other than agriculture, which meant that fewer people produced food for a larger population. In addition, natural disasters cannot be overlooked, since they have been frequent in Mexican history.

The lesson that can be learned from this transition is that, through trial-and-error, people found an adequate diet after a long period of time. It is likely that many plant and animal products, agricultural techniques, and cooking processes, were tried and rejected. The strategies that seem to have worked were the use of a wide variety of foods, both wild and domesticated, and the introduction of certain agricultural techniques and methods of food preparation. Some of the most successful examples are the use of corn, amaranth, beans, squash, tomatoes, algae, wild fowl, *chinampa*, agriculture, and preparation of *tortillas* and of fermented drinks that fix nitrogen from the air.

THE CONQUEST AS A PERIOD OF TRANSITION

Many pages have been written about the Conquest of Mexico. It is certainly one of the most interesting epics in the history of humankind. Two different and very complex civilizations met and rapidly gave birth to a new culture. From a biological point of view, the Conquest meant: (1) hybridization between human groups; (2) contact between isolated populations with a consequent exchange of infective and parasitic agents that caused high morbidity and mortality due to lack of antibodies; and (3) natural and manmade situations that brought forth hunger and more deaths.

The Epidemics

The impact of the new illnesses on the Native American populations was nearly immediate. Sahagun (1974) collected a description of the first great "pestilence" that killed a great number of Indians. It seems to have been smallpox and is described as follows:

> While the Spaniards were in Tlaxcala, a great plague broke out here in Tenochtitlan. It began to spread during the thirteenth month and lasted for seventy days, striking everywhere in the city and killing a vast number of our people. Sores erupted on our faces, our breasts, our bellies; we were covered with agonizing sores from head to foot.
>
> The illness was so dreadful that no one could walk or move. The sick were so utterly helpless that they could only lie on their beds like corpses, unable to move their limbs or even their heads. If they did move their bodies, they screamed with pain.
>
> A great many died from the plague, and many others died of hunger. They could not get up to search for food, and everyone else was too sick to care for them, so they starved to death in their beds.
>
> Some people came down with milder forms of the disease; they suffered less than the others and made a good recovery. But they could not escape entirely. Their looks were ravaged, for wherever a sore broke out, it gouged an ugly pock mark in the skin. And a few of the survivors were left

completely blind.

The first cases were reported in Cuatlan. By the time the danger was recognized, the plague was so well established that nothing could halt it, and eventually it spread all the way to Chalco. Then its virulence diminished considerably, though there were isolated cases for many months after. The first victims were stricken during the fiesta of Teotlecco and faces of our warriors were not clean of sores until the fiesta of Panquetzaliztli. (Leon Portilla 1962:92–93)

After this first epidemic, many followed. Malvido (1973) has published a detailed chronology of them. She lists sixteen for the sixteenth century, twenty-seven in the seventeenth century, and seventeen for the eighteenth century. Most of the diagnoses concerning the etiology of these epidemics are subject to speculation, but it is almost certain that the most important causes were smallpox, cholera, parotiditis, typhus, and measles.

Despite the considerable amount of historical information that has been recorded about these episodes, there is very little biological evidence concerning them. This is due to the dearth of archaeological studies of colonial churches and cemeteries. In the last fifteen years some excavations have been made of colonial sites, such as the convent of Huejotzingo, Puebla, the Cathedral of Mexico (Marquez Morfin 1984a), and the Convent of San Jeronimo in Mexico City.

A site that has a great potential for the osteological study of an epidemic is a cemetery in Cholula, Puebla, in which a large number of early colonial burials have been found. They all seem to date from a very short time span. The preliminary conclusion is that these are people who died in one of the epidemics. Unfortunately the study of these skeletons has not yet been completed.

One of the few convents for which there is a good internal chronology of burials is San Jeronimo in Mexico City. There it may be possible to study the variation of nutrition-related lesions in a large number of skeletons of nuns, over several centuries. This convent is beginning to be thoroughly studied.

On the other hand, skeletal series of the Late Postclassic are also now being analyzed. One example is the large collection coming from the city of Tiatelolco, which can be considered Tenochtitlan's twin. The immediate period of the Conquest is also becoming better known through materials that are being found in the excavations for the construction of the subway or Metro in Mexico City (Salas Cuesta 1982).

While information from the skeletal material of the years around the Conquest is still scanty, historical sources also offer possibilities for gaining an insight into the illnesses of this period and into how people and society viewed their diseases.

Hunger

In this period, epidemics were not the only cause of high mortality. Hunger made an important contribution. In the same article cited above, Malvido counts twenty-eight episodes that caused hunger in the sixteenth century; the number goes to forty-one in the seventeenth century and to forty-six in the following one hundred years. The episodes were caused by drought, invasions of locusts, heavy rains, hail, high prices of maize, and other factors.

One of the most moving descriptions of hunger is from the siege of Tenochtitlan, as told by an unknown Nahuatl poet quoted in Lopez Austin (1975:127–38)

> Broken spears lie on the roads;
> we have torn our hair in our grief.
> The houses are roofless now, and their walls
> are red with our blood.
>
> Worms are swarming in the streets and plazas,
> and their walls are splattered with gore.
> The water has turned red, as if it were dyed,
> and when we drink it,
> it has the taste of brine.
>
> We have pounded our hands in despair
> against the adobe walls,
> for our inheritance, our city, is lost and dead.
>
> We have chewed dry twigs and salt grasses;
> we have filled our mouths with dust and bits of adobe;
> we have eaten lizards, rats and worms. (Leon Portilla 1962:127–38)

A striking example of the effects of hunger comes from a study done in the archives of the city of Cholula, Puebla (Malvido 1975). Different illnesses affected the Cholulans in diverse ways. Smallpox and measles caused high mortality among children under five years of age without regard to social status. When more than fifteen years passed between epidemics, pregnant women were also affected, which led to spontaneous abortions and premature births. In contrast, *matlazahuatl* ("blotches that form a net") caused higher mortality among poor young adults. Hunger affected the poor and especially their children. Through the analysis of baptism, marriage, and death certificates, Malvido could reconstruct the ways in which the diverse epidemics and economic crises affected the demography of the region.

One of the major aspects by which to understand the effects of the Conquest on health is the way that the food supply changed. The Spaniards brought new plants and animals to Mexico, which had to compete for land and labor with the native foods. In some cases the adoption of new foods was very rapid. One of the conquerors, Andres de Tapia (1971), wrote that at the time when Cortes had taken Tenochtitlan and was in the neighboring town of Coyoacan, he received some rice from Veracruz. Mixed with it were three grains of wheat. Cortes had a Black man plant them. Two grains died, but one produced forty-seven spikes.

By 1539 Tapia found an abundance of good wheat and could buy a supply at a low price. He claimed that all the wheat that grew in the provinces came from the original grain that Cortes had ordered to be planted. He also states that Cortes brought various kinds of cattle, which became a successful enterprise, judging from the number of regulations for the control of slaughterhouses and meat markets that appeared during the sixteenth century (Dusenberry 1948) and the number of testimonies on how Indians in small and isolated villages accepted this new meat from cattle, pigs, and goats.

The shift in agricultural activities and cattle growing, plus the amount of land devoted to new plants such as sugar cane, had an impact on the native foods. But equally important causes of hunger were natural catastrophes, which, together with the new type of economy, gave rise to hoarding, state intervention, exploitation of those goods that Spain needed, and other disruptive conditions.

We have an idea about the magnitude of the impact of the Conquest on morbidity and mortality, which caused the depopulation of great areas of Mexico. We can identify specific illnesses through historical and osteological sources, and we can also start to understand the ways in which individuals and society suffered their diseases. The Nahuatl poem about the siege of Tenochtitlan is a gripping example of the despair caused by hunger. The description of the smallpox epidemic demonstrates acute clinical and epidemiological observational skills, together with a sensibility for the social effects of the plague.

New and Old Ideas About Disease

One of the most important consequences of the Conquest was its effect on the concepts of disease and its causes. Pre-Hispanic Mexicans lived in a universe where the gods were responsible for their fate, but they also used the observation of nature to guide their conduct. The European view was similar in many ways, although its origin was in a completely different cosmovision. Many texts have been written analyzing this situation. The most important ones on the Nahuatl view are found in references Lopez Austin (1975, 1984), Martinez Cortez (1965), Ortiz de Montellano (1979), and Viesca (1979).

Humans had to be healed in all their complexity, since they were understood as both bodies and souls immersed in their society, burdened with duties toward their gods. Pre-Hispanic medicines were based on this idea and gave consideration to all those aspects which today we would call "magical" and "rational" remedies. It is fascinating to see how complex this situation was and to view the biomedical effectiveness of some of the natural remedies that were used centuries ago. Some of them have already been incorporated into the Mexican pharmacopoeia and are part of the basic medical products used by the national health system.

The Europeans introduced the concept of sin as an explanation of disease. Some interpreted the calamities that came with the Conquest as the fair punishment for people who had worshipped the Devil, away from the true God. In this way, some thought of Mexico as an equivalent of Sodom and Gomorrah or ancient Greece or Rome, destroyed by an angry God. The promotion of the Virgin of Guadelupe as restorer of the Indian's lost health was an important component in this transitional period.

It is interesting to recall how New Spain viewed the diseases of epidemics. A *Coloquio* by Fernan Gonzalez de Eslava (Hernandez Rodriguez 1960) illustrates these ideas. In it there is a dialogue among Clemency, Knowledge, Health, and several characters related to disease and epidemics. Health states that Pestilence should leave the Indians in peace, because:

> Their disease grave and long-lasting,
> is suffered by us
> and it is true, as we see it,
> that God discharges in them,
> what we all deserve. (quoted in Hernandez Rodriguez 1960)

The dialogue also shows that disease can be fought not only with prayers, devotion, hope, and charity, but also with herbs, holy water from the church of the Virgen de los Remedios, and other remedies.

Research for the Future

The transition of the Conquest has left us with much more information than we have about earlier transitions, but we still know relatively little. More research has to be done. The materials contained in archives, such as those of the Inquisition, have to be explored further. Personal diaries, collections of medical prescriptions, ex-votoes in churches, personal letters, and other such documents can be a valuable source of information.

My current research has to do with understanding the magnitude and direction of the changes in the food supply and nutrition that started with the Conquest. There is an abundance of information, but it has not been gathered together and analyzed completely, although some interesting books have been published (e.g. Corcuera 1981; Farga 1980; Novo 1979; Rodriquez Rivera 1965). Some types of historical sources have not yet been effectively utilized, among them: the osteological evidence already cited and that will be available soon, lists of food items that were imported from Spain and the Philippines and those that were exported; price of foods in different places and times; and books of cooking recipes, restaurant menus, and personal diaries.

In our present time of transition and crisis, in which some of the changes that occurred as a consequence of the Spanish Conquest are being replicated, the knowledge of past adaptations can be useful. Today we hear that our Mexican foodways are being lost due to the intense contact with the European world. People fear that hamburgers, hot dogs, junk food, and such will replace traditional dishes such as *tacos* and *tamales*. What is not taken into consideration is that this same process occurred in the past. One has only to imagine an Aztec priest crying in despair that the new wheat, cattle, sugar cane, will lead to the demise of his cherished dishes. Mexican foods, such as the famous *moles* (sauces with hot pepper), *pan dulce* (sweet wheat bread), *carnitas* (deep fried pork meat), *albondigas* (meat balls), and *ates* (sweet pastes made from Mexican fruits), are truly hybrid foods that could not exist without the mixture of pre-Hispanic and Europoean contributions. Something similar can be said for many European cuisines of today that would not be the same without Mexican tomatoes, chocolate, peanuts, or maize. The adaptive strategies that developed with the Conquest may hold an answer for Mexico's transition to the future in a highly connected world with a global economy.

THE TRANSITION TO THE FUTURE

The Mexican Revolution of 1910 can be considered as the beginning of present-day Mexico. From this date, the whole world changed, and this transition has had and will continue to have an impact on the health of Mexico.

Before 1910, Mexico contained a series of relatively isolated regions. The human movements brought about by war started an intense migration within the country. Later, this movement included not only massive migration of people into large cities but also migration to the United States. Today, a greater proportion of Mexicans live in urban areas than in rural areas. Moreover, it is easy to travel from one part of the country to another by bus, train, car, or plane. Very few villages remain isolated. Poor Mexicans often travel to important pilgrimage centers, while middle-class Mexicans visit the United States or Europe. Radio and television reach nearly every corner of the country and carry their messages about new foods and new ways of life. Thus urbanization, ease of transportation, and communication networks are all affecting Mexican diet.

"Old" and "New" Pathology

At the same time, Mexico continues to be a pluralistic country, where one can find the very rich walking in the same street with people who do not even have a minimal living standard. There are still rural Indian communities in which people speak only their native language and cannot understand Spanish. These contrasts are related to patterns of illness. Physicians have identified two types of pathology in Mexico among Mexicans. There are the "new pathology" that can be found in industrialized countries and an "old pathology," often referred to as the "pathology of the poor," which are the diseases linked to poverty, bad sanitation, crowding, underemployment, high birth rate, and so on. A recent study (Larraza Hernandez et al. 1983), comparing diagnoses based on autopsies at the Hospital General de Mexico in 1953 and 1980, shows that the old pathology has remained unchanged, but the new pathology is increasing. The former includes infections, rheumatic fever, the long-term effects of alcoholism, and so on. The second type of pathology, which is similar to that of developed countries, includes hypertension, atherosclerosis, certain types of cancer (particularly those linked to the exposure to industrial toxins), aplastic anemias, and interstitial pulmonary fibrosis.

Transition and Diet

The presence of the two types of pathology is linked to the transformation Mexico is experiencing, which involves the continuation of a traditional way of life (albeit significantly altered) and an increasing industrialization with dramatic changes in the food patterns. The economic crisis has affected the way people live and what they eat.

Miriam Munoz de Chavez (1984) has identified two main trends in the Mexican diet, which she labels "polarization of foods" and "transnationalization of the diet." Polarization refers to a process in which certain foods are sent to specific parts of the country where they have wide acceptance and people can buy them. These are, of course, large cities or towns. This leaves small villages mainly dependent on their own resources. Transnationalization refers to the way that "international" foods are promoted by the media so that they come to be a need by the community. These foods include the broad category of "junk food," industrialized breads and pastries, flavor-giving products, canned juices, beer, wine, and the like. Most of them provide little or low quality nutrients for a very high price, which includes the cost of their distribution, packaging, and propaganda.

These trends are well established and are responsible for a sharp division in Mexican foodways. Some people eat too much and are obese, consuming extra calories in the form of fat and carbohydrates; others have insufficient nutrition and experience chronic malnutrition. Moreover, with the current economic crisis, cases of starvation are beginning to appear.

Directions of Future Work

There is a great concern for the country's future if these trends continue. At the same time, Mexican scientists are beginning to explore potential resources for improving the nutritional status of Mexicans. Old and new sources of foods and of cooking techniques are being studied. The past is being reexamined and reinterpreted in the search for a Mexican way of solving our problems.

We still do not have a clear picture of how contemporary Mexicans perceive their diseases. A group of physicians and anthropologists is starting to explore a series of important issues. We expect that a single illness entity can produce different effects in different people. Social class may influence the response to diabetes, for example. Dietary management and recommended weight reduction may lead to loss of access to low-cost sources of carbohydrates such as *tortillas*; weight reduction may cause social and psychological strain, since, at least in certain strata of our society, being plump is interpreted as a sign of health or as an element of sexual attraction. But these issues may change in accordance with each patient's biography and way of life. To explore these questions further, we plan to study the following diseases: rheumatoid arthritis, diabetes mellitus, and breast cancer.

Another subject of study is the analysis of how Mexican cultures can affect diseases, particularly those associated with stress. Our study includes rural and urban Mixtecos, a people with a tightly knit culture that seems to offer protection from larger society through the maintenance of common food patterns, social networks, a sense of belonging to a community, and other features. Our hypothesis is that cultures similar to that of the Mixtecos protect individuals against diseases that are caused by or that cause stress. This idea will be used to examine patterns of drug and alcohol consumption.

In conclusion, the study of disease in relation to ancient and modern transitions can help Mexico find a way to adapt better to economic and social changes and to face the future with hope for a better life.

NOTE

The author thanks Emily McClung de Tapia and Gretel Pelto for their valuable suggestions for improving this text.

REFERENCES

Aquirre Beltran, G. 1963. Medicina y magia. *Coleccion de Antropologia Social.* vol. 1. Mexico: Instituto Nacional Indegenista.

Casillas, L. E., and L. A. Vargas. 1984. La Alimentacion entre los Mexica. In *Historia General de la Medicina en Mexico.* vol. 1. Mexico Antiquo, F. M. Cortez, ed. Mexico: Academia Nacional de Medicina and Facultad de Medicina, Universidad Nacional Autonoma de Mexico.

Corcuera, S. 1981. *Entre Gula y Templanza. Un Aspecto de la Historia Mexicana.* Mexico: Facultad de Filosofia y Letras, Colegio de Historia, Universidad Nacional Autonoma de Mexico.

Corruccini, R. A. 1982. Pathologies relative to subsistence and settlement at Casas Grandes. *American Antiquity* 48(3):609–10.

Dusenberry, W. H. 1948. The regulation of meat supply in sixteenth-century Mexico City. *Hispanic American Historical Review* 28:38–52.

Engel, George L. 1979. The biomedical model: A procrustean bed? *Man and Medicine* 4(4):257–75.

———. 1977. The need for a new medical model: A challenge for biomedicine. *Science* 196(4286):129–36.

Farga, A. 1980. *Historia de la Comida en Mexico.* 2d ed. Mexico: Litografica Mexico.

Haviland, W. A. 1967. Stature at Tikal, Guatemala: Implications for ancient Maya demography and social organization. *American Antiquity* 32(3):316–25.

Hernandez Rodriguez, R. 1960. Epidemias Novohispanas durante el siglo XVI. *Memorias de la Academia Mexicana de la Historia* 28:5–20.

Hunn, E. 1982. Did the Aztecs lack potential animal domesticates? *American Ethnologist* 9(3):578–79.

Ladurie, E. Le Roy. 1982. *Montaillou, Village Occitan de 1294 a 1324.* Paris: Editions Gallimard.

Larraza Hernandez, O., et al. 1983. Patologia del subdesarrollo. Analisis comparativo de la mortalidad en el hospital general. *Ciencia* 34:201–20.

Leon Portilla, M. 1962. *The Broken Spears: The Account of the Conquest of Mexico.* Boston: Beacon Press.

Lopez Austin, A. 1984. *Cuerpo Humano e Ediologia. Las Concepciones de los Antiquos Nahuas.* Mexico: Instituto de Investigaciones Antropologicas, Universidad Nacional Autonoma de Mexico.

———. 1975. *Textos de Medicina Nahuatl.* Mexico: Instituto de Investigaciones Historicas, Universidad Nacional Autonoma de Mexico.

McClung de Tapia, E. 1980. Interpretacion de restos botanico procedentes de sitios arquelogicos. *Anales de Antropologia* 17:149–65.

———. 1977. Recientes estudio paleotenobatanicos en Teotihuacan, Mexico. *Anales de Antropologia* 14:49–61.

———. m.s. Archaeobotanical research in tropical North America.

McClung de Tapia, E., M. C. Serra, and A. E. Limon de Dyer. 1986. Formative lacustrine adaptation: Botanical remains from Terremote-Tlaltenco, D. F. Mexico. *Journal of Field Archaeology* 13:99–113.

Malvido, E. 1975. Efectos de las epidemias y hambrunas en la poblacion colonial de Mexico (1519–1810). *Salud Publica de Mexico, Epoca.* V 17(6):793–802.

———. 1973. Cronologia de epidemias y crises agricolas en al epoca colonial. *Historia Mexicana* 89:96–101.

Marquez Morfin, L. 1984a. *Sociedad Colonial y Enfermedad.* Mexico: Instituto Nacional de Antropologia e Historia, Coleccion Cientifica 136.

———. 1984b. Distribucion de la estatura en colecciones oseas Mayas prehispanicas. In *Estudios de Antropologia Biologica.* II. *Memorias del Colquio de Antropologia Fisica Juan Comas 1982.* R. Ramos Galvan and R. M. Ramos, eds. Mexico: Instituto de Investigaciones Antropologicas, Serie Antropologica 75.

Martinez Cortez, F. 1983. *Enfermedad ky Padecer.* Mexico: La Medicina del Hombre en su Totalidad, La Prensa Medica Mexicana.

———. 1965. *Las Ideas en la Medicina Nahuatl.* Mexico: La Prensa Medica Mexicana.

Munoz de Chavez, M. 1984. Tendencias en la dieta por grupos y neveles socioeconomicos. Paper delivered in the seminar "El Desafio de la Alimentacion," organized by the Programa Universitario de Alimentos, UNAM, October 17.

Nickens, P. R. 1976. Stature reduction as an adaptative response to food production in Mesoamerica. *Journal of Archaeological Science* 3:31–41.

Novo, S. 1979. *Cocina Mexiana o Historia Gastronomica de la Ciudad de Mexico.* 5th ed. Mexico: Editorial Porrua S. A.

Ortiz de Montellano, B. 1979. The rational causes of illness among the Aztecs. *Actes du XLII Congres Internationial des Americanistes* (Paris): 6:287–99.

———. 1978. Aztec cannibalism: An ecological necessity? *Science* 200:611–17.

Pena Paez, I., and C. V. Trevino. 1979. Vida, enfermedad y muerte a traves de los cantos y posias nahuatl. *Actes du XLII Congres International des Americanistes* (Paris): 6:271–78.

Pina Chan, R. 1967. *Una Vision del Mexico Prehispanico.* Serie de Culturas Mesoamericanas 1. Mexico: Instituto de Investigaciones Historicas, Universidad Nacional Antonoma de Mexico.

Rodriguez Rivera, V. 1965. *La Comida en el Mexico Antiquo y Moderno.* Coleccion Pormaca 21. Mexico: Editorial Promaca, S.A. de C.V.

Sahagun, F. B. 1974. *Historia General de las Cosas de Nueva Espana.* Coleccion Sepan Cuanto 300. Mexico: Editorial Porrua.

Salas Cuesta, M. E. 1982. *La Poblacion de Mexico-Tenochtitlan, Estudio de Osteologia Antropologica.* Coleccion Cientifica 126. Mexico: Instituto Nacional de Antropologica e Historia.

Santley, R. S., and E. K. Rose. 1979. Diet, nutrition and population dynamics in the Basin of Mexico. *World Archaeology* 11(2):185–207.

Schoeninger, M. J. 1979. Diet and status at Chalcatzingo: Some empirical and technical aspects of Strontium Analysis. *American Journal of Physical Anthropology* 51:295–310.

Tapia, A. 1971. Relacion hecha por el Senor Andres de Tapia sobre la conquista de Mexico. In *Coleccion de Documentos para la Historia de Mexico.* vol. 1. Mexico: Primera Edicion Faccimilar, Editorial Porrua, Biblioteca Porrua, 48.

Vargas, L. A. 1984. La alimentacion de los Mayas antiguos. In *Historia General de la Medicina en Mexico.* vol. 1. F. M. Cortez, ed. Mexico: Academia Nacional de Medicina and Facultad de Medicina, Universidad Autonoma de Mexico.

———. 1978. Definiciones y caracteristicas de la relacion medico paciente. *Estudios sobre Etnobotanica y Antropologia Medica* 3:19–36.

Viesca, T. C. 1979. El concepto de enfermedad en mesoamerica. *Actes du XLII Congres international des Americanistes.* (Paris): 6:259–70.

Weaver, D. S. 1980. An osteological test of changes in subsistence and settlement patterns at Casas Grandes, Chihuahua, Mexico. *American Antiquity* 46(2):361–64.

9 INFANT MORTALITY IN MASSACHUSETTS AND THE UNITED STATES IN THE NINETEENTH CENTURY

Alan C. Swedlund

The trajectory of infant and childhood mortality in various regions of the United States has been of long-standing concern to economic historians, demographers, and health researchers. One of the central issues is the shape of the trajectory itself and whether mortality of the young increased, decreased, or remained relatively constant during the second half of the nineteenth century (Higgs 1973; Meeker 1972; Condran and Crimmins 1979, 1980; Haines 1977, 1979; Kunitz 1984). In addition, there has been more limited consideration of the differences between urban and rural areas (Higgs 1973; Crimmins and Condran 1983; Haines and Preston 1984). Sufficient data and analyses are now available so that the trends invite both generalization and closer scrutiny. Moreover, we have learned, as we should have expected, that regional variations and local flux in population, climate, and economic conditions defy any attempt to make singular statements that apply to all areas at any one time.

Between 1865 and 1895 the proportion of males engaged in agriculture in Franklin County, Massachusetts declined from almost 50 percent to less than 15 percent. At the same time the proportion of foreign-born in the population increased from approximately 8 to almost 17 percent according to the Massachusetts State Censuses. A rapid transition in population size and composition was occurring in the rural areas of western Massachusetts as a result of commercialization, industrialization, and migration. An instructive setting for an investigation of infant and child health under conditions of transition was thus created.

In this chapter I will (1) review some of the trends (and perhaps, lessons) from American demographic history; (2) discuss the development of models of causality; and (3) relate certain of the empirical findings that derive from work in Franklin County, located in the Connecticut River Valley of Massachusetts.

Massachusetts is an appropriate focus because it is generally agreed that the nineteenth-century data from this state surpass all others (Condran and Crimmins 1979; Smith 1983). I will argue that the causes of infant mortality in nineteenth-century Massachusetts are quite similar to the causes of high health risk of infants in developing countries today. I wish also to suggest that the substantive and methodological contributions made to infant and child health in the late nineteenth and the early part of this century are quite significant and no doubt relevant to other contexts today. In this regard I believe there has also been some "reinventing of the wheel," in terms of understanding the factors associated with high infant risk.

Infant and childhood mortality are useful summary measures of societal well-being. This was recognized by population researchers historically (see discussion in Haines and Preston 1984:4) and is frequently echoed today by researchers in diverse settings (e.g., DaVanzo, Butz, and Habicht 1983). Moreover, most societies are keenly aware of the relationship between social and environmental stress on the one hand and infant health on the other. While some societies may permit, under conditions of stress or economic necessity, a proportion of infant deaths that are avoidable (Scrimshaw 1978, 1984; Johannson 1984), with few exceptions most societies place a high premium on healthy children and believe in the prevention of infant deaths if possible (however, see Johansson 1986). This was no less true in early America, and a considerable literature exists on the concern for infant health and child welfare (e.g., see Meckel 1980). In some respects the United States provides an excellent opportunity for investigation of historical patterns because not only did an ideology of child welfare exist from an early point in time, but also the opportunity for access to necessary resources was perhaps notably improved over many other historical populations, at least during the earlier phases of colonization and settlement. By the nineteenth century the urbanization, industrialization, and large-scale immigration affected significantly the trajectory alluded to above. Massachusetts, in particular, because of its long history of vital statistics and health registration systems, provides a useful population through which to review past trends.

GENERAL BACKGROUND TO THE PROBLEM

Before turning to some of the specific issues involved in the Massachusetts and American cases, it may be useful here to review very briefly the larger issue of historical population growth and the contributions to this growth that have been attributed to changes in fertility and mortality. It is now widely held that substantial reductions in the rate of mortality have occurred during the time since the wide-scale adoption of agriculture and that the pace of mortality decline was accelerated during the European Industrial Revolution and afterward. Perhaps most notable of the proponents of this view have been Thomas McKeown and his associates (McKeown 1976). McKeown has long argued that the decline in mortality historically has not been a function of improved medical practices per se, but is due largely to changes in standard of living and the availability of food during the eighteenth century, followed by sanitation and public health measures in the late nineteenth century. William McNeill (1980) and others have pointed out that these transformations were not without costs, while Kunitz (1983), Schofield (1983), Wrigley and Schofield (1981), Fogel (1984), and several others have added resolution to the initial arguments or offered new insights into the processes involved.

McKinlay and McKinlay (1977) have explored the role of medical care in the decline of mortality in the United States specifically since 1900. They argue that approximately 3.5 percent of the decline, at most, can be attributed directly to medical intervention. This was due largely to the development of vaccines for poliomyelitis, typhoid, diphtheria, and so on. By extension we can assume the effects of direct medical intervention to changes in infant and childhood mortality in the nineteenth-century United States to have been virtually nil. Thus, an understanding of the changes during this period can be gained independent of medical intervention except in those instances where practicing physicians actually may have contributed to the maintenance or increase of mortality levels.

Population Trends

It is not my purpose here to review mortality trends in the United States or in Massachusetts except as they bear directly on the issue of changing causal relations in infant and child mortality. Countless efforts have been waged to disentangle the actual trends from those implied by data that, to say the least, are less than perfect. The reader is referred to the authors cited above for more detailed discussion of the problem. In the case of Massachusetts it is quite clear that improvements in the vital registration system occurred in the 1840s which, by about 1850, had reduced substantially the under-registration of deaths, and from mid-century onward the data are considered relatively reliable (Gutman 1958, 1959). While absolute figures are still debated the overall trends are not in dispute (Figure 9.1).

Kunitz (1984) has argued that wide fluctuations in colonial and early antebellum death rates were dampened by a growing population and increasing endemicity. The change from epidemic to endemic patterns of diseases like measles and smallpox supports this contention. Rural rates of infant and child mortality are consistently lower than urban in the eastern United States (including Massachusetts) throughout the historical period (Condran and Crimmins 1980). Once data problems, changing age structure effects, and rural-urban differences are controlled, it appears that the trend in mortality during the nineteenth century was characterized by little movement in death rates until after 1850 and that any real improvements in life expectancy were still modest until approximately 1880 (Meeker 1972). Virtually all researchers agree

Figure 9.1
**Infant Mortality Rates for Massachusetts, Franklin County, and the
Four-Town Study Area of Deerfield, Shelburne, Greenfield, and
Montague, Massachusetts, 1850–1910.[1]**

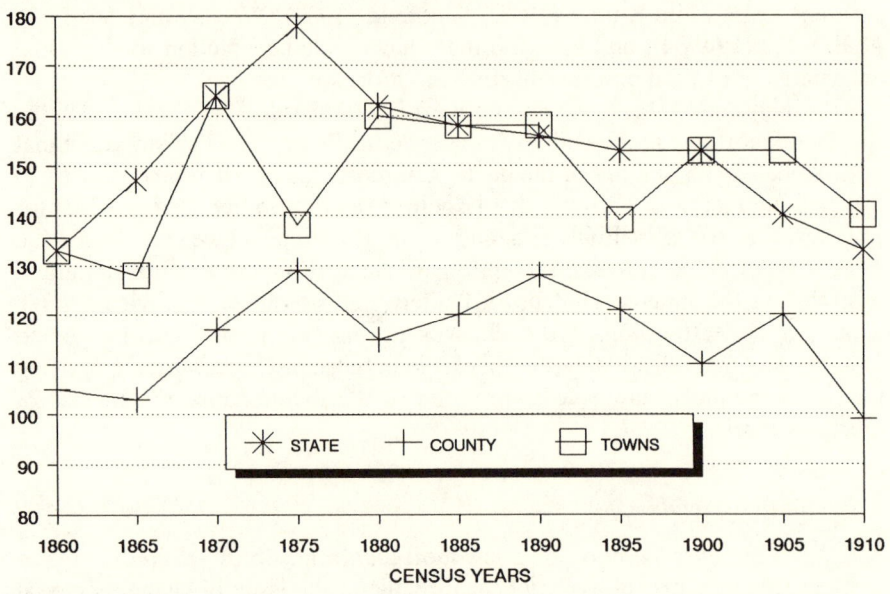

CENSUS YEARS

[1] Values based on three- or five-year averages.

Source: McArdle (1985).

that the principal causes of infant and childhood deaths were acute infectious diseases and that the "standard-of-living" argument and the health reform movement of the late nineteenth century were the major factors in reducing the effects of infectious disease (Meeker 1972; Petersen 1979). It is also apparent that, although adult survivorship may have been improving from 1850 onward, infant mortality was not declining and was probably increasing in many regions prior to 1880.

Principal correlates of infant mortality during the nineteenth century were those associated with nutrition and feeding practices, particularly during the earliest months of life and at weaning time. A host of intervening socioeconomic and ecological variables have been researched to clarify these associations further. Additional discussion will be focused primarily on this period of increased risk in infant mortality, the proximate causes including nutrition, some of the rural and urban correlates, and the development of models of causality.

History of Causal Inference

To observe that the medical establishment per se did not affect reductions in infant and childhood mortality in the United States in the nineteenth century is not to say that health professionals (including some physicians) were not making important contributions during this period. While the most noteworthy events were to take place in the late nineteenth and early twentieth centuries, throughout the 1800s there were progressive steps taken to understand more clearly the causal relations. That few effective measures were implemented until quite late should not obscure the fact that important insights had been gained and systematically studied. The major methodological changes are outlined here and summarizd in Table 9.1.

1820–1860

As Petersen (1979) and many others have noted, long before the contagionist view of disease was prominent there was ample and well-understood evidence for the fact that crowding, filth, "bad air," tainted food, and improper nutrition were associated with disease. Burnet and White (1972:106) point out that, if typhoid was historically attributed to the bad air around sewers rather than to the presence of the bacillus itself in the water, it did not diminish the impact of cleaning up the sewer and separating the drinking water from it. Prior to the wide-scale understanding of the germ theory of disease in the United States in the 1870s, midwives, some physicians, and no doubt many mothers advised women to get fresh air, exercise, and eat wholesome food when nursing their babies. Mothers were urged to keep the child clean, warm, and well fed. It is also true however, that the Health Reform Movement of the mid-nineteenth

Table 9.1

Changes in the Perception and Prevention of Infant and Child Mortality, 1800–Present.

Time	Substantive	Methodological
Pre-1861	Health reformers First boards of health	Theories of hygiene
1861–1880	Emergence of useful data Basic research	Germ theory Proximate causes
1881–1920	Public health measures (Sewage, drinking water, milk inspection, pasteuriza- tion)	Multifactorial causality
1920–Present	Antibiotic era, modern sys- tem of pre- and postnatal care	Multivariate approaches and interactions

century, despite promoting many aspects of hygiene, exercise, and diet, was also promoting a much exaggerated view of the emotional instability of women and their modern "habits" and the subsequent detriment to the mother's milk and health of their children (Meckel 1980; Apple 1981; Whorton 1982).

These problems were compounded by the American Industrial Revolution, which increasingly brought women into factory and commercial agricultural work outside the home. While it is true that the majority of these women were unmarried and without children; it is also true that many were women with infants and young children, particularly in urban areas, and especially the foreign-born women (Phelps 1912). Thus, the stage was set for a period in which nursing was often supplemented or abandoned altogether by a large number of women in the eastern United States.

Rural areas, especially in New England, were likewise affected by both trends in health knowledge and the increased risks to infants because of the tendency for manufacturing and commercial agriculture to exist side-by-side in many parts of the region. Moreover, unlike many contemporary rural settings in which infant mortality is high, a large proportion of the women in rural New England were literate and quite aware of "modern" social attitudes and the latest medical theories. Public schools were mandated in Massachusetts towns in the early 1700s. Vinovskis reports that school attendance in New England by children aged 5–19 years in 1840 was 81.8 percent (1981: 123–24). It dropped somewhat thereafter, probably due to urban growth and foreign immigration, but was still 73.8 percent of the population in 1860. From 1820 to 1860 it is not unreasonable to assume that rural infant mortality rates hovered around 130 per 1,000 births, perhaps rising one or two percent by 1860. Rates in Boston would more likely have been in the range of 160–175 per 1,000 and increasing somewhat over time.

1861–1880

By the end of this period the germ theory of disease had become widely known and, if not completely understood, at least partially integrated into the health knowledge of the study population. This is also a period of very substantial immigration into the eastern United States by many non-English speakers who found themselves in poorer areas of cities or on the commercial farms and small factories in the less-urbanized areas. American cities at this time are perhaps at their nadir from the standpoint of human health (Leavitt 1982; Petersen 1979; Rosenkrantz 1972; Condran and Cheney 1980). For virtually all of the large cities in the east and midwest at this time the following would hold true:

1. Few neighborhoods would have running water.
2. Garbage removal would be absent or infrequent, and quite probably dump pickers and pigs would be set free on the refuse to get rid of whatever possible.
3. Sewer systems would be rare, very inefficient, and drain raw sewage into the same rivers that provided drinking water.

4. Privys would be outdoor open pits or poorly designed septic systems adjacent to houses and tenements.

5. Cows' milk would most likely come from an urban dairy with little in the way of cooling or inspection practices, and cows would be fed on the swill from breweries or distilleries.

6. Fresh food would be available to those who could afford it but not kept under very sanitary conditions.

These circumstances, coupled with some particularly severe cholera epidemics, precipitated the highest levels of infant mortality ever experienced in the United States, and also brought about the establishment of boards of health in most cities and many smaller communities. At the same time, there were major breakthroughs in understanding of the correlates of infectious disease, and the proximate causes of infant and childhood mortality were

Table 9.2
Causes of Death in Infancy.

---

1. Premature birth

2. Difference of constitutional force (i.e., inherited factors)

3. Healthy districts (i.e., geographic differences)

4. Care in infancy
   a. First weeks
   b. Diseases of infancy and childhood
   (especially noted are gastrointestinal and respiratory)
   c. Food and nutrition
   (especially importance of mother's milk)
   d. Mother's temporary absence
   e. Effect of food on milk (i.e., mother's diet)
   f. Distillery milk

5. The poor (i.e., poverty)

6. Education and ignorance

7. Overlaid (that is, suffocation or infanticide (?))

8. Illegitimacy, foundlings, adopted children (see 4, d, 5)

9. Effect of cold (seasonality)

10. Country and city (i.e., urban problems, see 3)

Source: Massachusetts State Board of Health (1875).

becoming sufficiently well understood to inititate a period of comparatively effective health reform. Even so, Boston during these decades probably reached infant mortality rates of 200 per 1,000 births, while the average for the state as a whole would more likely have been 165 or 170 (Abbott 1897; Meckel 1980). Areas in rural western Massachusetts were probably below that, closer to 130-150 (Meindl 1979). Nevertheless, these high rates prompted general concern, collection of reliable data, and insights into the causes. For example, a listing of the principal causes of infant mortality in the State Board of Health Report for the State of Massachusetts in 1873 reports all of the major causes (Table 9.2).

Although the mutual exclusiveness of categories may be called into question, there is no major variable missing from this list. The proximate causes listed under "Diseases of Infancy and Childhood" include twenty-five childhood diseases that range from accidents, diphtheria, and typhoid to hydrocephaly and premature births. In other words, during this period the level of recognition of problems is sufficiently sophisticated and the biomedical and technological means adequate to the implementation of major public health measures.

1881–1920

These cut-off points are like those above, somewhat arbitrary, yet they still give a clear pattern of substantial reductions in infant and child mortality. By 1899, the rates of infant mortality had fallen from their high, 1870–1880 levels to their 1860 levels; by the 1920s, infant mortality was below 80 per 1,000 in most areas, and the urban and rural rates had pretty well converged.

The major factors associated with the reductions in mortality rates include the initiation of effective sewer systems and domestic water supplies, effective dairy and milk inspection, and many ordinances on the condition of housing, establishment of public parks, and food supplement programs, to name a few. Although pasteurization was developed and understood in the 1870s it was not until the 1920s that most states had enforceable laws requiring it. A great deal of political agitation on the part of child health reformers was also essential to the implementation of these programs (Strauss 1917; American Association for the Prevention of Infant Mortality; Meckel 1980).

It was during this period that the multivariate nature of infant and childhood mortality became clearly understood and could be acted upon. The relationship between infant feeding practices, hygiene, and poverty were spelled out, if in a somewhat implicit fashion, in numerous public documents and popular writings of the day. It is also clear at this time that while there was progress in the understanding of the problem there was also a contradictory process going on in the form of the wide-scale introduction of infant feeding formulas (see Nutrition below).

The Massachusetts Board of Health Reports after 1900, the writing of Phelps (1912), and the works of Robert Woodbury done under the auspices of the United States Children's Bureau (1926) make clear the quality of research that was being accomplished during this period. Woodbury reports the results of a comprehensive study of eight cities between 1911 and 1915. Information was collected on parents' income, occupation, age, and ethnicity for 22,000 live births and their outcome. The births were tabulated for their mother's parity, birth intervals, cause of death (if deceased), and for their complete history of feeding during the first year. The quality of the survey permitted an excellent example of case control studies using then up-to-date statistical procedures. Woodbury was able to show the excess mortality to artifically fed infants by cause and by month. He isolated the "intermediate causes" of poverty, ethnicity, and mother's nativity and looked at the interaction between father's earnings and availability of medical and nursing care on infant outcome. His conclusions were profound and ring true to this day. His observations on the roles of maternal age, breastfeeding, birth order, and economic status, for example, compare favorably with the findings in current studies on modern populations (Gortmaker 1979; DaVanzo, Butz and Habicht 1983).

By the 1930s modern patterns of maternal-child health were achieved. The major changes from this point on were those associated with the development and use of antibiotics and increasing accessibility of public health facilities and nutrition programs along with the development of sophisticated pre- and postnatal care programs. That poverty remained strongly associated with high risk is very clear (Gortmaker 1979; Miller 1985).

CONNECTICUT RIVER VALLEY: FRANKLIN COUNTY, MASSACHUSETTS

The seasons, local and endemic influences, and more than all, the means and manners of life in the family seem to be prominent as friends or foes, to aid or impair the infant constitution, in its struggle against the adverse influences that threaten it. (Massachusetts State Board of Health, 1873:195)

Given the vast amount of research and observations alluded to above it may be appropriate to ask what further historical research in a limited geographic area can add to the already richly detailed picture? To answer, I will discuss briefly current research involving the question of rural-urban differences and the issue of feeding practices and types of morbidity response. A third topic has to do with the structure and formation of the family as correlates of infant mortality. While exemplifying information to be gained in historical research, space does not permit a more detailed discussion here (Swedlund, Meindl, and Gradie 1980; Meindl 1980; Ginsberg 1983).

The communities discussed include Deerfield, Greenfield, Shelburne, and, to a lesser extent, Montague, in Franklin County, Massachusetts. The data have been collected from vital registrations, state and federal censuses, tax valuation lists, and a host of other primary and secondary sources and are described elsewhere (Swedlund, Temkin, and Meindl 1976; Swedlund, Meindl, and Gradie 1980; McArdle 1985).

Resources

A broad perspective on differences in infant and childhood mortality between urban and rural places focuses our attention on the specific resource and environmental correlates of regional differences. In the past there has been suspicion on the part of many historical demographers that the differences were associated with poor record-keeping in rural communities and that rural areas did not participate in the health reforms and improving standards of living during the late nineteenth and early twentieth centuries. Rural mortality was definitely lower in Massachusetts, and the above discussion points to some of the major reasons why. Even if underenumeration has been a factor, the levels of underenumeration in cities were probably far worse (Abbott 1897; Gutman 1958; Vinovskis 1981). A local town clerk in a community of 1,100 individuals would be far more likely to recover most of the annual births and deaths in the town as compared to the clerk of an urbanizing place with significant migration.

The estimate that rural infant mortality was probably about 30 percent lower than the urban rate, on average, is likely conservative. As Higgs (1973: 187) has pointed out, rural communities counted on shallow wells, springs, and cisterns for their water; their milk escaped pasteurization, "and the privy continued to provide the same primitive means of human waste disposal." But contrary to the notion that these were problems, one can easily envision the value of having one's own independent water source, whole milk produced fresh on the farm each day, rather than carted through the city in warm, contaminated containers, and using a privy designed for a family rather than a tenement. While family size might remain relatively high, the density of population was far lower and "crowding" much less of a problem.

The numbers of individuals who were occupied as farmers and who owned land is a good indicator of the ability to provide for children (Figure 9.2). It is also a reasonable proxy for standard of living in this population, since it reflects the ability to control property and provide fresh produce. Although one should not make too much of the relationship between childhood mortality and farm activity, it is temptimg to suggest that rural areas have compensating resources and environmental conditions which offset any lack of participation in explicit public health activities.

Another closely related factor apparent in rural areas during the nineteenth century is that, while there were distinct economic and class differences which had existed between individuals since colonial times, the range and variance in these differences is far less than found in urban areas of the same time period. This would account for additional reductions in risk stemming from resource limiting factors. A third factor is the level of female employment outside the home. Since the "putting out" system for home industry was more prevalent and

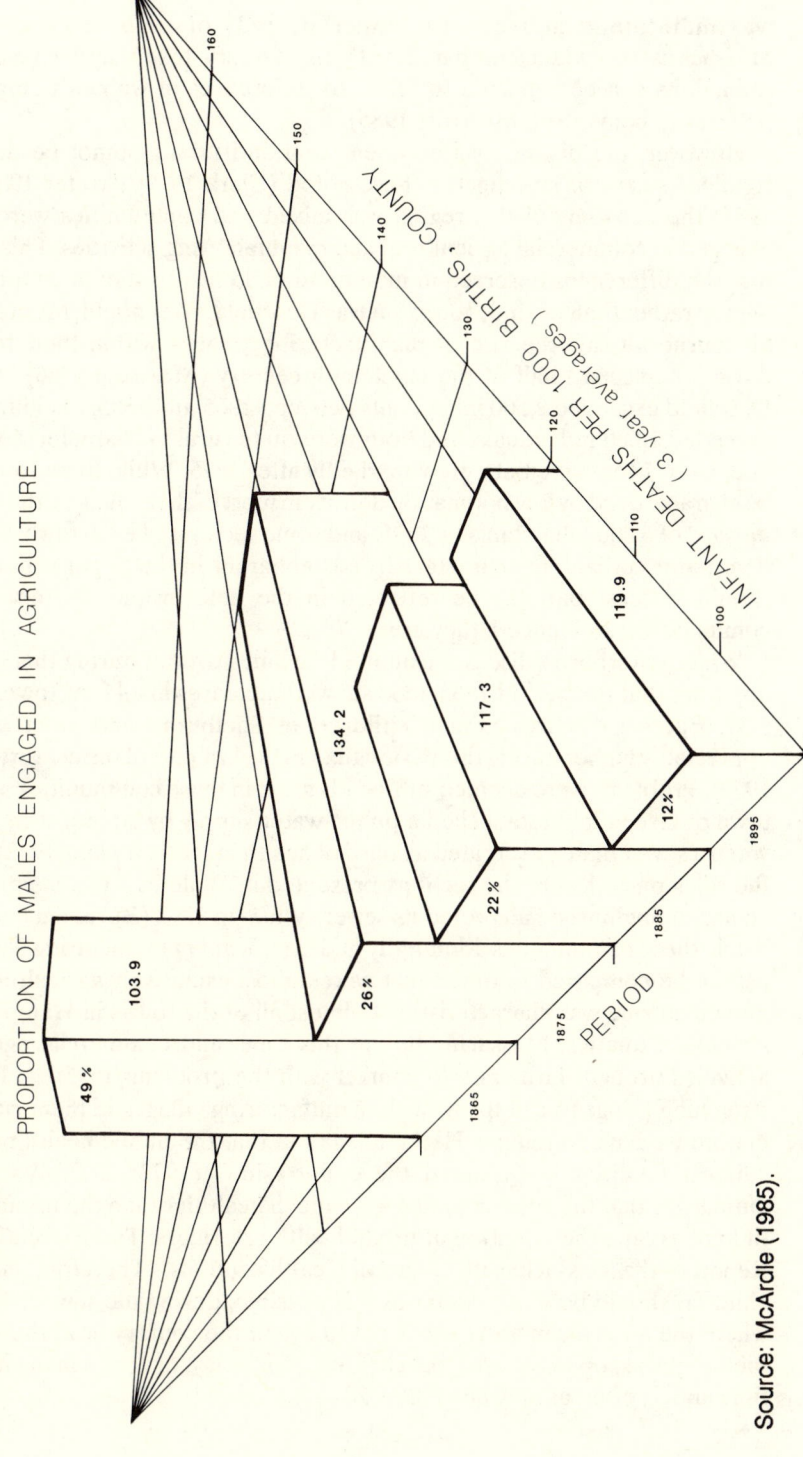

Figure 9.2
Proportion of Males Engaged in Agriculture and Infant Mortality Rate Over Four Periods in Nineteenth-Century Franklin County, Massachusetts.

Source: McArdle (1985).

was maintained actively for longer periods of time in rural western Massachusetts, when compared with the factory towns and cities, further reductions can be expected to relate to differences in women's employment patterns (Phelps 1912; McArdle 1985).

However, the distinctions between rural and urban cannot be drawn too rigidly. As several investigators have noted (Clark 1979; Paynter 1982; Pruitt 1984) the economy of this region was mixed and communities were actively engaged in commercial agricultural and manufacturing activities. This suggests that the differences observed in infant and child health should be a matter of degree rather than of kind. Towns such as Deerfield, Greenfield, Montague, and Shelburne all saw the rise of manufacturing villages within their townships during the second half of the nineteenth century (McArdle 1985). Although Deerfield exceeded 2,500 inhabitants between 1865 and 1895, Shelburne never exceeded 1,600 individuals, and both were quite rural in character. Greenfield and, later, Montague both grew markedly after 1875. While these towns could be characterized by low population density in most of their villages, they reached upward of 6,000 inhabitants by 1895, and some sections of each town were quite dense and "urban" in character. Trends apparent in the larger urban centers should at least partially be reflected in the demographic history of these communities, and indeed, they are.

While waterborne diseases exhibited declines overall during this time, it is apparent that the period 1865-1880 showed increases in all four towns (Figure 9.3). Enteric diseases among children in Shelburne and Deerfield were appreciably higher during this period than in the last part of the century (Meindl 1979). Problems were deemed sufficently great in these communities so that the town of Greenfield established a public water supply by aqueduct in 1869 and voted a sewer plan and created a board of health in 1880 (Jenkins 1982). Among the rules passed were the sections presented in Table 9.3. The manufacturing village of Shelburne Falls voted its sewer system in 1892 (Burnham et al. 1958). While these communities admittedly had significant manufacturing activity and cannot be compared to towns that were almost exclusively agricultural, some manufacturing was characteristic of almost all of the towns in Hampshire and Franklin Counties, Massachusetts, at this time, and commercial agricultural activities brought farmers into contact with the problems in cities. It may be stretching things to call towns with manufacturing villages in them rural, but I believe we have to temper Higgs' allegation that the public health movement "almost completely bypassed the countryside" (1973: 187). We also can emphasize that the rural counties were much healthier than the urban and this did not escape the attention of urban health reformers. The Eleventh Annual Report of the Massachusetts Board of Health cautions, "Therefore, infants and children should be taken, so far as it is possible, during the summer to places where the air is clean and cool: if not to live in the country or at the seashore, then to parks, open squares, beaches, etc., for a day, or for as many hours at a time and as often as may be" (1879: 20–21).

Figure 9.3
Deaths From All Waterborne Diseases in Deerfield, Shelburne,
Greenfield, and Montague, Massachusetts, 1850–1910.

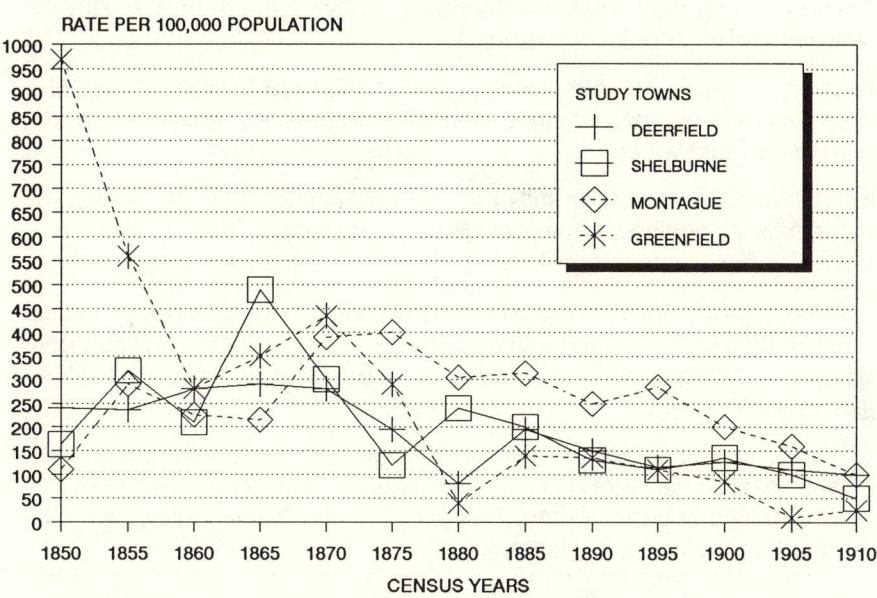

Source: Alan C. Swedlund

Thus far I have made only passing mention of seasonal peaks in mortality, but this was a significant feature of infant and childhood diseases, and it was well recognized by observers of the period (Massachusetts State Board of Health 1873). The pattern varied from region to region. In New Orleans the highest mortality tended to be in May, in Chicago and New York in July (Lentzner and Condran 1985), and in parts of Massachusetts the peaks were seen in August and September. While sharp annual increases are readily apparent in the larger cities, the rural areas would show more sporadic annual trends. Tests for periodicity in summer-fall epidemics in Franklin County are currently being investigated. Nevertheless, the seasonal epidemics were present and caused Dr. Charles Knowlton, a physician in the rural community of Ashfield, to write to the *Boston Medical and Surgical Journal* (1845) about the "autumnal fevers." Meindl (1980) has demonstrated the seasonality in dysenteric diseases for the towns of Deerfield and Shelburne.

These epidemics most severely affected infants and, secondarily, young children. The diagnoses tend to be of various gastroenteric diseases, and if one lumps the gastroenteric diseases along with "fevers" and "convulsions" (common symptoms of severe dehydration), the incidences can be staggering. The cause of death in such cases was probably the nonspecific pneumonia-diarrhea complex that is common

Table 9.3
Sections of the Rules of the Greenfield Board of Health, 1880.

Section 1. No person shall use the public street for the deposit of filth, sink-water, slops or offal of any kind.

Section 2. No person shall throw any dead animal or fowl into any public place or reservoir, road or stream in town, or cause any animal to be drowned in said waters.

Section 3. No person shall sell or offer for sale in this town any diseased meat, milk, or unwholesome provisions of any kind, or have such in his possession with intent to sell.

Section 4. Every householder in whose dwelling there shall occur a case of small pox, varioloid, diphtheria or scarlet fever shall immediately upon discovery thereof report such cases to the Board of Health, and receive instructions therefrom.

Section 5. No person from any dwellings wherein a case of contagious disease exists shall attend any school, church, or public gathering of any kind, or take any book or magazine to or from the public library without a permit from the Board of Health.

Source: Jenkins (1982:147).

in the Third World today and widespread historically (Kunitz 1984). Symptomatically the disease would take a similar course whether it be caused by E. coli, shigella, or salmonella, as Lentzner and Condran have noted (1985). The timing of these outbreaks corresponds to very warm times of the year when incubation of bacteria in food and milk would be at a very high level and when a new group of susceptibles (the past year's births) would be available. Cheney (1984) has been able to link the frequency and intensity of these periods to a number of health risks in the city of Philadelphia. These will be amplified somewhat below.

In sum, rural areas are perhaps distinctively different in the magnitude of their rates of disease, but they share many of the same experiences of their urban counterparts. That they were safer, better places to live cannot be disputed seriously; that they offered similar risks and complications is also apparently true. Similar contrasts are no doubt valid in Western Europe (McKeown 1976) as well as in America (Kunitz 1984). In contrast, many studies of rural-urban differentials in infant and childhood mortality in the Third World show that the rural areas have higher levels (e.g., DaVanzo, Butz, and Habicht 1983; Trussell and Preston 1982). The cause of these differences does not appear to be "rurality" per se, and when such variables as sanitation methods and mother's education (and, no doubt, poverty) are controlled, the differences disappear. In historical, rural New England, as we have noted, literacy and education were high, sanitation probably better than most cities, and poverty expected at least to show less variance. Modern cities in Latin America, Africa, and parts of Asia may have antiquated sewer and water systems and insufficient public health services, but many of them may compare favorably with the almost complete absence of such amenities in American cities of 1860.

Nutrition

Wray (1978) and others have pointed out that it is the artifically fed infant, both historically and in contemporary high mortality populations, who risks not only a higher likelihood of contamination, but also a higher chance of undernutrition or malnutrition that leaves him/her less able to withstand infection. The relationship between bottle feeding of cows' milk or infant formulas and infantile diseases was well known by health officials and many mothers, yet during the latter part of the nineteenth century and well into the twentieth, bottle feeding continued to be a very popular option. This pattern deserves some further comment, with emphasis on the systemic relationship between feeding practices and nutrition.

Apple (1981) has described in detail the conjugation of forces that produced a high incidence of formula feeding between 1870 and 1940. She describes the development of an ideology of "scientific motherhood" in which physicians and companies producing infant formulas taught that the modern solution to feeding one's child was by the bottle. Some of the major companies still in business today were producing a variety of food products as early as the 1860s and 1870s. Some were nothing more than wheat flour, or cereal and perhaps some sugar, but by the end of the nineteenth century many formulas did have nutritional ingredients. Mothers were frequently advised by physicians or early child care manuals to supplement breastfeeding with cereal or crackers dissolved in water. Apple also demonstrates that artificial feeding of infants was as popular among the well-to-do as the poor, but perhaps less so for middle-class women who were housewives or worked at home. The well-to-do would likely be better educated and have access to more hygenic circumstances than the poor. By 1889 it is estimated that the artificial food industry was an $8-10 million business and that 10,000,000 nursing bottles were produced in 1885 (Apple 1981: 315).

Also during the 1880s condensed milk was developed and became available in Europe and the United States. Since many physicians believed that boiling whole cow's milk would destroy its nutritive value, condensed milk afforded a cleaner, safer alternative to the milk available to many women, especially urban women. As noted above, although pasteurization was known during the late 1800s, and although some communities adopted milk inspection and pasteurization, most localities did not have effective pasteurization laws until the 1920s. Massachusetts made pasteurization a state requirement in 1928.

Thus, by the early twentieth century the alternatives to breastfeeding may have been reasonably safe and nutritious. The complications, of course, had to do with the conditions under which the formula or milk was prepared and also with the fact that little was known about the immune defenses transmitted to the child through breastfeeding.

Not only was there pressure of one sort to encourage adoption of artificial feeding or at least supplementaion, increasing numbers of women were working away from home and required safe alternatives to breastfeeding. It is reasonable to assume that many of these women worked in factories and shops by necessity of poverty rather than choosing to leave their young children in the care of others. We know that these factors combined to take their toll in urban areas:

> Recent statistics show that in Fall River the death rate among children from cholera infantum is 50 percent more than it is in Boston; and there is reason for the inference that this excess is due to the fact that the Fall River mothers wean their children very early, and feed them on cow's milk, to allow the mothers to resume their mill work. If the cows are tuberculous, the excess of cholera infantum through the infection of the mesenteric glands of the infants would be the natural explanation of excessive mortality. (Shumway 1895:53)

In a follow-up study of Fall River infant mortality conducted in 1908 by the Bureau of Labor (Phelps 1912), the conclusion was that mothers' work outside the home contributed only a small fraction to the total infant death rate. This study was done with considerable care and attention to a host of variables, yet the hypothesis offered by Shumway was not in fact tested. Phelps found that women at home had fewer infant deaths from gastroenteritis than those working but that it was still relatively high (34.6 versus 62.7 percent) and that women at home represented by far the largest portion of the sample. He also found that women at home tended to artifically feed or supplement the child as did working mothers. This would have been expected, given Shumway's perception of the problem. What Phelps was probably measuring was a significant fraction of poor mothers at home on "unpaid maternity leave."

To continue the comparison between urban and rural areas, the obvious hypothesis implied by the above quote is that, as industrialization progressed and increasing numbers of women became engaged in manufacturing and commercial agricultural activities, an increase in deaths associated with artificial feeding practices should be apparent, and this is supported by the Bureau of Labor study, quite expectedly. Overall, and in Franklin County, one should be able to detect a decline in the rates of waterborne diseases as public water supplies and sewage disposal were improved and an increase in diseases from cow's milk and infant formulas as industrialization increased. Although this research is still in an early phase, I believe the trends behave according to expectations. For example, the rates for waterborne infectious diseases declined

Figure 9.4
Tuberculosis Death Rates by Age Group in the Towns of Deerfield, Shelburne, Greenfield, and Montague, Massachusetts, 1850–1910.

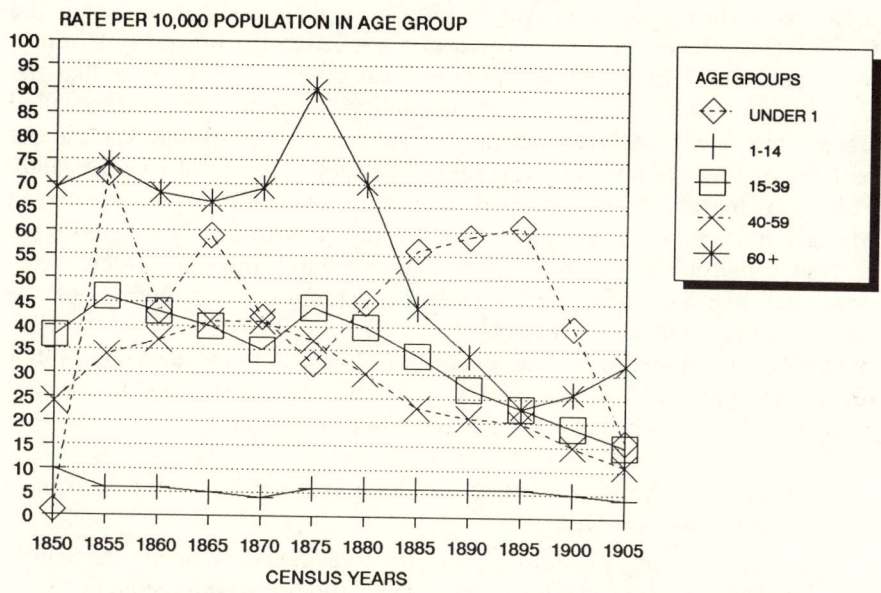

Source: McArdle (1985).

noticeably from 1865 onward. They also remained lowest in the most agricultural of the target communities, Deerfield, and declined most slowly in the latest of the industrializing communities, Montague (Figure 9.4).

The rates of tuberculosis for children under one year of age show a noticeable increase from 1875 to 1895 (McArdle 1985; Meindl 1979). While the registered cases may not be dramatic, I believe we cannot discount the fact that there was much misdiagnosis of tuberculosis at this time. If, for example, some were misclassified as pneumonia or other respiratory diseases we could expect much higher rates. In addition, bovine tuberculosis, which is most likely to be contracted from cow's milk, often infected the alimentary system in children and produced symptoms resembling other gastroenteric infections (Shumway 1895). It is believed that many of the cases of hydrocephaly reported in the historical literature are actually meninginal tuberculosis. Even in 1912 the English physicican George Still reported that 29 percent of the cases of tuberculosis he observed in childhood were due to alimentary infection (1912: 47). The patterns in Franklin Country communities correspond to those in urban areas in direction of trend if not in magnitude.

CONCLUSION

In this somewhat broad review of infant and childhood mortality in the nineteenth century it has been my purpose to describe overall trends, to define the patterns in Massachusetts from 1850 to 1910 and to further delineate the urban-rural differences one can identify by making comparisons with the Connecticut River Valley and, more specifically, Franklin County, Massachusetts. I believe it is apparent that research in an area like the Connecticut Valley can, indeed, add resolution to the already richly detailed story of nineteenth-century mortality. We still have a great deal to learn about patterns and associations in the rural but developing areas of New England. Further research should confirm, however, that rural areas in western Massachusetts shared in the ills of their urban counterparts. This is not to say that the "quality of life" was not appreciably better, and even nineteenth-century observers like Shumway (1895) were conscientious in pointing out the advantages of being in the country.

Many of the observations and associations found in the Connecticut Valley are preliminary and remain to be tested more rigorously, but the general patterns of infant mortality in rural areas with mixed economies seem clear:

1. There was an important health transition in western Massachusetts in the nineteenth century.

2. Contrary to some previous reports, the transition developed relatively late in the century, was not strictly linear, and was counteracted by the experience of infants and young children.

3. Health professionals of the late nineteenth and early twentieth cen-turies, despite their limited diagnostic capabilities, were acutely aware of most of the proximate causes and many of the intervening variables in infant and early childhood mortality.

The models, rudimentary though they were, resemble closely those postulated by epidemiologists working in developing areas today. Future research should delineate more accurately: (1) the secular trends of the principal infectious diseases associated with mortality; (2) the role of family formation variables, including fertility decline, that contribute to high risk families, and their subsequent attenuation; and, (3) the relationship between historical processes of development and contemporaneous ones with respect to changing health patterns.

It is reasonable to expect that then, as now, poverty and the differential access to resources were major intervening variables. Meindl (1980) has already demonstrated the advantages in survivorship to age 15 that were gained by being born of parents in the upper 50 percent wealth class in nineteenth-century Deerfield. Also 62.6 percent of that same upper wealth class consisted of farmers who owned their own land and presumably raised much of their own food. This was true of only 31.5 percent for the lower wealth class. Moreover, most of the mortality difference in relation to wealth is explained by maternal age differences between the class groupings—with lower wealth class mothers being significantly younger (Meindl: 1980 246–47). It would appear that the explanations sufficient to account for the well-documented and multivariate nature of infant mortality during the nineteenth century are indeed germane to contemporary case studies.

It is tempting to ask what further analogies are possible between the experience in the historical United States and the developing world today. Preston (1985) has recently presented a good case for the use of historical data from the United States as a control in measuring the contribution of resources and knowledge on current infant mortality levels in developing countries. Wray (1978: 213–15) has observed that, with respect to our understanding of the importance of breastfeeding, the experiences in the western world of 50 to 100 years ago is very appropriate to what is happening in developing areas today. The combined effects of risk of contamination in artificial feeding, lower nutritional value of some food supplements, and loss of transmitable immunoglobulins have taken their toll in Thirld World countries much the same way they did in Europe and America during the Industrial Revolution. If the recent experience with companies producing infant formulas is compared with Apple's review (1981, 1987) of nineteenth- and early twentieth-century marketing practices, it seems that history has repeated itself in this respect as well.

One should be cautious in extending these analogies too far, however, and especially with respect to the region described here. Nineteenth-century rural Massachusetts achieved literacy levels and standards of living that were not shared in many parts of the United States. The early establishment of vital registration systems and boards of health acted as a catalyst to effective responses to health problems at the local and state levels. Massachusetts historically, as today, enjoyed one of the lowest levels of infant mortality in the United States. The level of documentation permits detailed observation of the historical process, but Massachusetts no doubt reflects somewhat favorable levels of mortality at any point in time and in both rural and urban settings, when contrasted with other regions of the United States.

NOTE

Many people have made constructive comments on an earlier version of this paper. I would especially like to thank Gerald Friedman, Nancy Folbre, Sheila Ryan Johansson, Stephen Kunitz, Alan McArdle, and Richard Meindl. Drs. Meindl and McArdle have contributed very substantively to the data and their interpretation.

REFERENCES

Abbott, S. W. 1897. The vital statistics of Massachusetts: A forty years' summary (1856–1896). *28th Annual Report of the Massachusetts Board of Health.* Boston.

American Association for the Prevention of Infant Mortality. Annual Meeting Reports, 1910–1913. Boston.

Apple, R. D. 1987. *Mothers and Medicine: A Social History of Infant Feeding, 1890–1950.* Madison: University of Wisconsin Press.

———. 1981. "How shall I feed my baby?" Infant feeding in the United States, 1870–1940. Ph.D. diss., University of Wisconsin-Madison.

Burnham, W. F., E. H. Taylor, H. P. Ware, and T. W. Watkins. 1958. *History and Tradition of Shelburne, Massachusetts.* Springfield, Mass.: Pond-Eckberg.

Burnet, M., and D. O. White. 1972. *Natural History of Infectious Disease.* 4th ed. Cambridge: Cambridge University Press.

Cheney, R. A. 1984. Seasonal aspects of infant and childhood mortality: Philadelphia, 1865–1920. *Journal of Interdisciplinary History* 14(3):561–585.

Clark, C. 1979. The household economy, market exchange, and the rise of capitalism in the Connecticut Valley, 1800–1860. *Journal of Social History* 13:169–189.

Condran, G. A., and R. A. Cheney. 1980. Mortality trends in Philadelphia: Age and cause-specific death rates, 1870–1930. *Demography* 19(1):97–123.

Condran G. A., and E. Crimmins. 1980. Mortality differentials between rural and urban areas of states in the northeastern United States, 1890–1900. *Journal of Historical Geography* 6(2):179–202.

———. 1979. A description and evaluation of mortality data in Federal Census: 1850–1900. *Historical Methods* 12(1):1–23.

Crimmins E., and G. A. Condran. 1983. Mortality variation in U.S. cities in 1900: A two-level explanation by cause of death and underlying factors. *Social Science History* 7(1):31–60.

DaVanzo, J., W. P. Butz, and J.-P. Habicht. 1983. How biological and behavioural influences on mortality in Malaysia vary during the first year of life. *Population Studies* 37:381–402.

Fogel, R. W. 1986. Nutrition and the decline in mortality since 1700: Some preliminary findings. In *Long-term Factors in American Economic Growth.* S. L. Engerman and R. E. Galloway, eds. Chicago: University of Chicago Press.

Ginsberg, C. A. 1983. Sex-specific mortality and the economic value of children in nineteenth century Massachusetts. Ph.D. diss., University of California, Berkeley.

Gortmaker, S. L. 1979. Poverty and infant mortality in the United States. *American Sociological Review* 44(2):280–97.

Gutman, R. 1959. Birth and death registration in Massachusetts, III: The system achieves a form, 1849–1869. *Millbank Memorial Fund Quarterly* 37(3):302–10.

———. 1958. Birth and death registration in Massachusetts, II: The inauguration of a modern system, 1800–1849. *Millbank Memorial Fund Quarterly* 36:373–402.

Haines, M. R. 1985. Inequality and childhood mortality: A comparison of England and Wales, 1911, and the United States, 1900. *Journal of Economic History* 65(4):874–913.

———. 1979. The use of model life tables to estimate mortality for the United States in the late nineteenth century. *Demography* 16(2):289–312.

———. 1977. Mortality in nineteenth-century America: Estimates from New York and Pennsylvania census data, 1865 and 1900. *Demography* 14(3):311–31.

Haines M. R., and S. H. Preston. 1984. Cities, ethnicity, and child mortality in the United States in 1900. Paper presented at the SSHA Meetings, Toronto, Canada, October.

Higgs, R. 1973. Mortality in rural America, 1870–1920: Estimates and conjectures. *Explorations in Economic History* 10(2):177–95.

Jenkins, P. 1982. *The Conservative Rebel: A Social History of Greenfield, Massachusetts.* Greenfield, Mass.: Town of Greenfield.

Johansson, S. R. 1987. Centuries of childhood/centuries of parenting: Phillipe Aries and the modernization of privileged infancy. *Journal of Family History* 12:343–65.

————. 1984. Deferred infanticide: Excess female mortality during childhood. In *Infanticide in Animals and Man.* G. Hausfater and S. Hrdy, eds. New York: Aldine.

Knowlton, C. 1845. The autumnal fevers of New England. *Boston Medical and Surgical Journal* 32:69–73.

Kunitz, S. J. 1984. Mortality change in America, 1620–1920. *Human Biology* 56(3):559–82.

————. 1983. Speculations on the European mortality decline. *Economic History Review* 36:349–64.

Leavitt, J. W. 1982. *The Healthiest City: Milwaukee and the Politics of Health Reform.* Princeton: Princeton University Press.

Lentzner, H., and G. Condran. 1985. Paper presented at the Annual Meeting of the Population Association of America, March. Boston.

McArdle, A. 1985. Occupational mortality in nineteenth century Franklin County Massachusetts. Ph.D. diss., University of Massachusetts, Amherst.

McKeown, T. 1976. *The Modern Rise of Population.* New York: Academic.

McKinlay, J. B., and S. M. McKinlay. 1977. The questionable contribution of medical measures to the decline of mortality in the United States in the twentieth century. *Millbank Memorial Fund Quarterly* 55:405–28.

McNeill, W. H. 1980. *The Human Condition: An Ecological and Historical View.* Princeton: Princeton University Press.

Massachusetts State Board of Health. 1873. *Fourth Annual Report, Infant Mortality.* Public Document, 30:194–233. Boston: Wright & Potter.

Massachusetts State Board of Health. 1879. *Eleventh Annual Report.* Public Document, 30. Boston: Band, Avery & Co.

Meckel, R. A. 1980. The awful responsibility of motherhood: American health reform and the prevention of infant and child mortality before 1913. Ph.D. diss., University of Michigan.

Meeker, E. 1972. The improving health of the United States, 1800–1915. *Explorations in Economic History* 9(4):353–73.

Meindl, R. S. 1980. Family formation and health in nineteenth century Franklin County, Massachusetts. In *Genealogical Demography.* B. Dyke and W. Morrill, eds. New York: Academic.

————. 1979. Environmental and demographic correlates of mortality in nineteenth century Franklin County, Massachusetts. Ph.D. diss., University of Massachusetts, Amherst.

Miller, C. A. 1985. Infant mortality in the U.S. *Scientific American* 253(1):31–37.

Paynter, R. S. 1982. *Models of Spatial Inequality.* New York: Academic.

Petersen, J. 1979. The impact of sanitary reform upon American urban planning, 1840–1890. *Journal of Social History* 13(1):83–103.

Phelps, E. B. 1912. *Infant Mortality and its Relation to Women's Employment: A Study of Massachusetts Statistics.* Pts. I and II. *Report on Condition of Woman and Child Wage-Earners in the United States*, vol. 13. Washington, D.C.: Bureau of Labor.

Preston, S. H. 1985. Present patterns of demographic change in light of past experience. Proceedings of the IUSSP (Florence, Italy).

Pruitt, B. 1984. Self-sufficiency and the agricultural economy of eighteenth-century Massachusetts. *William and Mary Quarterly* 41:333–64.

Rosenkrantz, B. G. 1972. *Public Health and the State: Changing Views in Massachusetts, 1842–1936.* Cambridge: Harvard University Press.

Schofield, R. S. 1983. The impact of scarcity and plenty on population change in England, 1541–1871. *Journal of Interdisciplinary History* 14(2):265–91.

Scrimshaw, S. 1984. Infanticide in human populations: societal and individual concerns. In *Infanticide in Animals and Man.* G. Hausfater and S. Hrdy, eds. New York: Aldine.

————. 1978. Infant mortality and behavior in the regulation of family size. *Population and Development Review* 4:383–403.

Shumway, H. 1895. *A Hand-Book on Tuberculosis Among Cattle.* Boston: Roberts Brothers.

Smith, D. S. 1983. Differential mortality in the United States before 1900. *Journal of Interdisciplinary History* 13:735–59.

Still, G. F. 1912. *Common Disorders and Diseases of Childhood.* London: Oxford Medical Publications, Oxford University Press.

Strauss, L. G. 1917. *Disease in Milk: The Remedy Pasteurization: The Life Work of Nathan Strauss.* New York: E. P. Dutton.

Swedlund, A. C., R. S. Meindl, and M. I. Gradie. 1980. Family reconstitution in the Connecticut Valley: Progress on record linkage and the mortality survey. In *Genealogical Demography.* B. Dyke and W. Morrill, eds. New York: Academic.

Swedlund, A. C., H. Temkin, and R. S. Meindl. 1976. Population studies in the Connecticut Valley: Prospectus. *Journal of Human Evolution* 5:75–93.

Trussell, J., and S. H. Preston. 1982. Estimating the covariates of childhood mortality from retrospective reports of mothers. *Health Policy and Education* 3:1–36.

Vinovskis, M. A. 1981. *Fertility in Massachusetts from the Revolution to the Civil War.* New York: Academic.

————. 1972. Mortality rates and trends in Massachusetts before 1860. *Journal of Economic History* 32:184–213.

Whorton, J. C. 1982. *Crusaders for Fitness.* Princeton: Princeton University Press.

Woodbury, R. 1926. *Infant Mortality and its Causes.* Baltimore: Williams & Wilkins.

Wray, J. D. 1978. Maternal nutrition, breast-feeding, and infant survival. In *Nutrition and Human Reproduction.* W. H. Mosley, ed. New York: Plenum.

Wrigley, E. A., and R. S. Schofield. 1981. *The Population History of England, 1541–1871.* Cambridge: Harvard University Press.

10 HISTORICAL EPIDEMIOLOGY OF SMALLPOX IN KITEE, FINLAND

L. B. Jorde, K. Pitkänen, J. H. Mielke, J. O. Fellman and A. W. Eriksson

Most epidemiologic studies are confined to a relatively short time period. Yet much can be learned about the characteristics of infectious diseases by studying their long-term behavior in well-defined, spatially subdivided populations. Studies of measles epidemics, for example, have shown that their duration and periodicity are strongly affected by population size and density (Black 1966; Cliff and Haggett 1984; Cliff et al. 1981). The insights gained in these analyses aid not only in furthering an understanding of infectious disease epidemiology but also in making public health policy decisions (Frauenthal 1981).

Such studies can also help to answer important questions in historical demography. In particular, a great deal of debate exists regarding the importance of medical intervention in the decline of mortality rates during the past two centuries. Some researchers have concluded that medical intervention has played a major role in mortality reduction (Cherry 1980; Preston 1976), while others assign it much less importance (Collins 1982; McKeown 1976, 1979; McKinlay and McKinlay 1977). Smallpox is an especially good candidate for historical analysis of this question. It was a major cause of death in much of Europe during the late seventeenth and eighteenth centuries (Hopkins 1984). It was comparatively easy to diagnose, ensuring the reliability of historical disease records. And a specific form of intervention, Jennerian vaccination, was introduced at well-documented points in time.

In a previous study (Mielke et al. 1984), smallpox mortality was analyzed in the Åland Islands, Finland. Spectral analysis of a 140-year time series of smallpox deaths demonstrated a strong seven-year periodicity, reflecting the amount of time necessary to build up a cohort of nonimmune individuals through whom the virus could spread. Vaccination, introduced in Finland in 1803, considerably reduced the number of annual smallpox deaths and changed

Figure 10.1
A Map of Finland, Showing the Location of Kitee.[1]

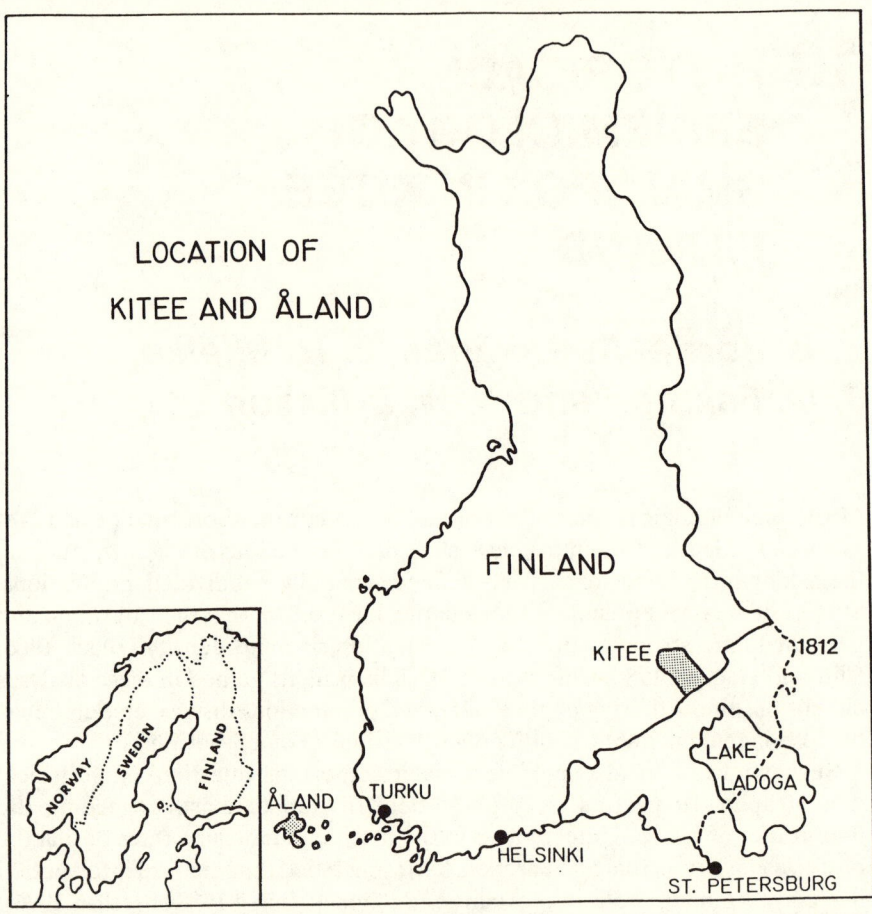

[1] In southeastern Finland the inner boundary is that of 1743 and the outer boundary is 1812.

the periodicity from seven to eight years. In addition, the age distribution of smallpox deaths changed. Prior to vaccination, smallpox had been almost exclusively a childhood disease; those who did not die from the disease acquired a lifelong immunity. After the introduction of vaccination, a much larger portion of the smallpox deaths consisted of adults. This was due in part to the fact that many people were not periodically revaccinated and thus lost their immunity later in life. Examination of population sizes and migration rates in Åland's fifteen parishes showed that the probability of a parish's being affected by an epidemic was highly correlated with its overall migration rate and population size.

This chapter presents an analysis of a 170-year time series of smallpox deaths in two municipalities located on the Finnish mainland, Kitee and Rääkkylä. The time series begins more than fifty years before the introduction of vaccination and continues until the last smallpox epidemic occurred in this population. The purpose of the analysis is to compare the spatial and temporal patterns of smallpox deaths in this mainland population with those of the more isolated population of Åland. It will be shown that many of the observed differences in epidemiologic patterns can be attributed directly to the highly contrasting ecological settings of the two populations.

Until the late nineteenth century, Kitee and Rääkkylä composed a single unit, with Kitee being the Lutheran "mother parish" and Rääkkylä a subsidiary chapelry. Unless stated otherwise, the two municipalities will be referred to together as Kitee. Kitee is located in the province of Northern Karelia in eastern Finland (Figure 10.1). Since Karelia lies on Finland's border with the Soviet Union (Russia), Kitee's ownership has alternated between Russia, Sweden, and Finland. During much of the Middle Ages, Kitee was ruled by Russia, but, along with much of Karelia, it was ceded to Sweden in 1617. During the seventeenth and early eighteenth centuries, most of the original population of this area, who were members of the Greek Orthodox Church, migrated to Russia. They were replaced by Lutherans who originated in other parts of eastern Finland. In 1721, Sweden lost territory to Russia, including the eastern part of Kitee. Kitee was then a border parish until 1812, when parts of Karelia were placed under Finnish rule. From 1809 to 1917, Finland was an autonomous state under Russian rule. Finland became independent in 1917, but much of Karelia was lost to the Soviet Union after World War II, making Kitee a border parish again.

After the Great Northern War (1700–1721), Kitee's population numbered only about 2,700, but it grew rapidly during the eighteenth century (as did most of Finland). By 1800, 10,000 people lived in Kitee, and the population reached 14,200 by 1850 and 17,700 by 1900. Today, the municipalities of Kitee and Rääkkylä consist of 15,400 individuals. The annual population growth rate from 1722 to 1800 was high, averaging 1.6 percent. Growth slowed to 0.9 percent from 1800 to 1850 and to 0.4 percent from 1850 to 1900. Much of the reduction in growth rate during the nineteenth century was due to emigration to other parts of Finland and to Russia.

MATERIALS AND METHODS

The primary source of data for this study is parish records kept by Lutheran ministers. A Swedish ecclesiastical law formulated in 1686 (Finland was a territory of Sweden at this time) dictated uniform instructions for keeping records of baptisms, burials, marriages, and interparish migration. By the mid-1700s, the death records included the dates of death and burial, the name of the individual, the individual's occupation (parent's occupation was given for children), the place of residence at death, the age at death, and the cause of death. Information on vaccination was obtained from written reports of the

Figure 10.2
Smallpox Deaths per Year in Kitee.

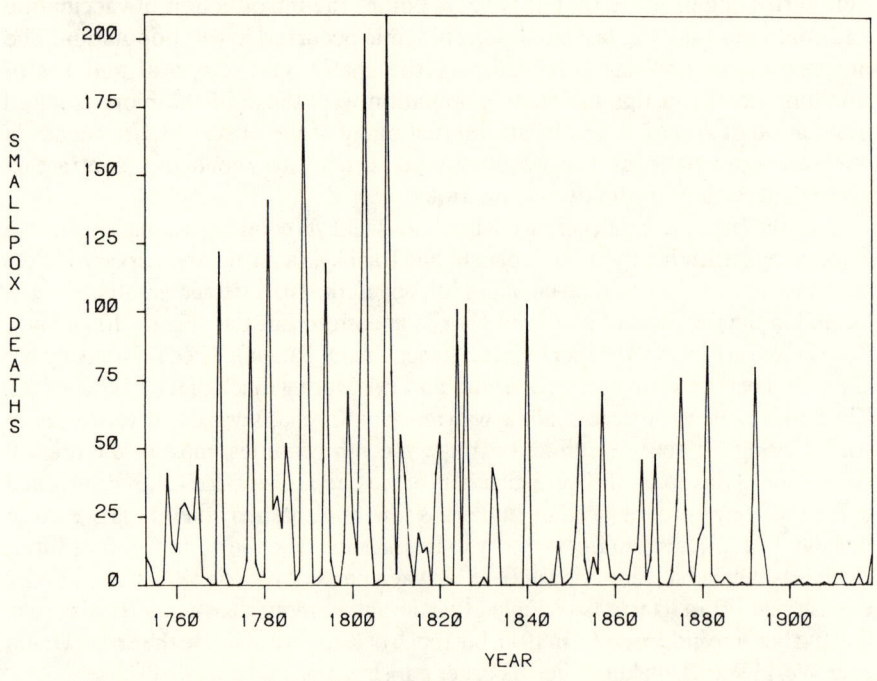

district physicians and vaccinators for Kitee and from published sources for the entire country of Finland (Björkstén 1908; Fagerlund 1924).

Since cause of death was recorded by parish priests, caution must be exercised when considering their diagnoses (Pitkänen 1977). Vague or conflicting causes of death were sometimes given. Although smallpox is one of the more easily diagnosed diseases, it seems to have been confused occasionally with other ailments, in particular, measles or scarlet fever. In this study, most conflicts of diagnosis were resolved by consulting reports of the district physicians.

Comparative data on smallpox deaths in the Åland Islands were taken partly from Mielke et al. (1984). Some additional material from Åland is presented here. Smallpox deaths for the entire country of Finland for the years 1774–1920 were taken from Fagerlund (1924), and their rates were estimated from a sample of parish death records for the years 1751–1773.

To assess the relative impact of smallpox on total mortality in Kitee, proportionate mortality ratios (PMRs) were calculated for each twenty-five- year time period. The PMR is simply the percentage of the total number of deaths in a time period that are attributed to a specific cause (Mausner and Bahn 1974). Age-specific PMRs were also computed by dividing the sample into discrete age groups.

Age-standardized PMRs were then calculated using the deaths in Kitee from 1750 to 1877 as a standard schedule.

Age-specific death rates due to smallpox were also calculated for Kitee and the Åland Islands. For standardization by age, the standard population used was that of Finland in 1880.

Vaccination figures are based on the number of children vaccinated each year. Children were generally vaccinated at about one year of age, and adult revaccinations are not included in the figures. The proportion of individuals vaccinated (PV) is estimated as

$$PV = \frac{v_t}{b_{t-1} - i_t} \times 100$$

where v_t is the number of children vaccinated in year t; b_{t-1} is the number of births in year t-1; and i_t is the number of infant deaths in year t.

To examine seasonal variation, smallpox deaths were grouped into monthly intervals for the total time period and for the separate periods 1750–1809 and 1830–1919. The transitional period 1810–1829, during which vaccination was introduced, was omitted. Edwards's (1961) test for seasonality was used to determine whether the observed variation was statistically significant. Edwards's test also fits a sine curve to the data. The ratio of the maximum point of this curve to the minimum point yields a numerical index of the degree of seasonality.

Periodicity in the time series of smallpox deaths was evaluated using spectral analysis. This technique produces a spectral density function, which specifies the amount of amplitude (variance) in the time series at each frequency, f. Frequency is measured in cycles per year. A large value for the spectral density function at $f = 0.25$, for example, would indicate that a large portion of the variance in the series can be expressed as a wave that repeats itself every four years. Further details on spectral analysis can be found in standard textbooks (Chatfield 1975; Jenkins and Watts 1968; Koopmans 1974).

Before estimating the spectral density function, long-term trends were removed from the time series by applying a polynomial regression in which the dependent variable was number of deaths and the independent variable was year. The residuals from the regression analysis formed the input series for spectral analysis. The input series was tapered to reduce the interference of estimates from one frequency band upon those from another frequency band. A triangular-shaped weighting function was used in smoothing the spectral density estimates.

RESULTS

Figure 10.2 shows the yearly distribution of smallpox deaths in Kitee from 1750 through 1919. As expected, the number of deaths per year decreases substantially after the period 1810–1830, when Jennerian vaccination was introduced into Kitee. This decrease is especially noteworthy when one considers the appreciable increase in population size during this period. Table 10.1, which gives the percentages of children vaccinated for smallpox in each five-year interval, demonstrates that vaccination became common in Kitee and Rääkkylä during and after the 1826–1830 time interval. After the epidemics of the 1870s, which were especially virulent throughout Europe (Hardy 1983; Mercer 1985), compliance increased substantially. For comparison, data are also given for the Åland Islands and for Finland. Among these populations, Åland clearly had the highest vaccination rates. In general, however, compliance appears to have been quite high in all populations, with the overall vaccination rate ranging from 88.2 percent in Rääkkylä to 99.9 percent in Åland. The average duration of the epidemics changed substantially after the introduction of vaccination. The mean duration for the 1750–1809 period was 474 days. It decreased to 368 days for the years 1810–1829 and to 320 days in the 1830–1919 period.

The impact of smallpox on mortality rates relative to other causes of death is shown by the PMRs in Table 10.2. Before vaccination (i.e., prior to 1825), the PMRs in Kitee ranged from 7 percent to 12 percent, while the PMRs after 1825 ranged from less than 1 percent to 5 percent. The age-standardized PMRs for Åland are considerably higher than those of Kitee prior to vaccination (14 percent to 16 percent). After vaccination was introduced, however, the PMRs for Åland were consistently lower than those of Kitee.

Table 10.2 also gives cause-specific death rates for smallpox, standardized by age. The picture here is somewhat different from that given by the PMRs. The death rate for Kitee is higher than that of Åland in the 1775–1799 period and thereafter. During the 1750–1774 period, smallpox deaths in Kitee were probably underestimated somewhat, due to the confusion of smallpox with measles. Thus, in this first time period, the rates for Kitee and Åland are probably quite similar.

Age-specific PMRs for Kitee are given in Table 10.3. In general, PMRs are considerably higher for children under age 15 than for older individuals. Smallpox was especially common among the 3–10 year age group, accounting for one-fifth to one-third of all deaths prior to the advent of vaccination. It is especially interesting to examine the way in which the PMRs changed in different age groups after vaccination was introduced. For all groups under age 15, PMRs underwent a dramatic reduction after 1825 (the reduction for the < 1 year age group is less substantial because vaccination usually took place at about one year of age). However, for those over age 15 — particularly the 16–25 and 26–40 year groups — PMRs increased substantially, going from less than 2 percent to 3–4 percent in the 16–25 year group. Vaccination thus converted smallpox from a childhood disease to one that affected both adults and children.

The age-specific PMRs for Åland are given in Table 10.4. The PMRs are much higher in the first two time periods in Åland than in Kitee, with smallpox

Table 10.1
Percentage Vaccinated in Kitee, Rääkkylä, Åland, and Finland, 1811–1920.[1]

Time Interval	Kitee	Rääkkylä	Åland[2]	Finland
1811–1815	35.4 (425)	4.3 (26)	96.2	49.7
1816–20	58.0 (655)	52.7 (314)	97.2	62.7
1821–25	11.0 (135)	8.5 (61)	52.3	55.7
1826–30	129.6 (1,713)	138.3 (1,199)	73.2	96.5
1831–35	55.9 (664)	70.0 (427)	117.8	83.3
1836–40	103.4 (1,068)	80.3 (439)	101.2	87.5
1841–45	119.5 (1,573)	101.5 (613)	95.8	92.0
1846–50	98.6 (1,343)	79.2 (471)	126.9	95.3
1851–55	94.4 (1,459)	77.9 (472)	103.4	90.6
1856–60	98.8 (1,359)	125.1 (708)	108.3	89.8
1861–65	88.8 (1,466)	106.0 (776)	100.9	90.7
1866–70	81.7 (1,086)	79.3 (486)	97.7	86.7
1871–75	111.2 (1,771)	101.8 (796)	101.8	97.8
1876–80	92.2 (1,316)	93.4 (684)	94.1	90.7
1881–85[3]	102.6 (921)	100.6 (497)	107.6	98.2
1886–90[4]	105.6 (1,273)	116.7 (718)	96.9	105.6
1891–95	108.5 (1,224)	108.5 (667)	107.6	101.5
1896–1900	96.8 (1,564)	110.0 (994)	101.5	96.6
1901–1905	107.1 (1,303)	87.9 (727)	102.0	92.3
1906–10	95.7 (1,690)	89.1 (985)	101.4	92.3
1911–15	96.1 (1,572)	89.8 (887)	104.8	94.2
1916–20[5]	98.4 (1,254)	94.7 (571)	97.3	81.4
TOTALS	91.2	88.2	99.9	90.2

[1] Actual number of vaccinated children for Kitee and Rääkkylä in parentheses. Some percentages are greater than 100 because of vaccinations of individuals older than 1 year of age and because of vaccinations of children who died before their first birthday.

[2] These figures differ slightly from the ones given in Mielke et al. (1984) because of the inclusion here of some new data.

[3] Number of vaccinated children in Kitee and Rääkkylä are not known for 1882–83.

[4] Number of vaccinated children in Kitee and Rääkkylä are not known for 1887, 1893, and 1905.

[5] Number of vaccinated children in Rääkkylä are not known for 1918.

Table 10.2
Age-Standardized Proportionate Mortality Ratios (Per 1000 Deaths)
and Cause-Specific Death Rates (Per 10,000 Population) for
Smallpox in Kitee and Åland.

Time Interval	Death Rates[1]		PMRs[2]	
	Kitee	*Åland*	*Kitee*	*Åland*
1750–74	19.8 (371)[3]	27.7	73.0	162.2
1775–99	36.4 (924)	26.2	120.8	142.4
1800–24	32.3 (999)	9.7	105.4	51.1
1825–49	9.6 (321)	2.9	47.1	11.0
1850–74	9.4 (374)	5.6	35.9	22.0
1875–99	6.2 (264)	0.5	29.9	3.2
1900–19	0.8 (29)	0.0	4.9	0.0

[1] The standard population used for estimation of cause-specific death rates was that of Finland in 1880.

[2] The standard age schedule used for estimation of PMRs was based on deaths in Kitee from 1750–1877.

[3] Actual number of smallpox deaths in Kitee are given in parentheses.

accounting for nearly half the deaths in the 3–10 year age group. It is also important to note that the PMRs for the 10–15 and 15–25 age groups are quite high in Åland during these time periods, while they are rather low in Kitee. Once vaccination commences, however, the rates fall more rapidly in Åland than in Kitee.

Tables 10.5 and 10.6 give the age-specific death rates due to smallpox for Kitee and Åland. Most of the patterns seen in the age-specific PMRs are observable in the age-specific death rates. As in Tables 10.3 and 10.4, the data in Tables 10.5 and 10.6 show that the age shift in death rates after vaccination is much more pronounced in Åland.

Figure 10.3 shows the monthly distribution of smallpox deaths for the total time period. There is clearly a predominance of deaths during the spring, with the highest percentage occurring in May. Application of the test for seasonality shows that this spring peak is highly significant (chi-square = 145, $p < 0.000001$). The monthly distributions for the 1750–1809 and 1830–1919 time periods are given in Figure 10.4. Although both time periods have clear peaks in the late spring and early summer (both significant at $p < 0.000001$), seasonality is much more pronounced for the later time period. The ratio of the maximum point of the fitted curve to the minimum point is only 1.3 for the 1750–1809 period, while it increases to 3.9 for the 1830–1919 period. Also the peak shifts from May in the early period to June in the later period.

Figure 10.5 is a spectral density plot for the total Kitee time series of smallpox deaths. The highest peak is seen at a frequency of 0.23 cycles per year, corresponding to a periodicity of 4.4 years. A secondary peak occurs at a frequency of 0.15 (period = 6.7 years). The results of a division of the time series into pre- and postvaccination time periods (1750–1820 and 1821–1919) are given in Figures 10.6 and 10.7, respectively. The peak in Figure 10.6 is seen at a frequency of 0.22 (period = 4.5 years), and the peak in Figure 10.7 is seen at a frequency of 0.15 (period = 6.7 years). The peak in the later time period is somewhat more pronounced than that of the earlier period. The spectral density for the total time period is a composite of the early and later periods, since it contains both of the principal peaks of the two periods.

As one might expect, the frequency of epidemics in Åland and Kitee affects the age distribution of deaths prior to the introduction of vaccination. The age-specific PMRs and death rates (Tables 10.3, 10.4, 10.5 and 10.6) tend to be higher in Åland than in Kitee in the 15–40 year age groups. With less frequent epidemics, older individuals are more likely to be nonimmune and thus die of the disease.

For comparison with Kitee and Åland, spectral density estimates of smallpox deaths for the entire country of Finland (1751–1920) are given in Figure 10.8. Although several peaks exist, the highest one occurs at a frequency of 0.125 (period of eight years). The data were then divided into two time periods, 1751–1824 and 1825–1920. Spectral analysis of these time series (results not shown) indicates a shift from a shorter periodicity (five years) in the earlier time period to a longer one (eight years) in the later time period.

DISCUSSION

As is shown by the PMRs, smallpox accounted for a substantial proportion of deaths in Kitee prior to the introduction of vaccination. In addition, the age-adjusted death rates show that the actual probability of dying of smallpox was moderately high before vaccination became available. The comparison of PMRs and death rates in Kitee and Åland (Table 10.2) presents an interesting puzzle. Why were PMRs higher in Åland than Kitee before vaccination when the age-specific death rates were lower? In part, this reflects the fact that the epidemics in Åland were less frequent than in Kitee. This clearly lowers the probability of dying from smallpox. However, in competition with other causes of death, smallpox was quite "successful" in Åland, as evidenced by the high PMRs. This may be related to the fact that smallpox appears to have greater virulence when individuals are exposed to larger quantities of the virus (Dixon 1962). With less frequent epidemics, a larger proportion of the population was

Table 10.3
Age-Specific Proportionate Mortality Ratios in Kitee (per 1,000 Deaths).

Time Interval	Age Group							
	<1	1–2	3–9	10–14	15–24	25–39	40–59	60+
1750–74	40.3	163.4	198.6	67.2	17.9	3.0	0.0	0.0
1775–99	77.5	256.9	322.2	187.2	12.2	1.8	0.0	0.0
1800–24	97.3	206.0	272.2	112.3	10.1	0.0	0.8	0.0
1825–49	33.8	88.1	119.4	65.4	48.1	3.2	0.0	0.0
1850–74	48.7	70.7	58.3	43.3	39.0	12.6	0.0	0.0
1875–99	38.6	51.0	50.4	47.1	31.1	16.4	2.7	0.4
1900–19	5.5	9.2	3.3	12.0	6.2	9.3	1.7	0.0

Table 10.4
Age-Specific Proportionate Mortality Ratios in Åland (per 1000 Deaths).

Time Interval	Age Group							
	<1	1–2	3–9	10–14	15–24	25–39	40–59	60+
1750–74	55.7	436.0	574.5	269.0	82.0	31.5	1.3	3.3
1775–99	57.2	262.5	423.1	289.5	72.8	1.7	0.0	0.0
1800–24	25.5	91.2	126.7	70.3	79.4	25.3	0.7	0.0
1825–49	11.4	13.8	8.2	68.2	41.2	7.1	1.6	0.0
1850–74	28.9	24.5	13.1	32.5	35.3	48.4	17.8	2.1
1875–99	3.1	2.9	5.7	0.0	4.0	1.4	4.1	1.0
1900–19	0.0	0.0	0.0	0.0	0.0	0.0	0.0	0.0

Table 10.5
Age-Specific Death Rates for Smallpox in Kitee (per 10,000 Average Population).

Time Interval	Age Group							
	<1	*1–2*	*3–9*	*10–14*	*15–24*	*25–39*	*40–59*	*60+*
1750–74	48.7	104.9	67.3	7.0	1.4	0.4	0.0	0.0
1775–99	115.8	176.5	120.0	26.2	1.1	0.2	0.0	0.0
1800–24	151.3	159.0	101.0	14.5	0.8	0.0	0.2	0.0
1825–49	45.1	45.8	26.9	5.2	2.9	0.4	0.0	0.0
1850–74	93.8	46.3	15.1	3.3	3.5	1.8	0.0	0.0
1875–99	70.5	26.6	7.5	2.8	2.3	1.9	0.6	0.3
1900–19	6.9	2.7	0.3	0.5	0.5	0.9	0.3	0.0

Table 10.6
Age-Specific Death Rates for Smallpox in Åland (per 10,000 Average Population).

Time Interval	Age Group							
	<1	*1–2*	*3–9*	*10–14*	*15–24*	*25–39*	*40–59*	*60+*
1750–74	162.2	159.4	68.4	10.8	4.1	2.0	0.0	0.0
1775–99	243.7	111.6	58.7	15.9	4.1	0.2	0.0	0.0
1800–24	87.4	37.9	15.8	4.3	6.0	2.8	0.2	0.0
1825–49	32.1	4.1	0.7	2.6	2.7	0.7	0.3	0.0
1850–74	65.2	8.8	1.8	1.9	2.6	5.3	3.5	1.6
1875–99	4.6	0.7	0.5	0.0	0.2	0.1	0.5	0.6
1900–19	0.0	0.0	0.0	0.0	0.0	0.0	0.0	0.0

Figure 10.3
Monthly Distribution of Smallpox Deaths in Kitee, 1750–1919.[1]

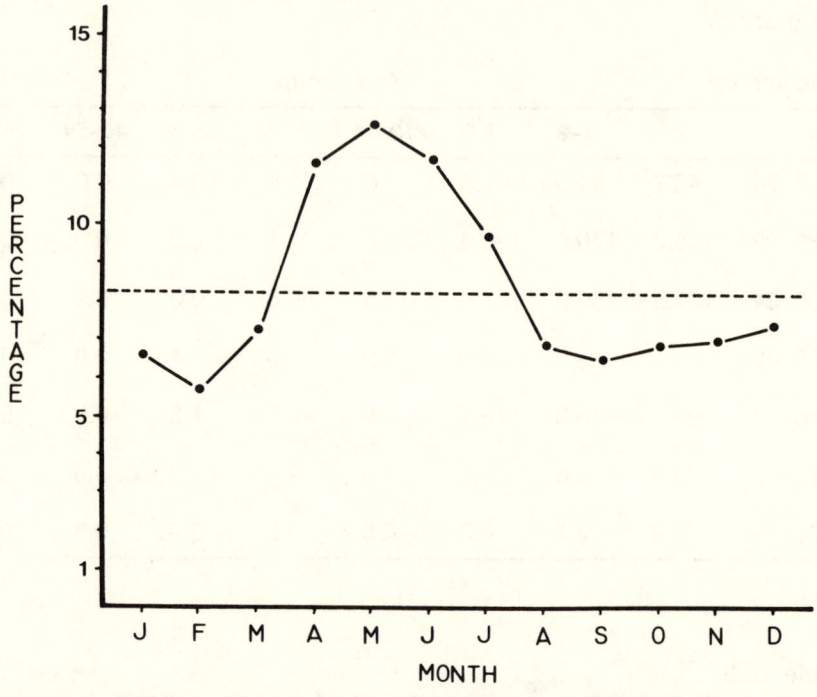

[1] The ordinate gives the percentage of the total number of deaths occurring in each month.

likely to be affected during an epidemic in Åland, resulting in greater exposure levels. Thus, the disease, when it did strike in Åland, was more lethal than in Kitee.

A comparison of PMRs and death rates in the two populations also shows that vaccination had a less dramatic impact in Kitee than in Åland. This is due in part to the lower vaccination rate in Kitee, but it might also reflect the greater exposure level of the mainland population.

In assessing the effects of vaccination on the reduction of smallpox mortality, one must also consider the fact that different epidemics had different levels of virulence. For example, the smallpox epidemic of the 1870s, which affected both Kitee and Åland, was noted to have been especially lethal in many other parts of Europe (Hardy 1983; Mercer 1985). The change in age-specific mortality, in which adults are more commonly the victims of smallpox after the introduction of vaccination, has been observed in England (Hardy 1983; Mercer 1985) as well as Kitee and the Åland Islands (Mielke et al. 1984). This age shift was caused by at least two factors. First, not everybody was vaccinated. Those who were not vaccinated would be less likely to be exposed to the virus during childhood, since

Figure 10.4
Monthly Distribution of Smallpox Deaths in Kittee for Pre- and Postvaccination Time Periods.[1]

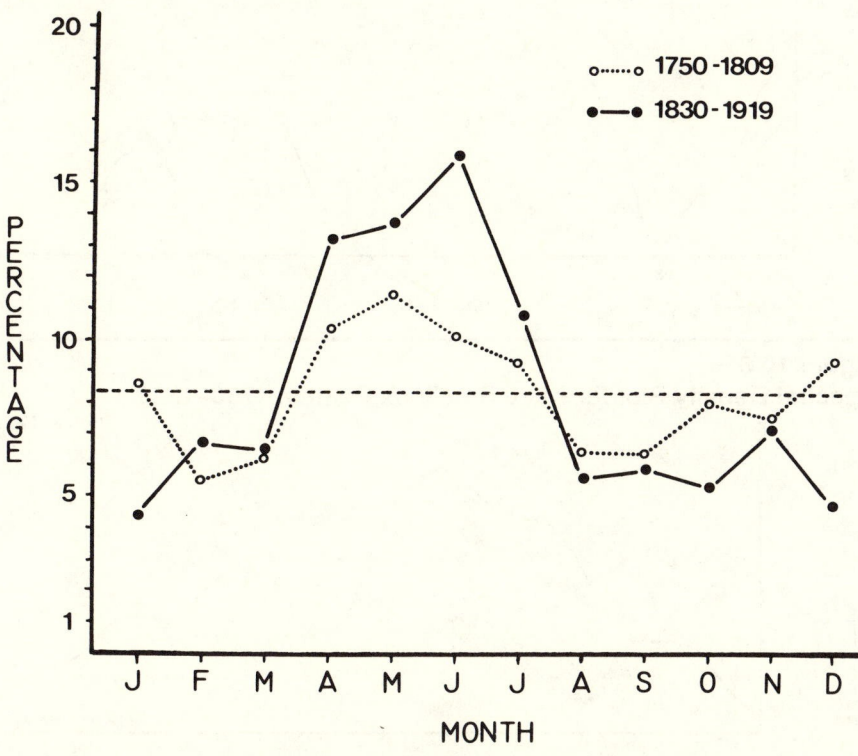

the frequency and duration of epidemics were reduced after vaccination became common. Second, many individuals were not aware that revaccination later in life was necessary in order to preserve immunity, and revaccination was not widely promoted by the authorities until late in the nineteenth century. Thus, many adults were not revaccinated and lost their immunity.

The pattern of seasonality seen in Kitee was also found in Åland. In these two populations, smallpox was primarily a spring disease, which conflicts somewhat with an earlier conclusion that smallpox in Finland was a winter disease (Jutikkala and Kauppinen 1971). The spring peak could reflect a reduced resistance to disease because of food shortages in this season. However, smallpox susceptibility appears to be largely independent of the economic or nutritional status of a population (Mercer 1985; Turpeinen 1977; Utterström

Figure 10.5
Spectral Density Plot for Kitee Smallpox Deaths, 1750–1919.

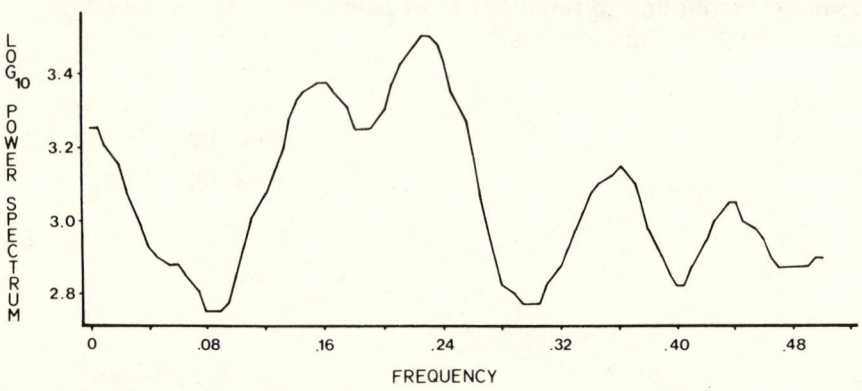

Figure 10.6
Spectral Density Plot for Kitee Smallpox Deaths, 1750–1820.

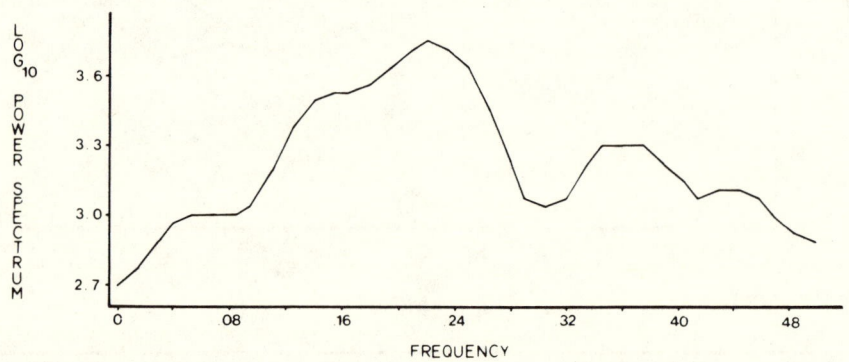

Figure 10.7
Spectral Density Plot for Kitee Smallpox Deaths, 1821–1919.

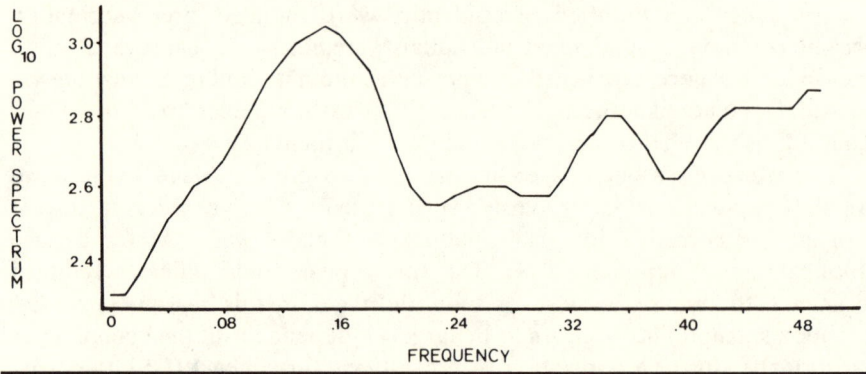

Figure 10.8
Spectral Density Plot for Finnish Smallpox Deaths, 1751–1920.

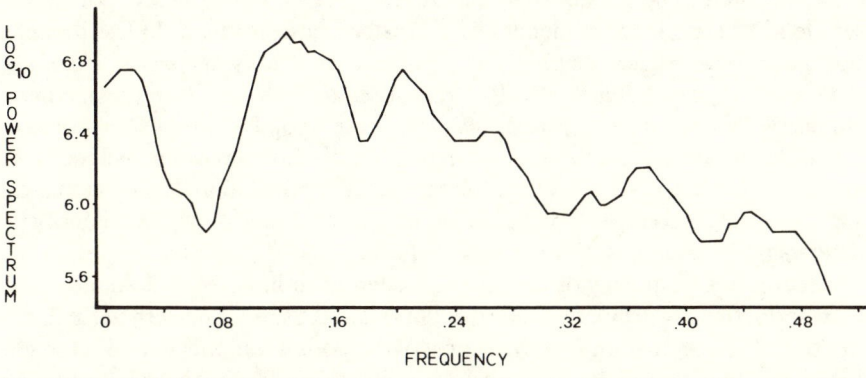

1954). Another factor might be the increased travel which takes place in the late spring, allowing a virus to spread more easily.

Both Kitee and Åland show a stronger seasonality after the introduction of vaccination (the ratios of maximum to minimum points of the fitted seasonality curve for Åland were 4.2 and 19.6 for the pre- and post-1801 samples). It is difficult to pinpoint the causes of this transition, but it could reflect increases in population density and migration rates in both populations in the later time periods, rather than actual effects of vaccination. A more densely populated area with higher population mobility might have epidemics of shorter duration, concentrating them in a particular season. Vaccination itself could play a role in concentrating the epidemics in one season by reducing the reservoir of susceptible individuals. Also, vaccination was performed during the summer months, which would mean that the largest number of susceptible persons would be available during spring.

The spectral analysis of smallpox deaths indicates that epidemics occurred with a somewhat regular frequency in Kitee, although the periodicities in Kitee are not nearly as pronounced as the seven-year periodicity seen in the Åland Islands. The periodicity of smallpox deaths in Kitee (4.4 years for the total time period) is also much shorter than that of Åland. Both of these results can be attributed to features of the mainland parish versus the island parishes. Because Kitee was much less isolated than Åland, its population was exposed much more frequently to the smallpox virus. Also, Kitee consisted of only one mother parish and its chapelry, Rääkkylä, during most of the time period under consideration. Thus, there was much contact between most members of the total population through religious functions. This stands in contrast to Åland, which consisted of fifteen separate parishes, five of which were separated from the others by large expanses of the Baltic Sea. Marital migration rates in Kitee were substantially higher than in Åland (Mielke et al. 1976; Pitkänen et al. 1988). This is a reflection of more frequent interpopulation contact in Kitee and would again facilitate the recurrent spread of the virus. Finally, one would expect the population density of Kitee to be greater than that of Åland, since more densely populated areas tend to experience epidemics with greater frequency than do less densely populated areas (Black 1966). Kitee's population density increased from 1.6 persons per square kilometer to 9.6 from 1721 to 1900 (land and water area combined). When considering land area only, Åland's population density increased from 4.2 to 14.0 during this time period. However, it is more proper to include both land and sea area for Åland. When this is done, the population density increases from 0.6 to 2.0 persons per square kilometer. Thus, a lower population density in Åland might be another factor responsible for less frequent epidemics.

A decreased frequency of epidemics is seen both in Kitee and Åland after the introduction of vaccination. Hardy (1983) noted a similar pattern in England after the 1853 Vaccination Act. With most of the population vaccinated, a longer period of time would be required to build up a large enough group of nonimmune persons to enable the virus to spread. Although the population density of both Kitee and Åland increased after vaccination, the density of susceptible individuals decreased, causing more infrequent epidemics. This interpretation is further supported by the postvaccination reduction in frequency of epidemics that occurred in Finland as a whole.

SUMMARY AND CONCLUSIONS

Smallpox was clearly an important cause of childhood mortality in Kitee. The introduction of vaccination in the early nineteenth century appears to have reduced the smallpox death rate substantially. To some extent this is in accord with the findings of Mercer (1985), who examined the effects of vaccination on death rates in several European countries. However, the effects of vaccination are limited primarily to childhood mortality. The effects on overall mortality are more modest.

Several useful comparisons can be made between the patterns of smallpox deaths in this population and those of the Åland Islands. Because of higher vaccination rates in Åland than in Kitee, a more pronounced reduction in smallpox deaths was seen in Åland. This comparison lends additional credence to the claim that vaccination was an important medical factor in smallpox mortality reduction.

Kitee and Åland experienced a similar age shift in smallpox mortality after the advent of vaccination. The fact that *both* populations exhibited the same type of age shift helps to affirm its epidemiologic importance and reality.

Another similarity in the two populations is the seasonal distribution of smallpox deaths. In both populations, smallpox was primarily a spring disease, and the seasonality became more pronounced after vaccination. This is due both to the effects of vaccination itself and to changes in population density and migration rates.

The analysis of periodicity in Kitee shows that smallpox deaths were less strongly periodic here than in Åland. The periodicities seen in Kitee occurred with greater frequency than those in Åland. This reflects differences in population density, social organization (two versus many parishes), migration rates, and geographic location. The shift from a shorter to a longer periodicity after vaccination was seen in Kitee, in Åland, and in the entire country of Finland. That this same pattern was seen in all three populations, in spite of increases in population density, helps confirm the impression that a longer period of time was required to build up a cohort of susceptible individuals after vaccination was introduced.

Future studies of these populations will focus on other determinants of smallpox mortality, such as specific intervillage and interparish migration patterns. Similar analyses of other infectious diseases (measles, scarlet fever, cholera, and typhus) are under way. Population data such as these, in which spatial and temporal variation in mortality rates can be analyzed in detail, can provide useful insights into both the epidemiology and historical consequences of infectious diseases.

NOTE

We wish to thank Mrs. Margareta Damsten for aid and advice. Drs. Barry Edmonston and Stephen Kunitz provided valuable discussion. This research was supported by NSF grants BNS–8319448 and BNS–8319057 and by grants from the Sigrid Juselius Foundation and the Academy of Finland. Part of this research was conducted while Jorde and Mielke were at Samfundet Folkhälsans Genetiska Institut, Helsinki, Finland.

REFERENCES

Björkstén, J. I. 1908. *Vaccinationens Historia i Finland*. II. Helsinki, Finland.
Black, F. L. 1966. Measles endemicity in insular populations: Critical community size and its evolutionary implication. *Journal of Theoretical Biology* 11:207–11.
Chatfield, C. 1975. *The Analysis of Time Series: Theory and Practice*. New York: Halsted.
Cherry, S. 1980. The hospitals and population growth: The voluntary general hospitals, mortality and local populations in the English provinces in the eighteenth and nineteenth centuries. *Population Studies* 34:59–75.
Cliff, A. D., and P. Haggett. 1984. Island epidemics. *Scientific American* 250:138–47.
Cliff, A. D., P. Haggett, J. K. Ord, and G. R. Versey. 1981. *Spatial Diffusion: An Historical Geography of Epidemics in an Island Community*. Cambridge: Cambridge University Press.
Collins, J. J. 1982. The contribution of medical measures to the decline of mortality from respiratory tuberculosis: An age-period-cohort model. *Demography* 19:409–27.
Dixon, C. W. 1962. *Smallpox*. London: J. & A. Churchill.
Edwards, J. H. 1961. The recognition and estimation of cyclic trends. *Annals of Human Genetics* 25:83–87.

Fagerlund, L. W. 1924. Om dödligheteni smittkopperi Finland och nyttan af vaccination. *Official Statistics of Finland*. XI. New Series, vol. 37. National Board of Health. Helsinki, Finland.

Frauenthal, J. C. 1981. *Smallpox: When Should Routine Vaccination Be Discontinued?* Boston: Birkhaeuser.

Hardy, A. 1983. Smallpox in London: Factors in the decline of the disease in the nineteenth century. *Medical History* 27:111–38.

Hopkins, D. R. 1984. *Princes and Peasants: Smallpox in History.* Chicago: University of Chicago Press.

Jenkins, G. M., and D. G. Watts. 1968. *Spectral Analysis and Its Applications.* San Francisco: Holden-Day.

Jutikkala, E., and M. Kauppinen. 1971. The structure of mortality during catastrophic years in a pre-industrial society. *Population Studies* 25:283–85.

Koopmans, L. H. 1974. *The Spectral Analysis of Time Series.* New York: Academic.

McKeown, T. 1979. *The Role of Medicine: Dream, Mirage or Nemesis?* Princeton: Princeton University Press.

———. 1976. *The Modern Rise of Population.* New York: Academic.

McKinlay, J. B., and S. M. McKinlay. 1977. The questionable contribution of medical measures to the decline of mortality in the United States in the twentieth century. *Milbank Memorial Fund Quarterly* 55:405–28.

Mausner, J. S., and A. K. Bahn. 1974. *Epidemiology: An Introductory Text.* Philadelphia: Saunders.

Mercer, A. J. 1985. Smallpox and epidemiological-demographic changes in Europe: The role of vaccination. *Population Studies* 39:287–307.

Mielke, J. H., L. B. Jorde, P. G. Trapp, D. L. Anderton, K. Pitkänen, and A. W. Eriksson. 1984. Historical epidemiology of smallpox in Åland, Finland: 1751–1890. *Demography* 21:271–95.

Mielke, J. H., P. L. Workman, J. Fellman, and A. W. Eriksson. 1976. Population structure of the Åland Islands, Finland. In *Advances in Human Genetics*. vol. 6. H. Harris and K. Hirschhorn, eds. New York: Plenum.

Pitkänen, K. 1977. The reliability of the registration of births and deaths in Finland in the eighteenth and nineteenth centuries: Some examples. *Scandinavian Economic History Review* 25:138–59.

Pitkänen, K., L. B. Jorde, J. H. Mielke, J. O. Fellman, and A. W. Eriksson. 1988. Marital migration and genetic structure in Kitee, Finland. *Annals of Human Biology* 15:23–34.

Preston, S. H. 1976. *Mortality Patterns in National Populations with Special Reference to Recorded Causes of Death.* New York: Academic.

Turpeinen, O. 1977. Causal relationship between economic factors and mortality. *Yearbook of Population Research in Finland* 15:31–45.

Utterström, G. 1954. Some population problems in pre-industrial Sweden. *Scandinavian Economic History Review* 2:103–65.

11 PARASITIC LOAD IN SOUTH AMERICAN TRIBAL POPULATIONS

Francisco M. Salzano

HOST-PARASITE RELATIONSHIPS AT DISTINCT SOCIOCULTURAL SETTINGS

The relationship between humans and their parasites is as old as our species and involves subtle interactions. Dunn (1968) has aptly classified this relationship using two dichotomies. First, we can consider whether the infections occurred by sexual or asexual organisms and, second, whether they need a vector or not (indirect or direct infections, respectively). Asexual infections may be introduced into a population by a single dose in a single individual, and multiplication in the community occurs most readily if the agent is rare. Examples of indirect asexual infections are malaria and yellow fever; direct asexual infections are measles and smallpox.

Sexual infections cannot normally be introduced into new populations by single doses, and the agents multiply more readily if they occur in large numbers. Indirect sexual infections involve many of the helminthiases; direct sexual infections are not numerous, but they include the well-known helminth *Enterobius vermicularis* (pin worm). Asexual infections are generally more immunogenic than sexual ones.

The study of the effects of infection in bones and mummified tissues, as well as of archeological data, can be of value in assessing prehistoric relationships (Fonseca 1969; Ferreira, Araujo, and Confalonieri 1982). On the other hand, it should be borne in mind that the host-parasite relations evolve and the view that commensalism (peaceful coexistence) should be the ideal evolutionary end point for both host and parasite was recently questioned by Ewald (1983). After considering several pieces of evidence he concludes: (1) diseases transmitted by biting terrestrial arthropods are more severe than those transmitted without vectors; and (2) among vector-transmitted parasites, severity is positively associated with the degree to which humans are used as vertebrate hosts.

Another angle is considered by Damian (1964). He examines in what way antigen sharing by parasite and host ("molecular mimicry") could influence their coevolution. This author introduces the term "eclipsed antigen" for an antigenic determinant of parasite origin which resembles an antigenic determinant of its host and reviews cases of such antigens in helminths, bacteria, and viruses.

Fix (1984) develops a Monte Carlo simulation, based on Semai Senoi of Malaysia, similar to that seen among unacculturated South American Indians (small nomadic groups, with frequent fissions and fusions; see Neel and Salzano 1967). He verified how epidemics of infectious diseases would affect the genetic microdifferentiation of these groups and, therefore, their rate of evolution.

In what way could cultural practices influence the pattern of diseases seen in a given group? This question has been considered by many investigators, examples of them being Alland (1966) and Garruto (1981). The former stresses the importance of considering the cognitive system as it relates to disease theory, as well as the role of the medical practitioner. The latter examines the natural history of several types of diseases in isolated groups: infections (endemic and epidemic), nutritional, toxic or deficiency states, genetic disorders and congenital anomalies, and culturally specific psychoses.

The different factors involved in the acculturation process have been classified by Salzano (1985), who also discusses some specific cases among South American Indians. The interactions between nutrition and infection have been considered by Dubos (1965) and Holmes (1984), the latter presenting specific examples from Venezuela. The need for global evaluations was stressed by Ross (1978), who discusses food taboos, diet and hunting strategies among the Ecuadoran Jívaro. This ecological approach was followed in an investigation of four Brazilian tribes (Mekranoti, Xavante, Bororo, and Kanela), described by Gross et al. (1979), Werner et al. (1979) and Flowers et al. (1982). It is clear that only through such integrated studies will we be able to at least partially understand the many factors which influence disease patterns at this sociocultural level.

DATA FROM SOUTH AMERICA

Although the literature on the health of South American Indians is already voluminous, few attempts have been made to interpret them in more general terms. In what follows I will review some of these data, with the hope of providing background for more meaningful analyses. The extensive investigations of F. L. Black and co-workers will not be presented, since it is presented in Chapter 4 of this volume. The data on the prevalence of tuberculosis among these Indians was reviewed recently (Salzano 1985) and will not be considered again.

General Health Surveys

General observations about the Amerindian health, without quantitative data, are numerous, and one such study can be traced to as early as the end of the last century (Ranke 1898). Table 11.1 summarizes the twelve studies I could find in which a more systematic and comprehensive approach was followed. They involved fifteen tribes and one group of tribes (the Xingu Indians of Brazil), in six countries, and included 3,555 individuals. If the items of a thorough physical examination are classified in thirteen categories, it will be seen that not all of these individuals were examined with equal detail; however, in twelve of the fourteen samples the number of items examined systematically was seven or more. Skin tests were concomitantly performed in eight of the fourteen surveys, and almost eleven of them involved at least one laboratory study on blood. Stool and urine studies were also done in six of them.

While the majority of the tribes lived in a tropical environment, one (the Aymara) inhabited the highlands of Chile, and three others (Alacaluf, Ona, Yamana) the cold southern tip of this same country. The types of pathologies observed among these four tribes, however, did not show marked departures from those seen in the other groups. Moreover, Damionovic (1948) observed differences in the state of health of the Ona and Yamana on one hand, and the Alacaluf on the other, at the time of his investigation. The latter showed lower frequencies of caries and tuberculosis infection, but higher prevalences of syphilis, scabies, and pyoderma.

The most important disease in the majority of the tropical tribes is malaria. Tuberculosis infection was documented in most of them also, with and without the occurrence of active forms of the disease. The immunological system of individuals from these groups is being subjected to a constant challenge, and this is manifested by high gamma-globulin levels, observed in several of them. Other health problems mentioned frequently are epidemics of influenza, measles, and whooping cough.

I have personally participated in the investigations in the Xavante and Cayapo and can attest to the difficulty of establishing generalizations about the health of these populations. For instance, 12 percent of the 209 Xavante Indians seen at the village of Simoes Lopes presented a diffuse, nontoxic goiter, completely absent in the seventy-eight inhabitants examined in another community (Sao Domingos) of the same tribe. The marked difference in the prevalence of diseases in men and women found among the Xavante, on the other hand, did not occur among the Cayapo. The latter showed skin problems of varying degrees of magnitude (about one-half had scabies or a dermatitis-like condition), ailments practically absent among the Xavante.

Intestinal Parasites

Results related to eighteen studies which investigated the prevalences of intestinal parasites in South American Indian populations, including 2,071

TABLE 11.1
General Health Surveys Performed in South American Indians.

Observations	2 tribes Surinam 184 (1)	3 tribes French Guiana 257 (2)	Waorani Ecuador 293 (3)	Campa Peru 589 (4)	Cayapo Brazil 184 (5)	Kren-Akorore Brazil 79 (6)	Xingu Indians Brazil 254 (7)	Xingu Indians Brazil 600 (8)	Karajá Brazil 117 (9)	Xavante Brazil 287 (10)	Aymara Chile 636 (11)	Alacaluf Chile 19 (12)	Ona Chile 14 (12)	Yamana Chile 42 (12)
Physical examination														
Height / weight	+		+		+	+	+	+		+	+			
Eyes		+	+	+	+					+	+	+	+	+
Ears and hearing			+		+					+	+	+	+	+
Oral cavity		+	+	+	+				+	+	+	+	+	+
Thyroid			+				+			+	+			
Lymph nodes		+			+		+			+	+			
Cardiovascular system		+	+	+	+	+	+	+	+	+	+			
Pulmonary system	+	+	+		+	+			+	+	+	+	+	+
Spleen	+	+	+		+	+	+			+	+			
Liver		+	+		+	+	+			+	+			
Bone and joints		+	+	+	+					+	+	+	+	+
Skin and appendages		+	+	+	+					+	+	+	+	+
Central nervous system			+				+		+	+	+			
Skin tests	+		+	+				+		+		+	+	+
Hematological variables	+		+			+	+	+		+	+			
Blood parasites	+	+	+				+	+		+				
Antibody tests	+		+			+	+	+		+		+	+	+
Stool and urine tests			+	+		+	+	+		+				

Bibliographic references: (1) Schaad (1960); tribes studied: Oajana and Trio; (2) Cabannes, Lannovy, and Ruffie (1964): tribes studied: Oajana, Oyampi and Emerillon; (3) Larrick et al. (1979); Kaplan et al. (1980); (4) Eichenberger (1966); (5) Ayres and Salzano (1972); the height and weight data are given in Da Rocha and Salzano (1972); (6) Baruzzi et al. (1977); (7) Baruzzi (1970); (8) Hugh-Jones et al. (1972); (9) Oliveira (1952); (10) Neel et al. (1964); Weinstein et al. (1967); Neel et al. (1968a,b); (11) Díaz et al. (1978); (12) Damianovic (1948).

TABLE 11.2
Prevalences (in percent) of Intestinal Parasites Observed in South American Indians

Parasites found	Unknown Surinam 120 (1)	Yanomama Venezuela 125 (2)	Yanomama Venezuela 177 (3)	Rio Negro Indians Venezuela 173 (3)	Chocó Colombia 46 (4)	Ticuna Colombia 59 (5)	Ticuna Colombia 176 (6)	Waorani Ecuador 65 (7)	Aguaruna Peru 119 (8)	Campa Peru 405 (9)	Palikur Brazil 21 (10)	Galibi Brazil 55 (10)	Three tribes Brazil 53 (2)	Unknown Brazil 43 (11)	Surui Brazil 200 (12)	Kren-Akorore Brazil 35 (13)	Xingu Indians Brazil 139 (14)	Xavante Brazil 60 (15)
Helminths																		
Ascaris lumbricoides	—	89–99	73–80	52–76	74	60–85	76	3	62	28	76	78	46–67	70	53	15	18	70
Trichuris trichiura	—	68–92	9–53	0–29	30	92–95	77	2	92	20	19	49	46–100	91	5	76	—	20
Ancylostoma duodenale	—	76–79	39–67	6–22	30	60–100	83	46	93	45	90	80	60–96	95	43	97	81	97
Strongyloides stercoralis	—	3–11	0–1	0–12	—	—	25	—	7	11	10	10	0–20	26	33	30	11	5
Enterobius vermicularis	—	—	—	—	—	—	—	3	—	—	—	—	—	—	<1	—	13	2
Taenia Sp	—	—	—	—	—	—	—	—	—	—	—	—	—	—	6	—	—	—
Hymenolepis nana	—	—	—	—	—	—	—	—	—	—	—	—	—	—	4	—	—	—
Capillaria sp	—	—	—	—	—	—	—	—	—	—	—	—	—	—	1*	—	—	—
Protozoans																		
Entamoeba coli	53–63	91–100	70–84	16–47	50	—	69	51	49	37	14	31	20–69	42	—	24	87	67
Giardia lamblia	5–22	4–5	20	12–52	—	—	22	28	11	—	5	7	20–27	12	3	9	29	7
Entamoeba histolytica	9–38	28–77	—	—	61	—	55	20	—	21	10	16	0–29	23	1	18	61	48
Endolimax nana	19–39	24–39	—	—	—	—	26	—	—	—	33	14	0–12	51	—	12	38	28
Iodamoeba butschlii	7–17	21–66	—	—	28	—	20	—	—	—	14	11	0–29	12	—	24	39	25
Chilomastix mesnili	11–25	10–53	—	—	—	—	15	—	—	—	—	—	0–38	7	—	9	17	8
Trichomonas hominis	—	—	—	—	—	—	4	—	—	—	5	—	—	—	—	—	—	—
Balantidium coli	—	—	—	—	—	—	2	—	—	—	—	—	0–11	—	—	—	1	—
Entamoeba hartmanni	5–29	0–19	—	—	—	—	—	—	—	—	—	—	0–32	16	—	—	—	—
Enteromonas homini	—	—	—	—	—	—	—	—	—	—	—	—	0–6	—	—	—	—	—
Dientamoeba fragilis	—	—	—	—	—	—	—	—	—	—	—	—	0–2	—	—	—	—	—

*Subsequently confirmed by Coimbra (1982)

Bibliographic references: (1) Asin and van Thiel (1963); (2) Lawrence et al. (1980); (3) Holmes (1984); the Rio Negro Indians include the descendents of many intertribal crosses; (4) Duque et al. (1959); (5) Schwaner and Dixon (1974); (6) Restrepo (1962); (7) Kaplan et al. (1980); (8) Berlin and Markell (1977); (9) Eichenberger (1966); (10) Bruno (1978); (11) Knight and Prata (1972); (12) Coimbra and Mello (1981); (13) Baruzzi et al. (1977); (14) Baruzzi (1970); (15) Neel et al. (1968a).

individuals, are presented in Table 11.2. There is wide variation both among different tribes and among villages within a tribe. Considering first the helminths, it will be seen that six of the twenty-one values presented there for *Trichuris trichiura* (29 percent) lie in the interval between 91 percent and 100 percent. About half of those related to *Ancylostoma duodenale* occur in the range between 71 percent and 100 percent, while two-thirds of those dealing with *Ascaris lumbricoides* fall in the interval between 31 percent and 70 percent. *Strongyloides stercoralis* is much less frequent (highest prevalence of 33 percent among the Surui), while *Enterobius vermicularis*, *Taenia*, *Hymenolepis nana*, and *Capillaria* have been reported only sporadically.

Considering now the protozoans, Table 11.2 indicates that six species occur most frequently, the respective most common intervals of prevalences being as follows: *Entamoeba coli*: 62 percent of the percentages between 31 percent and 70 percent; *Giardia lamblia*: 95 percent in the interval between 1 percent and 30 percent; *Entamoeba histolytica*: 59 percent also between 1 percent and 30 percent; *Endolimax nana*: 85 percent between 11 percent and 30 percent; *Chilomastix mesnili*: 64 percent between 1 percent and 20 percent. The remaining species (*Trichomonas hominis*, *Balantidium coli*, *Entamoeba hartmanni*, *Enteromonas homini* and *Dientamoeba fragilis*) are much less common, and were detected in a few surveys only.

What generalizations can be presented related to these results? There has been some discussion about the presence of *A. lumbricoides* and *A. duodenale* in pre-Columbian Indians, the evidence for or against this presence being unfortunately mostly indirect and inconclusive. Allison et al. (1974) reported the presence of *A. duodenale* in a Peruvian mummy dating around 900 A. D., while Ferreira, Araujo, and Confalonieri (1980, 1983) also found indications of ancylostomids in archeological material and a Brazilian mummy about 3,500 years old. These observations, therefore, suggest that at least infections with *A. duodenale* could have existed in the continent before the Conquest, which raises an interesting question. Fonseca (1969) asserts that if this was true, the parasites could not have been carried by human migrations across the Bering Strait, since the larval forms could not have resisted the low temperatures of the soil.

The prevalence observed may have been influenced by many factors, such as:

1. Diagnostic methods.
2. Level of parasitemia.
3. Age structure of the subjects tested.
4. Nutrition.
5. Level of sanitation.
6. Cultural practices.
7. Treatment.

These factors may interact in complex ways, making generalizations difficult. But examples of meaningful approaches exist. Schwaner and Dixon (1974), for instance, consider the relevances of helminthiasis in two communities of Ticuna Indians as a measure of cultural change. Modernization in one of them contributed to a reduced incidence and worm burden in the inhabitants. On the other hand, they mention that the Cofan Indians of eastern Ecuador use a hallucinogenic drug (prepared from the plant *Banisteriopsis rusbayana*) that was shown to contain antihelminthic properties. Holmes (1984) was surprised to find that intestinal parasitism did not significantly affect the nutritional status of the Rio Negro and Yanomama Indians she studied. What is still lacking, however, are more analytical analyses relating types and levels of parasitism to other quantifiable indicators of cultural change. It is still unclear, for instance, whether hunter-gatherers with rudimentary agriculture are less or more infected than agriculturalists, in the absence of therapeutic measures, although we could guess that they would probably have lower burdens.

As an example of the investigation of bacterial intestinal parasites, mention can be made of the study of Eveland, Olver, and Neel (1971). They found a wide spectrum of known pathogenic and nonpathogenic strains of *E. coli* among Yanomama Indians living in northern Brazil, but in addition thirteen serotypically unique 0 strains. This is a striking finding, since only 147 previously recognized 0 serotypes of this micro-organism have been found in a very large number of isolates from samples obtained in all parts of the world.

Filariasis

Search for microfilaria was performed in eighteen samples, including a total of 13,073 individuals (Table 11.3). As would be expected, since *Mansonella ozzardi* is the only autochthonous filaria species in the continent, this parasite is the most common of the microfilariae found in South American Indians. The prevalences vary from zero to as high as 96 percent, without a clear clustering of values. It should be pointed out, however, that part of this variation may be due to technical problems. For instance, Lawrence et al. (1979a) obtained higher prevalences of this filaria in villages of Amazonian Indians examining peripheral blood lymphocyte culture preparations not specifically designed for the purpose of detecting the parasite than with conventional smears. This was probably due to the concentration effect inherent in the lymphocyte method. *Dipetalonema perstans* occurs in some populations together with *M. ozzardi*, but their detection (and that of *Wuchereria bancrofti*) is made more difficult because they migrated to the peripheral blood circulation at night only (while *M. ozzardi* do not show this periodicity). Skin biopsies also furnish underestimates of the true prevalence of this last parasite (Moraes et al. 1978).

Since both *D. perstans* and *W. bancrofti* were probably introduced in the continent through individuals of African ancestry, their presence may be an indicator of contacts with people of this extraction. But the situation, in each

TABLE 11.3
Prevalences (in percent) of Microfilariae among South American Indians.

Tribe	Country	Sample size	Bibliographic reference	Dipetalonema perstans	Wuchereria bancrofti	Mansonella ozzardi	Onchocerca volvulus
Several	Guyana	9,506	1	11	0	1	—
Several	Surinam	881	2	47	<1	89	—
Oajana	Surinam	51	3	—	—	0	—
Trio	Surinam	71	3	—	—	0	—
Piaroa	Venezuela	28	4	18	0	14	—
Yanomama	Venezuela	159	4	0	0	11	—
Several	Colombia	18	5	11	0	39	—
Several	Colombia	332	6	0	0	96	—
Ticuna	Colombia	197	7	—	—	14	—
Yanomama + Makiritare	Brazil	258	8	—	—	0	0–61
Içana River Indians	Brazil	124	9	—	—	54–64	—
Baniwa	Brazil	24	10	0	0	87	—
Ticuna	Brazil	198	10	0	0	46–93	—
Kanamari	Brazil	30	10	0	0	20	—
Katukina	Brazil	30	10	0	0	0	—
Ticuna	Brazil	290	11	0	0	29	—
Ticuna	Brazil	800	12	—	—	33–57	0
Xavante	Brazil	76	13	—	—	0	—

Bibliographic references: (1) Orihel (1967); (2) Fros (1956); (3) Schaad (1960); (4) Beaver et al. (1976); (5) Marinkelle (1973); (6) Marinkelle and German (1970); (7) Restrepo (1962); (8) Rassi et al. (1976); (9) Lage (1964); (10) Lawrence et al. (1979b); (11) Rachou (1957); (12) Moraes et al. (1978); (13) Neel et al. (1964).

Table 11.4
Prevalences (in Percent) of Malaria Parasites in Two Groups of South American Indians.

Parasites Found	Tribe, Country, Sample Size, Bibliographic Reference, and Date of Study				
	Xingu Indians, Brazil			Campa, Peru	
	223 (1) 1966/1967	303 (2) 1968	97 (3) 1970	123 (4) 6/1973	123 (4) 9/1973
Plasmodium vivax	28	13	6	6	–
Plasmodium falciparum	18	29	5	–	–
Plasmodium malariae	5	1	–	54	83
Plasmodium sp	–	–	–	1	2
Mixed infections -	1	3	–	3	1
Negative	48	54	89	36	14

Bibliographic references: (1) D'Andretta et al. (1969a); (2) D'Andretta et al. (1969b); (3) Baruzzi et al. (1976); (4) Sulzer et al. (1975).

case, should be examined considering the presence of vectors, they may be different in diverse regions. Another question that has been considered is whether a single species of vector may transmit more than one type of filaria (Orihel 1967). Time trends are also important. For instance, Orihel asserts that *D. perstans* and *M. ozzardi* are not as prevalent among Guyanese Amerinds now as they apparently were seventy years ago.

Onchocerciasis had never been found in Brazil until the end of the sixties and beginning of the seventies. In mid-1973 M. A. P. Moraes and colleagues discovered the infection among groups of Yanomama Indians living along the left bank of the Tootobi river. Since a pioneer highway that was being opened through the jungle passed near the region inhabited by these Indians, the possibility that the disease might rapidly spread became a reality, and work by Rassi, Lacerda, and Guimarães (1976) proved this to be true. They discovered two other foci of the infection in Brazil and its spread to the Makiritare Indians. Just to illustrate the rapidity of the spread of the disease, it might be mentioned that our team of investigators had performed in 1966–1967 thorough physical examinations (including eye observations) in villages situated in the regions of two of these foci, without finding signs of the disease (Salzano and Neel 1976). This situation is of extreme practical and theoretical interest, since documentation can be made of the way this disease may spread and how measures could be taken to eradicate it before it becomes a public health problem.

Malaria

Since, as was indicated before, malaria is one of the main health hazards faced by South American Indians (as well as by a very large fraction of non-Indians living in the tropics) it is surprising to find how little has been published on the prevalence and other aspects of this disease in these people. Table 11.4 lists the four studies I could locate. While *Plasmodium vivax* and *Plasmodium falciparum* are the most important infectious agents among the Xingu Indians, *Plasmodium malariae* is the most frequent parasite among the Campa. The latter finding is interesting since, in general, *P. malariae* is much less frequent than the other two species. The isolation of the Campa and conditions especially favorable to the reservoir (which may be animal) and vector of this micro-organism may be responsible for the finding. Since it is believed that *P. falciparum* was not present in the Americas before the fifteenth century, its occurrence among Indians reflects contact with people of European or African descent.

Baruzzi et al. (1976) investigated the role that malaria may play in the occurrence of the so-called Tropical Splenomegaly syndrome among the Xingu Indians. The syndrome is characterized by the presence of a persistently large spleen, hepatic sinusoidal lymphocytosis, and disproportionate elevation of serum Ig M levels, as well as malaria antibody titers. As a rule, the Indians with these characteristics do not demonstrate limitation of their physical activity, but after acute episodes of hemolysis they may present physical prostration and intense anemia, as well as increase in reticulocyte counts and bilirubin levels. Death may occur in the most severe cases.

Toxoplasmosis

Toxoplasma gondii has been shown to be almost cosmopolitan in distribution, and numerous serologic surveys have revealed that infection with this parasite is common in both humans and animals. The prevalences found in seven studies of South American Indians are presented in Table 11.5. The frequencies vary all the way from 25 percent to 100 percent. Among the Xavante, Weinstein, Neel, and Salzano (1967) found an adult with the type of inactive chorioretinitis often associated with congenital toxoplasmosis. The mode of transmission of this parasite is still obscure. Lovelace, Moraes, and Hagerby (1978) attributed the low prevalence found in some Ticuna communities to their dietary preference for fishing and the unimportance of hunting and animal husbandry to their culture and economy; other authors concur with the opinion that the ingestion of meat may be an important epidemiological factor in the spread of the infection.

Papovaviruses

Eight Brazilian and one Paraguayan Indian populations have been studied for the prevalences of JC and BK papovaviruses (Table 11.6). The frequencies

Table 11.5
Prevalences (in Percent) of Antibodies to *Toxoplasma Gondi* Among South American Indians.

Tribe	Country	Sample Size	Bibliographic Reference	% Infected with *Toxoplasma gondii*
Not indicated	Surinam	27	1	30
Wayana & Emerillon	French Guiana	237	2	37
Oyampi & Emerillon	French Guiana	134	2	72
Tiriyo	Brazil	200	3	43
Ticuna	Brazil	408	4	25–29
Xikrin	Brazil	118	3	46
Mekranoti	Brazil	175	3	52
Kren-Akorore	Brazil	70	5	89
Xingu Indians	Brazil	254	6	52
Xavante	Brazil	107	7	100

Bibliographic references: (1) Roever-Bonnet (1967); (2) Fribourg-Blanc et al. (1975); (3) Black (1975); (4) Lovelace et al. (1978); (5) Leser et al. (1977); (6) Baruzzi (1970); (7) Neel et al. (1968a).

range from 0 percent to 8 percent for the first and 0 percent to 28 percent for the latter. These values are much lower than those found in other populations, where frequencies as high as 75 percent were reported for JC and 89 percent for BK in apparently normal individuals (Brown, Tsai, and Gajdusek 1975). These viruses are interesting, because they can exist in humans as a latent infection. Transmission may be through urinary contamination, since urine has been the source of most isolations of the BK virus. The two types seem to behave independently at the population and individual level.

Hepatitis B Antigen

Shortly after the discovery of the Australia antigen (hepatitis B antigen, HB Ag), seroepidemiological studies in various parts of the world indicated that its prevalence among apparently healthy tropical African and Southeast Asian populations was generally between 5 percent and 20 percent, whereas in Europeans, North Americans, and Brazilians was less than 1 percent (Salzano

Table 11.6
Prevalences (in Percent) of Antibodies to the JC and BK
Papovaviruses Among South American Indians.

Tribe	Country	Sample Size	Bibliographic Reference	% Positive Antibodies	
				JC HI1	BK HI[1]
Tiriyo	Brazil	49	1	–	6
Kaxuyana	Brazil	18	1	–	28
Ewarhoyana	Brazil	9	1	0	0
Xikrin	Brazil	53	1	–	11
Kuben-Kran-Kegn	Brazil	47	1	–	6
Mekranoti	Brazil	60	1	8	2
Kren-Akorore	Brazil	66	2	0	6
Xingu Indians	Brazil	107	2	0–4	3–6
Guayaki	Paraguay	58	1	0	5

[1] Hemagglutination inhibition.

Bibliographic references: (1) Brown et al. (1975); (2) Candeias et al. (1977).

and Blumberg 1970). The results obtained among several South American Indian populations is shown in Table 11.7. The prevalences found ranged from 0 percent in the Quechua of Peru to 71 percent among the Brazilian Mekranoti, a Cayapo subgroup. It is curious that another subgroup of the same tribe, the Xikrin, also shows a high prevalence of the antigen (61 percent); the other tribe with a high frequency, however, lives farther apart in Ecuador (the Waorani, with 64 percent).

Experimental studies and clinical observations have shown that the serum hepatitis virus may be transmitted by a nonparenteral route. An oral transmission may be possible, since saliva may contain minute amounts of blood. The possibility that arthropods could be vectors has also been considered.

Skin Diseases

Pyoderma is one of the most common dermatologic morbid conditions in the tropics. But population surveys from remote populations are not numerous. Lawrence et al. (1979b) studied members of three Brazilian Amazonian tribes, while two other populations from the same general region but living further to the Southwest, were investigated by Tanus, Coimbra, and Santos (1984).

Table 11.7
Prevalences (in Percent) of Hepatitis B Antigen Among South American Indians.

Tribe	Country	Sample Size	Bibliographic Reference	% Positive for HB Ag
Yanomama	Venezuela	1635	1	0–31
Waorani	Ecuador	181	2	64
Quechua	Peru	102	3	0
Cashinahua	Peru	89	3	20
Several	Peru	363	4	1
Tiriyo	Brazil	200	5	5
Xikrin	Brazil	118	5	61
Mekranoti	Brazil	175	5	71
Kren-Akorore	Brazil	68	6	23
Xingu Indians	Brazil	Unknown	6	2

Bibliographic references: (1) Soyano et al. (1976, 1979); (2) Kaplan et al. (1980); (3) Blumberg et al. (1970); (4) Madalengoitia et al. (1975); (5) Black (1975); (6) Baruzzi et al. (1977).

Staphylococcus aureus was isolated in both studies; in the first, other micro-organisms found were *Streptococcus pyogenes* and *Corynebacterium diphtheriae*, while in the second *Staphylococcus epidermidis* was also observed. In both investigations resistance to some of the most common antibiotics were already detected.

A high prevalence of keloid blastomycosis was reported by Baruzzi et al. (1973) among a single tribe of the Xingu National Park, the Caiabi. Fifteen of the 180 individuals examined (8 percent) presented the condition. The observed lesions included papules, nodules, and verrucose formations that could be clearly distinguished histologically from the more common blastomycosis caused by *Paracoccidioides brasiliensis* and always showed the presence of *P. loboi*. Visceral impairment was not found, and the carriers were generally not much affected by the infection. No new cases, however, were discovered among the Caiabi after 1956, the date of their transfer to the Xingu National Park, despite the fact that no precautions were taken to avoid transmission of the disease. Therefore, this unusual aggregation of cases was due to conditions prevailing in the environment where they formerly lived.

Another epidemic, this time of leishmaniasis, was described by Carneri, Nutels, and Miranda (1963) in another tribe of the Xingu National Park, the Waura. Among fifty Indians of a village, twelve were affected by ulcers, in some cases multiple in number. The outbreak began a few months after the village had been moved from an earlier site situated four hours' canoe journey up the Rio Batovi. The epidemic started in 1962 but by late 1964 was over, and when a new medical team visited the tribe in 1968 there were no active lesions (Aston and Thorley 1970). The latter authors performed a detailed survey, using the Montenegro skin test, and verified a high prevalence of antibodies to *Leishmania brasiliensis* (present in 76 percent of 212 males and 47 percent of 188 females). This high percentage of positive reactions was not accompanied by the presence of active primary or secondary lesions, since none was found. This was in sharp contrast with the situation in a nearby neo-Brazilian *fazendae*, where they did find such lesions. The explanation given for the difference was better hygiene and nutrition among the Indians. As for the epidemic, two hypotheses can be advanced to explain it; either the area was a temporary focus of a higher concentration of infected flies, or there was a very localized strain of *Leishmania* which was significantly more virulent than the surrounding normal strain.

RETROSPECT AND PROSPECT

In global evaluations about the parasitic load of South American Indians, the obvious, first question to ask is whether the disease was present in the New World before Columbus. This is important because host-parasite adaptations require time, and for many of the pathogenic organisms considered here (*A. lumbricoides, A. duodenale, D. perstans, W. bancrofti, P. vivax,* and *P. falciparum*) no conclusive evidence exists for or against this view.

Time trends are intimately connected with these sources of origin, but other factors, such as the size and mobility of the populations, sociocultural practices, and preventive or curative measures, are undoubtedly important. Such trends were documented in relation to the prevalence of microfilariae in Guyana. The identification of situations in which a given parasite is in the process of colonizing new hosts and territories can be of the utmost importance for the understanding of the dynamics of host-parasite relationships, and such a situation is now happening for onchocerciasis in northern Brazil.

The importance of the general physical environment was made clear by the epidemics of blastomycosis among the Caiabi and of leishmaniasis among the Waura Indians. But host effects may be significant also. The benign effect of leishmaniasis among the Xingu Indians, compared to neo-Brazilian, was already mentioned. Nutels (1968) is also surprised at both the clinicoradiological and epidemiological aspects of tuberculosis in "virgin" populations like the Suia and Txukahamae Indians of central Brazil. He would have expected different patterns, such as the so-called infant type in adults and the rapidly evolving and military forms, similar to those found among the Senegalese soldiers taken to France during the First World War. Instead, he found a disease that in its clinical, radiological, and even epidemiological aspects could be equated with that of persons with a long experience with the bacillus. At the other end of the scale, Giglioli (1968) asserts that the high susceptibility of the Guyana Indians to malaria was without doubt one of the major causes of their decline over the past 150 years.

Diet factors are undoubtedly important when intestinal parasites are considered, but, as was indicated previously, they may have also influenced the epidemiology of toxoplasmosis.

Some of the populations considered here are quite isolated, and this may explain the peculiar composition of the *E. coli* strains found among the Yanomama Indians of northern Brazil. The low frequencies of the JC and BK papovaviruses, as well as of the hepatitis B antigen in some South American Indian populations, may result from this same isolation.

An alarming observation was the one that many strains of the micro-organisms responsible for pyoderma are already resistant to some of the most common antibiotics. This indicates a need for a more judicious use of these therapeutic agents.

Several ongoing medical investigations are being developed in Brazil, with the dual objectives of assisting the Indians and obtaining more scientific information about the factors responsible for their health and disease. The studies at the Xingu National Park performed by teams of the Escola Paulista de Medicina and headed by Dr. R. G. Baruzzi started in 1965 and continue up to the present. The program of tuberculosis diagnosis and control was started by Dr. N. Nutels in 1952, and is also fully active at present, now coordinated by Dr. J. A. N. de Miranda, from the National Service of Tuberculosis Control in Rio de Janeiro. Two other projects started recently: the first is under the responsibility of the Brazilian National School of Public Health, also located in Rio de Janeiro, and is headed by Dr. L. F. Ferreira; the other is being directed by Dr. H. V. Dourado, head of the Hospital of Tropical Diseases in Manaus. It is hoped that these systematic investigations may furnish in the future important additional data on the subject of the present chapter.

More meaningful insights on the many questions raised here may be obtained through efforts in the following lines:

1. More paleopathological studies, with an emphasis in areas (like the deserts of Chile) especially suited for the preservation of human remains.

2. Determination of the reservoirs and vectors of a series of pathogenic agents, some of them discussed above.

3. Experimental studies (like those of Wood 1975), with the objective of determining the factors responsible for the attraction of disease vectors to susceptible hosts.

4. Immunological profiles of individuals who, due to their genetic constitution in the chromosome region responsible for the immune response, may show differential susceptibility to a given parasite.

5. More detailed investigations about parasite cycles.

6. Development of statistical models responsible for a given host-parasite situation (for instance, the effects of population sizes, degree of isolation, sources of infections, and specific biological and cultural attributes).

The future of the South American Indian will depend to a great extent on the policies of the national governments of the countries where they live. For instance, the present emphasis of the Brazilian government in the building of huge dams for the production of energy has already affected many tribal territories, essential for their survival. A more disciplined control of contacts with non-Indians, especially those of the more isolated groups, is also very important. For example, it is known that the two most famous Brazilian Jesuit catechists of the sixteenth century, Manoel da Nobrega and Jose de Anchieta, were affected by tuberculosis and should have infected a large number of Indians, possibly with fatal consequences. A recent symposium held in Rio de Janeiro also considered the medical services presently offered by the Brazilian National Indian Foundation (Funai) and several alternatives. The difficulties of providing medical care to villages scattered over a vast territory of difficult access were examined. The recommendations stressed the importance of combining the scientific approach to medicine with the traditional methods of treatment.

There is a tendency, well established in Brazil, for the Indian leaders to take over the direction of their own affairs, until recently dealt with exclusively by nonIndians. This salutary move will enable them to best define their goals and to adopt firm measures that could reduce the level of morbidity in their populations, therefore contributing to a healthier and happier life.

REFERENCES

Alland, A., Jr. 1966. Medical anthropology and the study of biological and cultural adaptation. *American Anthropologist* 68:40–51.

Allison, M. J., A. Pezzia, I. Hasegawa, and E. Gerszten. 1974. A case of hookworm infestation in a precolumbian American. *American Journal of Physical Anthropology* 41:103–6.

Asin, H. R. G., and P. H. van Thiel. 1963. On intestinal protozoa in the urban and bushland population in Surinam. *Tropical and Geographical Medicine* 15:108–20.

Aston, D. L., and A. P. Thorley. 1970. Leishmaniasis in Central Brazil: Results of a Montenegro skin test survey among Amerindians in the Xingu National Park. *Transcripts of the Royal Society for Tropical and Medical Hygiene* 64:671–78.

Ayres, M., and F. M. Salzano. 1972. Health status of Brazilian Cayapo Indians. *Tropical and Geographical Medicine* 24:178–85.

Baruzzi, R. G. 1970. Contribution to the study of the toxoplasmosis epidemiology. Serologic survey among the Indians of the Upper Xingu River, central Brazil. *Revista Do Institudo de Medicine Tropical De Soa Paulo* 12:93–104.

Baruzzi, R. G., R. M. Castro, C. D'Andretta, Jr., S. Carvalhal, O. L. Ramos, and P. L. Pontes. 1973. Occurrence of Lobo's blastomycosis among "Caiabi" Brazilian Indians. *International Journal of Dermatology* 12:95–98.

Baruzzi, R. G., L. J. Franco, J. R. Jardim, A. Masuda, C. Naspitz, E. R. Paiva, and N. Ferreiro-Novo. 1976. The association between splenomegaly and malaria in Indians from the Alto Xingu, central Brazil. *Revista Do Institudo de Medicine Tropical De Soa Paulo* 18:322–48.

Baruzzi, R. G., L. F. Marcopito, M. L. C. Serra, F. A. A. Souza, and C. Stabile. 1977. The Kren-Akorore: A recently contacted indigenous tribe. In *Health and Disease in Tribal Societies*. K. Elliott and J. Whelan, eds. Amsterdam: Elsevier.

Beaver, P. C., J. V. Neel, and T. C. Orihel. 1976. *Dipetalonema perstans* and *Mansonella ozzardi* in Indians of southern Venezuela. *American Journal of Tropical Medicine and Hygiene* 25:263–65.

Berlin, E., and E. Markell. 1977. An assessment of the nutritional and health status of an Aguaruna Jívaro community, Amazonas, Peru. *Ecology of Food and Nutrition* 6:69–81.

Black, F. L. 1975. Infectious diseases in primitive societies. *Science* 187:515–18.

Blumberg, B. S., W. T. London, A. I. Sutnick, and I. Millman. 1970. Australia antigen, hepatitis and susceptibility to leukemia. In *Comparative Leukemia Research*. R. M. Dutcher, ed. Basel: Karger.

Brown, P., T. Tsai, and D. C. Gajdusek. 1975. Seroepidemiology of human papovaviruses. Discovery of virgin populations and some unusual patterns of antibody prevalence among remote peoples of the world. *American Journal of Epidemiology* 102:331–40.

Bruno, A. A. G. 1978. Condicões sánitarias de escolares em zonas rurais do Território Federal do Amapá. M. Sc. thesis, Universidade Estadual de Campinas, Campinas, Brazil.

Cabannes, R., G. Larrouy, and J. Ruffié. 1964. Étude clinique et hématologique des Indiens du Haut-Oyapock et du Haut-Maroni (Guyane Francaise) Oyampi, Emerillon et Oayana. *Bulletin De La Societe De Pathologue Exotique, Et De Ses Filiales* (Paris) 57:307–25.

Candeias, J. A. N., R. G. Baruzzi, S. Pripas, and M. Iunes. 1977. Prevalence of antibodies to the BK and JC papovaviruses in isolated populations. *Revista De Saúde Publica*, São Paulo 11:510–14.

Carneri, I., N. Nutels, and J. A. Miranda. 1963. Epidemia de leishmaniose tegumentar entre os Índios Waurá do Parque Nacional do Xingu (Estado de Mato Grosso, Brasil). *Revista Do Institudo de Medicine Tropical De Soa Paulo* 5:271–72.

Coimbra, C. E. A., Jr. 1982. Notas para uma análise epidemiológica dos achados de ovos de capillaria sp em exames de fezes realizados entre os Suruís do Parque Indígena de Aripuanã, Rondônia. *Boletim do Centro de Estudos e Pesquisas em Antropologia Médica Brasília* 1:5–6.

Coimbra, C. E. A., Jr., and D. A. Mello. 1981. Enteroparasitas e *capillaria sp* entre o grupo Suruí, Parque Indígena Aripuanã, Rondônia. *Memorias Do Instituto Oswaldo Cruz*, Rio De Janerro 76:299–302.

Damian, R. T. 1964. Lecular mimicry: Antigen sharing by parasite and host and its consequences. *American Naturalist* 98:129–49.

Damianovic, J. 1948. Realidad sanitaria de la población indígena de la zona Austral Antártica. *Rev. Chil. Hig. Med. Prev.* 10:3–17.

D'Andretta, C., Jr., A. S. Ramos, I. Kameyana, L. C. Souza Dias, and H. Penteado Jr. 1969a. Nota preliminar sobre a prevalência de malária entre os Indígenas do Parque Nacional do Xingu. *Revista Paulista De Medicina* 74:331–32.

———. 1969b. Estudo da prevalência da malária em Índios do Parque Nacional do Xingu. Determinação dos índices parasitários e explênico. *Revista Da Sociedade Brasileira De Medicine Tropical* 3:12.

Da Rocha, F. J., and F. M. Salzano. 1972. Anthropometric studies in Brazilian Cayapo Indians. *American Journal of Physical Anthropology* 36:95–101.

Díaz, B., D. Gallegos, F. Murillo, E. Covarrubias, T. Covarrubias, R. Rona, W. Weidman, F. Rothammer, and W. J. Schull. 1978. The multinational Andean genetic and health program. II. Disease and disability among the Aymara. *Bulletin of the Pan American Health Organization.* 12:219–35.

Dubos, R. 1965. *Man Adapting.* New Haven: Yale University Press.

Dunn, F. L. 1968. Epidemiological factors: Health and disease in hunter-gatherers. In *Man the Hunter.* R. B. Lee and I. De Vore, eds. Chicago: Aldine.

Duque, O., G. Arcila, and H. Zuluaga. 1959. Estudio comparativo de la infección por *Entamoeba histolytica* y otros parasitos Iitestinales em Indios y Blancos del Chocó (Colombia). *Antioquia Medica* 9:365–85.

Eichenberger, R. W. 1966. Una filosofía de salud pública para las tribus indígenas Amazónicas. *America Indigina* 26:119–41.

Eveland, W. C., W. J. Olver, and J. V. Neel. 1971. Characteristics of *Escherichia coli* serotypes in the Yanomama, a primitive Indian tribe of South America. *Infection and Immunity* 4:753–56.

Ewald, P. W. 1983. Host-parasite relations, vectors, and the evolution of disease severity. *Annual Review of Ecology and Systematics* 14:465–85.

Ferreira, L. F., A. J. G. Araújo, and U. E. C. Confalonieri. 1983. The finding of helminth eggs in a Brazilian mummy. *Transcripts of the Royal Society for Tropical and Medical Hygiene* 77:65–67.

———. 1982. Os parasitos do homem antigo. *Ciência Hoje* 1(3):63–67.

———. 1980. The finding of eggs and larvae of parasitic helminths in archaeological material from Unai, Minas Gerais, Brazil. *Transcripts of the Royal Society for Tropical and Medical Hygiene* 74:798–800.

Fix, A. G. 1984. Kin groups and trait groups: Population structure and epidemic disease selection. *American Journal of Physical Anthropology* 65:201–12.

Flowers, N. M., D. R. Gross, M. L. Ritter, and D. W. Werner. 1982. Variation in swidden practices in four central Brazilian Indian societies. *Human Ecology* 10:203–17.

Fonseca, O. 1970. Parasitismo e migrações humanas pré-históricas. In *Estudos do Pré-História Geral e Brasileira.* P. Duarte, ed. São Paulo: Instituto de Pré-História, Universidade de São Paulo.

Fros, J. 1956. Filariasis in South American Indians in Surinam. *Docum. Med. Geogr. Trop.* 8:63–69.

Fribourg-Blanc, A., E. Bois, and J. Feingold. 1975. Bilan épidémiologique des Amérindiens de Haute-Guyane Francaise: Sérologie de la toxoplasmose. *Médecine et Maladies Infectieuses* 5:502–7.

Garruto, R. M. 1981. Disease patterns of isolated groups. In *Biocultural Aspects of Disease.* H. R. Rothschild, ed. New York: Academic.

Giglioli, G. G. 1968. Malaria in the American Indian. In *Biomedical Challenges Presented by the American Indian.* Pan American HealthOrganization. Scientific Publication 165:104–13.

Gross, D. R., G. Eiten, N. M. Flowers, F. M. Loei, M. L. Ritter, and D. W. Werner. 1979. Ecology and acculturation among native peoples of central Brazil. *Science* 206:1043–50.

Holmes, R. 1984. Non-dietary modifiers of nutritional status in tropical forest populations of Venezuela. *Interciencia* 9:386–91.

Hugh-Jones, P., D. L. Aston, M. I. D. Cawley, J. Guillebaud, H. I. Jones, R. A. Mills, P. H. Rees, and A. P. Thorley. 1972. Medical studies among Indians of the Upper Xingu. *British Journal Hospital Medicine* 7:317–34.

Kaplan, J. E., J. W. Larrick, J. Yost, L. Farrell, H. B. Greenberg, K. L. Herrmann, A. L. Sulzer, K. W. Well, and L. Pederson. 1980. Infectious disease patterns in the Waorani, an isolated Amerindian population. *American Journal of Tropical Medicine and Hygiene* 29:298–312.

Knight, R., and A. Prata. 1972. Intestinal parasitism in Amerindians at Coari, Brazil. *Transcripts of the Royal Society for Tropical and Medical Hygiene* 66:809–10.

Lage, H. A. 1964. Mansonelose em Índios do grupo Aruak, do Rio Içana. *O Hospital* 66:557–64.

Larrick, J. W., J. A. Yost, J. Kaplan, G. King, and J. Mayhall. 1979. Patterns of health and disease among the Waorani Indians of eastern Ecuador. *Medical Anthropologist* 3:147–89.

Lawrence, D. N., B. Erdtmann, J. W. Peet, J. A. Nunes de Mello, G. R. Healy, J. V. Neel, and F. M. Salzano. 1979a. Epidemiologic studies among Amerindian populations of Amazônia. II. Prevalence of *Mansonella ozzardi. American Journal of Tropical and Medical Hygiene* 28:991–96.

Lawrence, D. N., R. R. Facklam, F. O. Sottnek, G. A. Hancock, J. V. Neel, and F. M. Salzano. 1979b. Epidemiological studies among Amerindian populations of Amazônia. I. Pyoderma: Prevalence and associated pathogens. *American Journal of Tropical and Medical Hygiene* 28:548–58.

Lawrence, D. N., J. V. Neel, S. H. Abadie, L. L. Moore, L. J. Adams, G. R. Healy, and I. G. Kagan. 1980. Epidemiological studies among Amerindian populations of Amazônia. III. Intestinal parasitoses in newly contacted and acculturating villages. *American Journal of Tropical and Medical Hygiene* 29:530–37.

Leser, P. G., M. E. Camargo, and R. G. Baruzzi. 1977. Toxoplasmosis serologic tests in Brazilian Indians (Kren-Akorore) of recent contact with civilized man. *Revista Do Institudo de Medicine Tropical* 19:232–36.

Lovelace, J. K., M. A. P. Moraes, and E. Hagerby. 1978. Toxoplasmosis among the Ticuna Indians in the state of Amazonas Brazil. *Tropical and Geographical Medicine* 30:295–300.

Madalengoitia, J., N. Ishida, T. Umenay, T. Miyamoto, J. Mejía, W. Flores, S. Sánchez, and R. Méndez. 1975. The prevalence of hepatitis B antigen among hepatitis patients and residents of Peru. *Pan American Health Organization.* Bulletin 9:142–47.

Marinkelle, C. J. 1973. First finding of *Dipetalonema perstans* in Colombia. *Tropical Geographical Medicine* 25:51–52.

Marinkelle, C. J., and E. German. 1970. Mansonelliasis in the Comisaría del Vaupés of Colombia. *Tropical Geographical Medicine* 22:101–11.

Moraes, M. A. P., M. M. R. Almeida, J. K. Lovelace, and G. M. Chavez. 1978. *Mansonella ozzardi* entre Índios Ticunas do Estado do Amazonas, Brasil. *Boletin De La Oficina Sanitaria Panamericana* 85:16–25.

Neel, J. V., A. H. P. Andrade, G. E. Brown, W. E. Eveland, J. Goobar, W. A. Sodeman, G. H. Stollerman, E. D. Weinstein, and A. H. Wheeler. 1968a. Further Studies of the Xavante Indians. IX. Immunologic status with respect to various diseases and organisms. *American Journal of Tropical and Medical Hygiene* 17:486–98.

Neel, J. V., W. M. Mikkelsen, D. L. Rucknagel, E. D. Weinstein, R. A. Goyer, and S. H. Abadie. 1968b. Further studies of the Xavante Indians. VIII. Some observations on blood, urine, and stool specimens. *American Journal of Tropical and Medical Hygiene* 17:474–85.

Neel, J. V., and F. M. Salzano. 1967. Further studies on the Xavante Indians. Some hypotheses—generalizations resulting from these studies. *American Journal of Human Genetics* 19:554–74.

Neel, J. V., F. M. Salzano, P. C. Junqueira, F. Keiter, and D. Maybury-Lewis. 1964. Studies on the Xavante Indians of the Brazilian Mato Grosso. *American Journal of Human Genetics* 16:52–140.

Nutels, N. 1968. Medical problems of newly contacted Indian groups. In *Biomedical Challenges Presented by the American Indian*. Pan American Health Organization. Scientific Publication. 165:68–76.

Oliveira, H. C. 1952. O estado de Saúde dos Índios Karajá em 1950. *Boletim do Museu Paulista* 6:489–508.

Orihel, T. C. 1967. Infections with *Dipetalonema perstans* and *Mansonella ozzardi* in the aboriginal Indians of Guyana. *American Journal of Tropical and Medical Hygiene* 16:628–35.

Rachou, R. G. 1957. Distribuição geográfica das filarioses humanas no Brasil. *Revista Brasileira De Malariologia Doenças Tropicais.* 9:79–100.

Ranke, K. E. 1898. Beobachtungen über Bevölkerungsstand und Bevölkerungsbewegung bein Indianern Central-Brasiliens. *Correspondenz-Blatt der deutschen Gesellschaft für Anthropologie, Ethnologie und Urgeschichte* 29:123–34.

Rassi, E., N. Lacerda, and J. A. Guimarães. 1976. Study of the area affected by onchocerciasis in Brazil: Survey of local residents. *Bulletin of the Pan American Health Organization* 10:33–45.

Restrepo, M. 1962. Estudio parasitológico de una región del Amazonas Colombiano. *Antiquia Medica* 12:462–84.

Roever-Bonnet, H. 1967. Toxoplasmosis in Surinam (Netherlands Guyana). A serological survey. *Tropical Geographical Medicine* 19:221–28.

Ross, E. B. 1978. Food taboos, diet and hunting strategy: The adaptation to animals in Amazon cultural ecology. *Current Anthropology* 19:1–36.

Salzano, F. M. 1985. Changing patterns of disease among South American Indians. In *Diseases of Complex Etiology in Small Populations: Ethnic Differences and Research Approaches*. R. Chakraborty and E. J. E. Szathmary, eds. New York: Alan R. Liss.

Salzano, F. M., and B. S. Blumberg. 1970. The Australia antigen in Brazilian healthy persons and in leprosy and leukemia patients. *Journal of Clinical Pathology* 23:39–42.

Salzano, F. M., and J. V. Neel. 1976. New data on the vision of South American Indians. *Bulletin of the Pan American Health Organization* 10:1–8.

Schaad, J. D. G. 1960. Epidemiological observations in Bush Negroes and Amerindians in Surinam. *Tropical Geographical Medicine* 12:38–46.

Schwaner, T. D., and C. F. Dixon. 1974. Helminthiasis as a measure of cultural change in the Amazon Basin. *Biotropica* 6:32–37.

Soyano, A., Z. Layrisse, M. Layrisse, and J. V. Neel. 1979. Hepatitis-Bs antigen in an isolated population of Southern Venezuela: A family study. *Journal of Medical Genetics* 16:201–5.

Soyano, A., I. Malavé, R. Walder, Z. Layrisse, and M. Layrisse. 1976. Hepatitis-B antigen in an isolated Indian population (Yanomama Indians), southern Venezuela. *Revista Brasileira Pesquisas Medicas e Biologicas* 9:247–53.

Sulzer, A. J., R. Cantella, A. Colichan, N. N. Gleason, and K. W. Walls. 1975. A focus of hyperendemic *Plasmodium malariae-P. Vivax* with no *P. falciparum* in a primitive population in the Peruvian Amazon jungle. Studies by means of immunofluorescence and blood smear. *Bulletin of the World Health Organization* 52:273–78.

Tanus, R., C. E. A. Coimbra, Jr., and R. V. Santos. 1984. Pesquisa de portadores inaparentes de *Staphylococcus aureus* entre os grupos indígenas Suruí e Karitiana, Rondônia. Abstracts, XX *Congresso da Sociedade Brasileira de Medicina Tropical*:136.

Weinstein, E. D., J. V. Neel, and F. M. Salzano. 1967. Further studies on the Xavante Indians. VI. The physical status of the Xavantes of Simões Lopes. *American Journal of Human Genetics* 19:532–42.

Werner, D., N. M. Flowers, M. L. Ritter, and D. R. Gross. 1979. Subsistence productivity and hunting effort in native South America. *Human Ecology* 7:303–15.

Wood, C. S. 1975. New evidence for a late introduction of malaria into the New World. *Current Anthropology* 16:93–104.

12 MORTALITY AND MORBIDITY CONSEQUENCES OF VARIATION IN EARLY CHILD GROWTH

Jere D. Haas

As human populations undergo social change associated with migration, urbanization, and economic transition they often express concomitant alterations in diet which result in changes in nutritional and health status. Also, the associated alterations in the physical and biotic environment of these populations in transition may result in new physiological stresses which affect human nutritional requirements. As a result malnutrition often is a common characteristic of "changing" populations. This malnutrition is usually expressed in the form of protein and energy deficiencies as well as iron and vitamin A deficiency diseases such as anemia and xerophthalmia. Protein-energy malnutrition (PEM) usually manifests itself during periods of human growth and results in growth retardation.

The most vulnerable stages of growth are the prenatal period, when maternal malnutrition results in fetal growth retardation, and the early postnatal period, from birth to about six years, when the child is experiencing major biological, psychological, and social changes. For this reason retarded fetal and early child growth is often used as an important indicator of poor nutritional status in human populations. Although malnutrition may affect growth, it is not growth retardation itself that is of primary importance to the clinician, epidemiologist, or health planner. It is that malnutrition may lead to increased susceptibility to infectious disease and ultimately to death — the worst case. If growth retardation is to be used as an indicator of malnutrition and malnutrition in turn is considered an important contributing factor to increased morbidity and mortality, then a clear relationship must be established between growth retardation and the risk of increased morbidity and mortality.

This chapter reviews the literature on prenatal and infant growth as it relates to morbidity and mortality. The review focuses on populations living in developing countries where social, economic, and physical environmental changes are ever-present factors affecting human health and well-being. Growth retardation is viewed here as an important indicator of poor health. There is a need, however, to improve the diagnostic power of specific growth indicators so as to identify children at risk of poor health and death. A human adaptability approach is taken in an effort to place the study of population variation into the context of public health while at the same time expanding upon the adaptive significance of phenotypic variation.

FUNCTIONAL CONSEQUENCES OF VARIATION IN INFANT GROWTH

The examination of functional consequences of subnormal growth has significance to human adaptability theory as well as to the practical application of anthropometry for nutritional status assessment. By functional consequence we mean that gradations in the deviation of a child's growth from the pattern of normal growth will result in increasing limitations of the child to function physically or to accomplish mental tasks. This increasing disfunction with increasing growth retardation can be expressed in several ways, depending on the parameter of growth being measured and the nature of the function that is of relevance to the investigator. For example, the functional consequence of weight loss or failure to gain adequate weight reflects short-term insults to the growth of the child. When weight loss is severe as the result of dehydration from diarrhea, risk of death may be high (Gomez et al. 1956). Thus, increased mortality is a functional consequence of this type of growth failure. On the other hand, reduced statural growth throughout childhood and adolescence may result from chronic undernutrition. This leads to a shortened adult stature. One documented functional correlate of short adult stature, presumed to be the result of childhood undernutrition in women, is reduced reproductive performance and lower offspring birthweight (Thomson and Billewicz 1963).

FUNCTIONAL CORRELATES OF HUMAN GROWTH AND HUMAN ADAPTABILITY

Anthropometric diagnosis of nutritional status relies on the assumption that form reflects function, at least from the point of view that the greater degree of deviation from growth normality, the greater the risk of disfunction. A similar paradigm exists in the biological anthropological theory of human adaptability. Baker (1966) outlines an approach to test the significance of human biological variation in the context of responses to environmental stress. This approach provided the framework for much of the human adaptability research of the past twenty years. It sought to explain the source of biological variation within and between populations, such as body morphological variation through an analysis of adaptive responses to specific environmental stress. By definition, adaptive responses are fundamentally beneficial to the individual. Mazess (1975) expresses this well in his critical review of the high altitude adaptation literature. Unless a trait can objectively be ascertained to "benefit" an individual, it cannot be deemed adaptive.

In an effort to provide a systematic examination of adaptation, Mazess proposed that the benefit of an individual phenotypic characteristic should be observed within one of several "adaptive domains." These include physical performance, growth and development, reproduction, health, nutrition, intellectual ability, central nervous system functioning, cross-tolerance to stress, and affective functioning. Mazess notes that benefit is rarely demonstrated for most phenotypic characteristics that anthropologists call adaptive.

However, benefit may go unrecognized if it is measured out of the context of the total environment in which it became adaptive. Herein lies a major methodological problem of biological anthropology in its effort to discern the adaptive significance of characteristics that may have had their evolutionary origin in past and extinct environments where selection pressures are no longer recognizable.

MALNUTRITION, GROWTH FAILURE, AND MORTALITY AND MORBIDITY RISK IN CHILDREN

One approach to the study of growth that is of particular relevance to the problem of "adaptation and benefit" as suggested by Mazess (1975) is the estimation of the best anthropometric indicators and their appropriate cut-off points for assessing nutritional status. This approach quantifies the relationship between a growth measure such as weight or height, and a functional outcome measure, such as mortality, morbidity, or mental development. In the case of mortality or certain morbidity events, it is possible to dichotomize the classification into alive-dead or well-sick for the purpose of identifying two subpopulations. The anthropometric characteristics of the two subpopulations can be described and, in the case of well-sick the degree of overlap in the distributions can be analyzed to identify areas of overlap. In addition, the two population distributions can be tested for the sensitivity and specificity of a given cut-off point to correctly identify sick and well or alive and dead children. A more detailed description of the procedure will be presented later. At this point, it is important to discuss nutritional status assessment in somewhat more detail so that the application of this analytical approach can be better understood, both in the context of nutritional anthropometry and human adaptation theory.

Poor nutritional status or malnutrition can be assessed in young children in several ways:

1. Dietary intake of specific nutrients.
2. Biochemical evaluation of nutrients and metabolites in urine and blood.

3. Clinical evaluation of the symptoms and signs of nutritional diseases.

4. Anthropometric assessment of nutritional effects on body morphology.

While all of these methods have broad application, each measures different aspects of human nutrition. Probably the most widely used method is nutritional anthropometry. It is relatively easy to do, can be readily used in large surveys as well as clinical situations, and is relatively sensitive to change in nutriture of young children.

The assessment of nutritional status by anthropometry is based on the fact that malnutrition affects child growth and that leads to some degree of deviation from normal growth patterns. The more severe the malnutrition, the greater the effect on growth and the greater the deviation from normal. The deviation of individual children from a healthy population reference standard (a common definition of "normal") can be expressed as a percent of the reference median or mean, a percentile standing, or a Z-score which is based on the reference population mean and standard deviation. By far the most commonly used expression is the percent of standard. This approach has been used to classify children by degrees of wasting or weight retardation (Gomez et al. 1956) and by degrees of stunting or height retardation (Waterlow 1972). The classification devised by Gomez and colleagues (1956) describes four classes or grades of weight relative to a reference standard. Children above 90 percent of the reference weight for a given age (WA) are considered normal, those from 75 to 89 percent of the reference WA are considered first degree malnourished, 60 to 74 percent of WA are second degree malnourished, and less than 60 percent WA are third degree malnourished. A classification for stunting reported by Waterlow (1972) also has four catagories, with children above 95 percent of reference height-for-age (HA) considered normal. Kanawati and McLaren (1970) present four catagories of wasting or low weight-for-height (WH), which permits a further distinction into acute versus chronic growth failure.

Similar classification schemes have been applied to other anthropometric indicators such as skinfolds, mid-upper arm circumference, and weight-for-height (Jelliffe 1966). What is striking about these classifications of PEM is that there is no rational basis for the exact cut-off points used to distinguish the various grades of PEM. While the more severe levels may coincidently correspond to the first or third percentile or minus 2 standard deviations for the reference populations, less severe levels are much more arbitrary. Rarely has the use of a statistically derived cut-off such as this been scrutinized in regard to what it means biologically.

Recently, there have been several attempts to improve upon the use of nutritional anthropometry to assess nutritional status. This research has focused on such questions as: What are the best indicators to use under specific situations (Habicht 1980; Habicht, Meyers, and Brownie 1982)? What are the appropriate reference standards to use in different countries or with different ethnic groups (Habicht et al. 1974; Goldstein and Tanner 1980; Haas 1981)?

What are the appropriate cut-off points for classifying children at different grades of malnutrition (Brownie and Habicht 1984)?

The research on the determination of best indicators of nutritional status assessment is conditioned by the intended use for the information to be derived from an assessment. Some indicators may be better suited for screening and identifying children who need immediate medical care or for estimating the prevalence of malnutrition in a community. Other indicators may be better suited for targeting and monitoring nutrition and health programs or for their later evaluations. It seems that studies of human population biology could benefit most from an improvement in the estimation of true prevalence of a disease by anthropometric methods. This would greatly improve our ability to ascribe functional consequences to morphological variation and thus clarify two points that plague our interpretation of cross-population growth studies: Are there substantial differences in growth patterns of children living in different environments that are not confounded by nutrition and disease differences, and are the functional consequences of deviation from a common growth curve similar in populations living under different environments? For both questions, traditional versus modernizing populations provide a good contrast of environments, while prospective risk of death and morbidity serve as important and convenient measures of functional consequence.

STUDIES OF GROWTH FAILURE AND IMPAIRED FUNCTION IN INFANTS AND YOUNG CHILDREN

In order to demonstrate the state of knowledge in the area of growth and function, as well as to provide an introduction to some of the methods used, this section will selectively review the literature on the topic. The two aspects of impaired function to be discussed are death and morbidity.

Neonatal Mortality and Birthweight

The prospective risk of death as a function of degree of growth retardation has been the most widely studied parameter in this area. The relationship between mortality (infant, neonatal, and perinatal) and birthweight has been the most frequently studied example of the consequences of growth retardation. From the early studies of Karn and Penrose (1951) a methodology was developed to analyze the effects of selection on birthweight. This analytical method fits a parabolic distribution to the relationship of birthweight (BW) and neonatal mortality, expressed as the natural log of the ratio of survivors/nonsurvivors (ln s/d), to determine such parameters as the optimal birthweight or the weight associated with the lowest mortality (highest ln s/d). This approach was later used by Jayant (1964, 1966) for Indian and London infants, Hollingsworth (1965) for Ghanaian infants, and Fracarro (1956) for Italian infants. A major feature of these earlier studies was the clear demonstration of the increased risk of neonatal death with decreasing birthweights below the population mean and with very heavy infants as well, thus suggesting a condition of balancing selection for this morphological characteristic. Van Valen and Mellin (1967) criticized this approach on statistical grounds and reanalyzed previously published data along with those of births from New York City to derive new critical weights as well as "selective mortality" or the excess death rate for the entire sample over that observed at the optimal birthweight class. Finally they computed the "effective mortality," the proportion of all mortality that is selective for birthweight. Their analysis of previously published data indicates that populations with high mortality have more intense selection but less effective mortality for birthweight.

Sansing and Chinnici (1976) introduce the concept of "lower discriminating birthweights" to distinguish those infants whose weights fall below the level where risk of death is equal to risk of surviving. There is also an upper discriminating birthweight which defines comparable risk for very heavy infants. Of particular significance in this paper is the introduction of another analytical procedure to describe the birthweight-mortality relationship that is based on conditional probabilities of surviving, dependent upon the probability of achieving a certain birthweight.

O'Donald (1968, 1970) provides a method for estimating the intensity of natural selection for birthweight by analyzing the change in the population mean and variance mean that resulted after selection (death) had occurred. Population fitness is calculated before and after selection, and the increase in relative fitness can be computed as the ratio of the change in fitness over the mean fitness across birthweight catagories. Beall (1981) uses this approach to show that reduced mean birthweights at high compared to low altitudes in Peru are accompanied by reduced optional birthweights and reduced selection intensity at high altitude.

Much of the aforementioned research is directed at problems related to natural selection for birthweight and is thus of relevance to the anthropological study of human evolution. Public health interests have also been served by this research, as high-risk newborns can then be identified for special care. Of particular interest is the work of Lubchenco, Searls, and Brazie (1972), who incorporate gestational age with birthweight to refine the "at risk" determination in Denver infants, and the work of Goldstein and Peckham (1976), who analyze the relative importance of birthweight versus gestational age on mortality risk in British infants. Thus, there are practical public health issues as well as theoretical evolutionary biology issues that can be addressed through similar analyses of the functional consequences of phenotypic variation. Even though the two general objectives require somewhat different methodologies, they are both concerned with documenting such parameters as *optimal phenotypic values* based on lowest risk of a deleterious outcome such as the birthweight with the lowest mortality risk, *discriminating values* that are associated with an acceptable or expected level of outcome such as the birthweight at which neonatal mortality risk equals survival risk, and the *best cut-off value* of an indicator that results in least misdiagnosis (false negatives and false positives) or lowest cost of misdiagnosis.

Recent research in these areas has focused on the interpretation of newborn body size and mortality risk in populations living in less developed countries where a paucity of research exists. While much of the neonatal mortality in developed countries can be attributed to the low end of the birthweight distribution, most of the low birthweight infants (under 2,500 grams) in these countries are small because they are delivered prematurely (Villar and Belizan 1982a). Relatively few of these fetuses suffer from growth retardation. However, in less developed countries, the prevalence of low birthweight is higher, and most of these small newborns do suffer intrauterine growth retardation (IUGR). Since the causes of low birthweight are quite different between more and less developed countries, it is reasonable to assume that the consequences of low birthweight in terms of mortality risk may also differ between these populations. Also, since intrauterine growth retardation, a reflection of maternal malnutrition, may be either chronic or acute in nature, the mortality risk in the newborn may vary by the type of IUGR. This problem is currently being investigated in several populations living in very different environments in Latin America. These include a heterogeneous urban population of broad socioeconomic status living in Rosario, Argentina (Caulfield 1989), high altitude and low altitude urban populations living in Bolivia (Haas, Balcazar, and Caulfield 1987; Conlisk 1987; Haas, Conlisk, and Frongillo 1989), and a lower socioeconomic class population from Mexico City (Haas, Balcazar, and Caulfield 1987; Balcazar 1988; Balcazar and Haas, in press). Some of the results from the Mexico City study are presented here to illustrate the kind of analysis which can produce better criteria for screening newborn infants so as to allocate more efficiently scarce medical resources to those infants at greatest risk of early neonatal death.

Balcazar (1988) analyzes birth records from the maternal and child health center "Maximino Avila Camacho" in Mexico City to determine the relationship between gestational age, birthweight, and recumbent length as these predict perinatal and early neonatal mortality risk. The data were analyzed using misclassification analysis and receiver operating characteristics (ROC) curves of specificity (Sp) and sensitivity (Se) of selected postnatal newborn risk characteristics to classify children who die in the first three days. Sensitivity is the proportion of newborns correctly identified by the indicator (birthweight, gestational age, or birthweight-for-gestational age) as dying. This is the ratio of true positives divided by all deaths. Specificity is the proportion correctly identified by the indicator as surviving, or the ratio of true negatives divided by all survivors. The positive predictive value (PV +) is the proportion of those predicted to die to those who actually die, or the ratio of true positives to all infants below the indicator's designated cut-off value. At different cut-off levels of an indicator there will be different values of Se, Sp, and PV +.

These characteristics of sensitivity and specificity reflect the discriminatory power of the indicator of risk. At varying values of the cut-off point of an

Table 12.1
Sensitivity and Specificity Analyses for Neonatal Mortality for Four Different Indicators (Mexico City Series).

	Cut-Off Value	Sensitivity (Se)	Specificity (Sp)	Sensitivity & Specificity	Positive Predicted Value (PV+)	Efficiency
Total Sample (n = 9,975; survivors = 9,867; deaths = 108)						
Birthweight (g)	2,200	0.629	0.965	1.594	16.5	96.1
Gestational age (wks)	35	0.490	0.968	1.458	14.7	96.3
Birthweight by gestational age[1]	85	0.657	0.867	1.524	5.1	86.5
Birthweight by gestational age[2]	-0.6	0.666	0.745	1.411	2.7	74.4
Preterm (n = 1,198; survivors = 1,138; deaths = 60)						
Birthweight (g)	2,000	0.900	0.896	1.796	31.3	89.6
Gestational age (wks)	34	0.833	0.817	1.65	19.3	81.8
Birthweight by gestational age[1]	80	0.783	0.875	1.658	24.8	87.0
Birthweight by gestational age[2]	-0.6	0.816	0.716	1.532	13.1	72.1
Term (n = 8,777; survivors = 8,729; deaths = 48)						
Birthweight (g)	2,500	0.395	0.914	1.309	2.4	91.1
Gestational age (wks)	39	0.562	0.518	1.08	0.6	51.8
Birthweight by gestational age[1]	85	0.416	0.877	1.293	1.8	87.4
Birthweight by gestational age[2]	-1.2	0.416	0.887	1.303	1.9	88.4

[1] % of standard.

[2] z score.

indicator for diagnosis, the value for sensitivity is inversely related to specificity. There are costs of misdiagnosis in that some cut-off points will yield fewer false positives at the expense of more false negatives. As sensitivity, and hence the ability to correctly identify all who will die, increases the discriminatory power to identify correctly those who will survive, or specificity, decreases. This approach underlies many of the techniques used in diagnostic medicine as applied to medical decision making (Weinstein and Fineberg 1980). The methods have been further modified by Swets et al. (1979) to evaluate diagnostic procedures using receiver operating characteristics (ROC) curves which are plots of specificity versus sensitivity across all cut-off values of the indicator.

Table 12.1 summarizes the results of this analysis for the total sample of Mexico City infants as well as for subsamples of preterm ($\leq$ 37 weeks) and full-term (> 37 weeks) infants. The best cut-off point (CP) to classify infants who will die is estimated in this case by the maximum sum of Se and Sp to be 2,200 grams for the full sample of 10,000 births, or 2,000 grams for preterm and 2,500 grams for full-term infants. Estimating birthweight relative to expected birthweight-for-gestational age does not improve the maximum sum of Se and Sp for either the subgroups or the whole sample. Figure 12.1 summarizes the results on ROC curves. From these curves it is clear that birthweight alone has a high Se at any level of Sp above 50 percent, compared to gestational age or birthweight-for-gestational age. These results agree with those reported by Hellier and Goldstein (1979) for perinatal mortality risk in three developed countries. We recognize, however, that the potential for measurement error of gestational age is probably much greater than for birthweight. The relatively poor sensitivity of gestational age as an indicator of mortality risk is probably due, in part, to this error. Subdivision of the sample into preterm and full-term results in a higher sum of Se and Sp for all indicators among the preterm subsample compared to the total sample or the full-term sample. Also, gestational age has no predictive power in the full-term infants who make up 93 percent of the total sample. We have expanded our analysis through the use of logistic regression procedures to model the risk of death from birthweight and gestational age. The results of the preliminary analysis suggest that when the entire sample is examined the best model of mortality risk includes only birthweight in the form of the equation

$$P\,(y = 1) = F\,(7.32 - 7.10BW + .094BW^2)$$

where $P\,(y = 1)$ is the probability of dying during the first three postnatal days, $F = 1/(1 + e^{\alpha + \beta x})$, and BW is birthweight.

When the sample is subdivided by gestational age the logistic regression models are quite different. For preterm infants the best model is simply a linear function of birthweight. For full-term infants the best model is one that includes a quadratic function for birthweight, gestational age, and an interaction term of birthweight with gestational age. We suspect that the inclusion of gestational age

Figure 12.1
Adapted ROC Probability Plot for Three Indicators of Early Neonatal Mortality in a Mexico City Population.

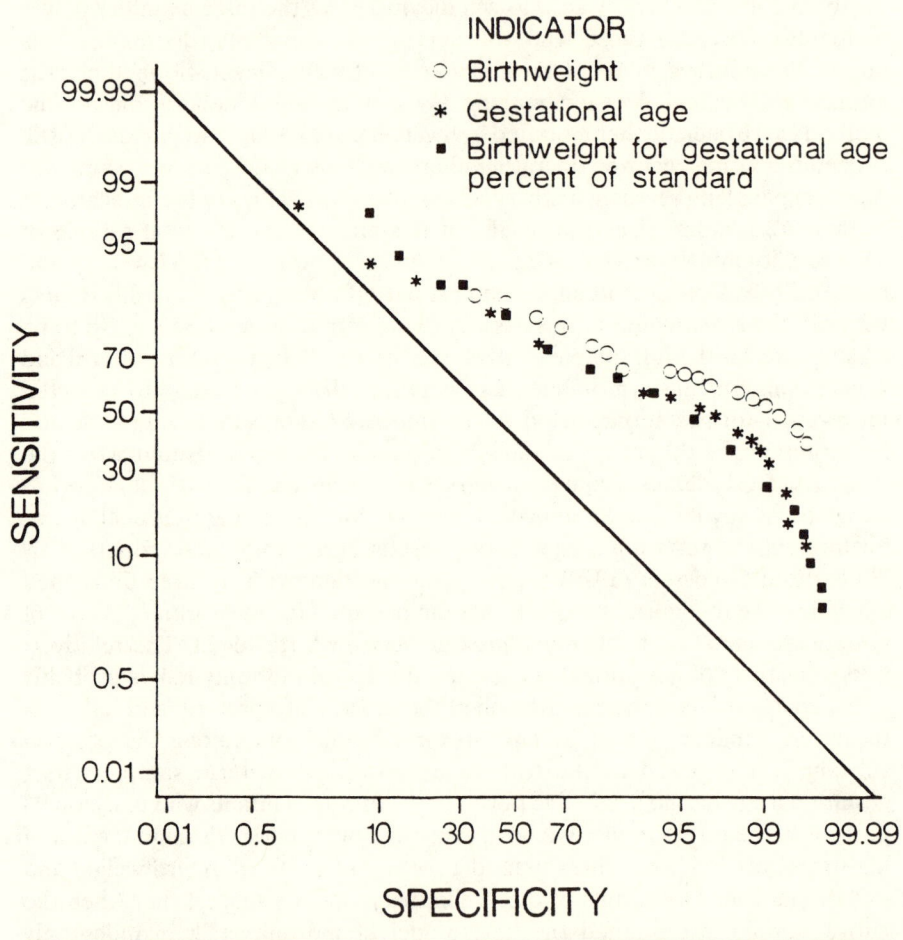

Source: Balcazar (1988).

in the full-term model may reflect the slight increased risk of death among post-term and very large infants.

Other anthropometric indicators such as recumbent length and head circumference were also evaluated as risk factors for mortality in this sample from Mexico City. The infants were classified as to the type of fetal growth retardation (acute or chronic) following a modified version of the scheme suggested by Villar and Belizan (1982b). This classification is based on identifying infants whose weights and crown-heel lengths fall below the tenth percentile levels for a given gestational age using the newborn reference standards developed by Lubchenco et al. (1966).

In this classification scheme all babies who are below the tenth percentile for weight at their specific gestational ages are classified as "small for gestational age" (SGA). Within this group of SGA infants it is possible to identify those whose recumbent or crown-heel length is also below the tenth percentile. These infants are classified as "proportionate" in their growth pattern, and this reflects a long-term or chronic form of growth retardation (CGR). SGA infants who have normal linear growth with recumbent length above the tenth percentile are classified as "disproportionate" in their growth pattern, which reflects an acute growth retardation (AGR). Table 12.2 presents the risks of dying during the early neonatal period for these six different classifications of newborns. A relative risk of 1.0 is represented by the full-term infant with normal birthweight. Relative to normal, term infants, all other groups carried at least a twofold increased risk of mortality. Of particular interest is the greater mortality risk observed in the SGA infants who were classified as proportionately growth retarded compared to those classified as disproportionately growth retarded. This is particularly striking for the full-term infants where the CGR group has nearly ten times the mortality risk of the AGR group.

It appears that these results conflict with those cited in Hoffman and Bekketeig (1984) where newborn infants have a greater mortality risk if they are suffering AGR. An examination of the birthweight distributions of survivors and nonsurvivors for each group of Mexican full-term SGA infants, however, reveals similar birthweight distributions (mean and standard deviation) for AGR

Table 12.2
Relative Risks for Neonatal Mortality by Gestational Age and Growth Retardation Classification.

Gestational Age Group	Weight Adequate for Gestational Age (AGA)	Weight Small for Gestational Age (SGA)	
		Chronic Growth Retarded (CGR)[1]	Acute Growth Retarded (AGR)[2]
Full-term, 37 wks	1.0[3]	26.0	2.7
(number)	(7,642)	(96)	(788)
Preterm, 37 wks	10.4	74.3	48.7
(number)	(1,066)	(24)	(44)

[1] Weight proportionate to length.

[2] Weight disproportionate to length.

[3] Reference category has mortality rate of 2.8 per 1000 deliveries. All other categories have mortality rates equal to the relative risk times 2.8.

nonsurvivors and CGR survivors. This suggests that at comparable birthweights the disproportionately growth-retarded infant is more likely to die, as suggested by Hoffman and Bekketeig. Also these authors and others who have examined the postnatal consequences of chronic and acute fetal growth retardation have used a different classification system which would result in different patterns of postnatal risk among groups of SGA infants. The more common classification scheme follows Villar and Bellizan (1982b) and uses a low Rohrer's ponderal index (weight x $100/\text{length}^3$) as an indication of disproportionate growth retardation. The application of this alternative scheme to the Mexican data suggests that more misclassification and inferior discrimination of infants at risk results from the use of ponderal index in place of recumbent length for gestational age (Balcazar 1988). Moreover, variations between studies in random and systematic measurement errors for gestational age, birthweight, crown-heel length and mortality are likely to contribute substantially to the differences in percentage distribution among classified groups, as well as the mortality risk within groups. The results presented here are preliminary, but they highlight two points: (1) heterogeneity in mortality risk does exist across infant subgroups; and (2) the exact magnitude of the risks is no doubt, influenced by errors in misclassification. This emphasizes the need for future evaluation of the classification scheme using data bases with accurate measurements of both crown-heel length and gestational age.

Childhood Mortality and Growth

Mortality risk has also been used as a criterion for evaluating anthropometric indicators of nutritional and health status in preschool children. In these cases the analysis has been quite different from that applied to birthweight. Mortality is a particularly appropriate outcome variable in the evaluation of indicators of malnutrition and adaptation for several reasons: (1) it can be easily categorized into two groups—living and dead; (2) it has functional meaning; and (3) it is relatively easy data to collect and tabulate. It has limitations as well which are associated with multifactorial causes of death and with bias in reporting deaths and their causes. Certain morbidity characteristics of a population may also be used as less severe outcomes. Morbidity also suffers from limitations similar to mortality data and must be used with caution.

Many researchers have reported on the relationship between reduced weight or height-for-age in hospitalized populations of preschool children. The "Gomez classification" of weight-for-age was established on Mexican children admitted to malnutrition wards (Gomez et al. 1956). Subsequent work by Garrow and Pike (1967), Kahn (1959), and McLaren et al. (1969) on other clinical populations provided insight and contradictory results regarding the relationship between weight and height deficits and mortality risk. Until recently few studies have been conducted on nonhospitalized and free-living populations.

Studies by Kielman and McCord (1978) in India and Sommer and Lowenstein (1975), Trowbridge and Sommer (1981), and Chen, Chowdhury, and Huffman (1980) in Bangladash use relative risk of death of malnourished children compared to "healthy" well-nourished controls to evaluate various anthropometric indicators in large free-living samples of children under demographic and health surveillance. All of these studies show increased mortality risk with decreasing values of weight, height, or mid-upper arm circumference. The most comprehensive of these studies is the one by Chen and colleagues (1980) which is further analyzed by Cogill (1982). While Chen, Chowdhury, and Huffman attempt to rank anthropometric indicators of nutritional status by the criteria of relative risk, Cogill employs a battery of analytical approaches that include sensitivity and specificity criteria; such as, the maximum sum of sensitivity plus specificity across various levels of an indicator, ROC curves. Cogill also uses various statistical procedures that evaluate the degree of difference between Se and Sp distributions (cf. Habicht, Meyers, and Brownie 1982; Brownie, Habicht, and Cogill 1986). These are analogous to normalized distances of various anthropometric indicators as they discriminate children who will survive from those who will die over a twenty-four-month period of surveillance. The normalized distance statistic proves to be the best criterion for ranking indicators due to its statistical efficiency and computational ease. Although the distance measures are useful for ranking indicators, they do not provide information on the best cut-off value of an indicator for identifying individual children. Maximum sum of Se plus Sp and ROC curves, however, can be used in this way. It should also be noted that the determination of best indicators and cut-off values of prospective risk of death are dependant on such factors as cause of death, length of surveillance, precision of measurement, number of deaths observed, and, perhaps, sex of the child.

Childhood Morbidity and Growth

Another approach to the application of these methods could employ consequences of growth failure that are less severe than death. Risk of hospitalization or specific morbid events such as diarrhea could also be studied under appropriate surveillance situations. It has been postulated that growth failure due to PEM and diarrheal disease are mutually causative in that an indirect relationship exists. While the effect of diarrhea on growth and PEM has been well documented (Martorell et al. 1975; Rowland, Cole, and Whitehead 1977), the reverse effect of PEM on increasing the risk of diarrhea is less conclusive. Chen, Hug, and Huffman (1981) provide one of the best attempts to test this reverse effect through a prospective field study of diarrheal risk in Bangladesh. They report no difference in diarrheal hospitalization rates over twenty-four months when children were classified by weight-for-age, height-for-age, and weight-for-height at the beginning of the surveillance period. Nor did they observe a relationship between diarrheal attack rates and previously achieved growth or growth rates. However, this result could be challenged on several grounds. The study only considers the number of diarrhea episodes and not their severity. For example, deaths due to diarrhea are not treated separately from milder diarrhea episodes. Furthermore, the data they report do suggest an effect of reduced height-for-age on diarrheal treatment rates in children of normal weight-for-height. Among children of normal weight-for-height the 493 with height-for-age between 85 percent and 89 percent of the Harvard standard have a 33 percent higher treatment rate than the 578 with normal height (above 90 percent of standard). It is possible that a two-year surveillance of diarrhea (or deaths) is too long a period to link to such a labile measure as weight taken at the beginning of the observation period. Height could be expected to be a better indicator of long-term prognosis due to its relative stability and reflection of chronic growth retardation.

Little has been done to convert information on growth failure and morbidity into an evaluation of anthropometric indicators of nutritional or health status. McDowell and King (1982) examine the sensitivity, specificity, and predictive values of arm circumference and weight in identifying clinically malnourished Zambian children. While they report higher specificity (.42 - .43) at a fixed sensitivity (.95) for arm circumference measures relative to weight measures (Sp = .30 - .36), they do not analyze height and provide Sp values for only one cut-off point for each indicator.

We have attempted to establish criteria for assessing mild-to-moderate growth failure using morbidity data from a semi-urban area of West Java in Indonesia. In that case it was felt that several issues were important to investigate. The first is whether healthy middle-class West Javan children grow as well as the international growth reference (WHO 1983) and thus follow the generalizations of Habicht et al. (1974) that populations of middle- and upper-class preschool age children around the world differ very little in weight and height or length. This observation has been used to justify a single universal international reference standard to evaluate child growth. The second is to determine whether the various nutritional status classification schemes of Gomez et al. (1956), Waterlow (1972), and Kanawati and McLaren (1970) have any validity for mild-to-moderately growth-retarded children. The third issue follows from the second; we wished to know what are the best cut-off values for weight-for-age, height-for-age, and weight-for-height to be used in screening moderately malnourished children in this population. The fourth issue is the choice of best anthropometric indicators of mild-to-moderate nutritional status.

The data used to explore these issues were obtained from records of a maternal-child health clinic in Bogor, Indonesia. This clinic provides primary and secondary health care to the semi-urban neighborhood and also provides a unique service of out-patient care to children who have been diagnosed as suffering from the most severe forms of protein-energy malnutrition, kwashiorkor and marasmus. From the health clinic records for the years 1976–1981 we identified 3,398 male children (aged 1 to 60 months) who were seen at least three times by clinic staff. From the records it is possible to assign each child to one of three groups according to a pediatrician's diagnosis:

1. "Healthy" well-nourished, middle socioeconomic class children with no history of major illnesses. (N = 1752)
2. "Sick" children who have had major and at times repeated bouts of illness such as upper- and lower-respiratory infections and gastrointestinal, skin, and eye infections. (N = 1489)
3. "Severely sick" children with clinical symptoms of kwashiorkor, marasmus, or marasmic kwashiorkor. (N = 157)

The results relative to the four issues presented above can be summarized. Figure 12.2 shows that the "healthy" Indonesian children generally track between the tenth and fifteenth percentile of the United States growth reference standards used by WHO (1983). Those children who are from the upper socioeconomic classes of Bogor and who are seen by private pediatricians track between the twenty-fifth and thirty-fifth percentile of the WHO reference.

Figure 12.2
Age Trends in Body Weight of Healthy U.S. and Indonesian Boys.

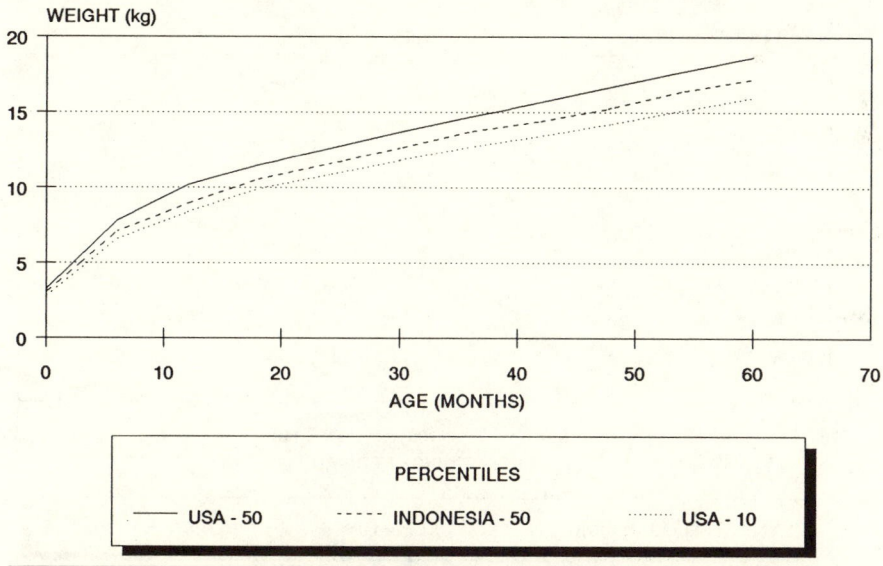

Source: U.S. curves redrawn from Hamill et al. (1977). Indonesian curve drawn from Y. Husaini, unpublished data.

Figure 12.3
Frequency Distributions of Weight for Three Subgroups of Indonesian Preschool Male Children.

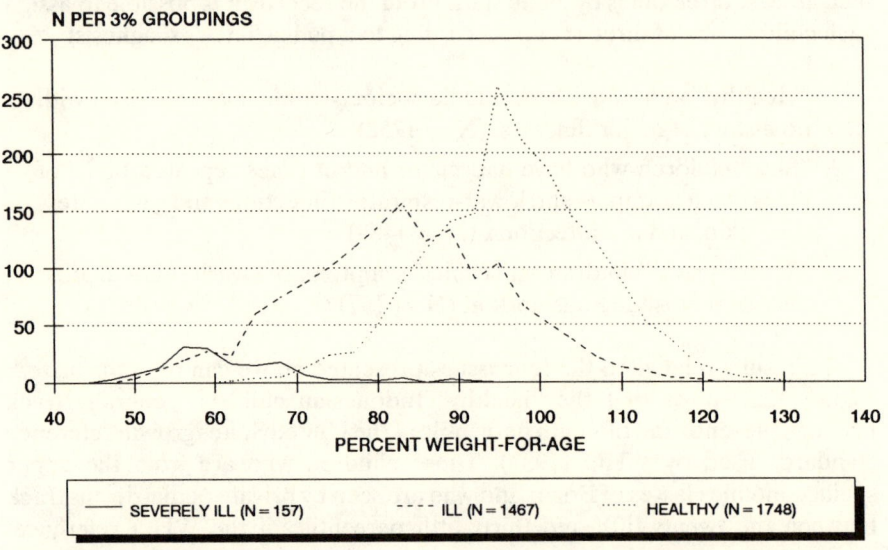

Figure 12.4
Frequency Distributions of Height (Length) for Three Subgroups of Indonesian Preschool Male Children.

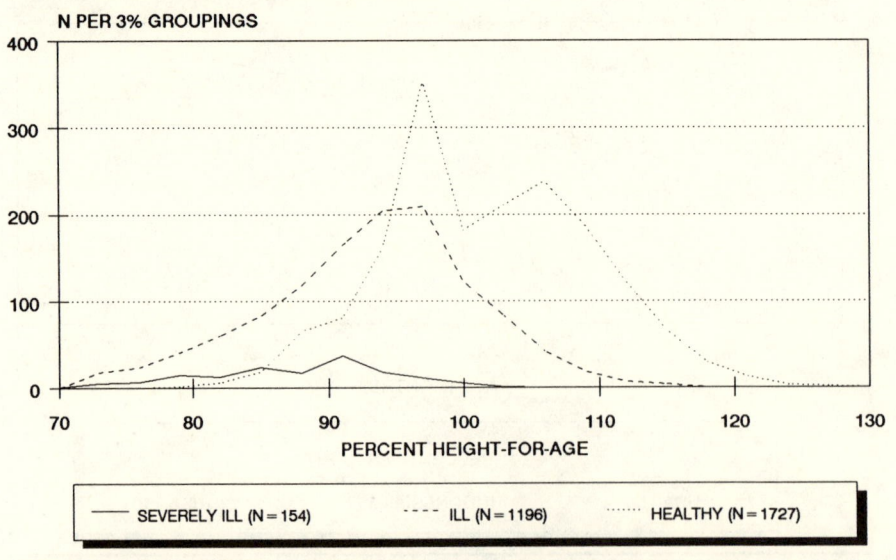

Source (Both Figures): Y. Husaini, unpublished data.

Therefore, the healthy Bogor middle-class children are still smaller than the Bogor upper class who in turn are smaller than American children.

Weights and heights for all children were standardized relative to mean values for healthy children of the same age. Each child is represented by a value for weight computed as

$$\text{weight-for-age} = \frac{\text{actual weight x 100}}{\text{mean weight of healthy boys of the same age.}}$$

Height-for-age was computed the same way. Figures 12.3 and 12.4 present the frequency distributions for the three diagnosed groups and show that weight seems to distinguish the three groups better than height. The best cut-off values for weight-for-age, height-for-age, and weight-for-age were determined by the maximum sum of sensitivity plus specificity to identify whether a child was likely to be diagnosed as "moderately sick" or "severely sick." The results of this analysis are summarized in Table 12.3. It is clear that diagnosis of "severely sick" is done with much more certainty than "moderately sick." The sum of Se plus Sp is consistently higher for all indicators at all ages for the severe classes. The higher Se plus Sp for weight-for-age compared to height-for-age supports the observation of better discriminatory power for weight at both levels of severity of illness. Examination of the cut-off values determined to be the "best" suggests that percent weight-for-age is substantially lower in severe than moderate groups but that percent height-for-age is only slightly lower in severe cases and then only after twelve months. This suggests that the progression from moderate to severe illness is an acute event superimposed on mild but chronic growth retardation. It is also important to note that the cut-off values for percent weight-for-age and height-for-age are not constant across all ages. Cut-off values tend to decrease with age, suggesting several explanations: True population variation (coefficient of variation) is not constant across ages; the type and severity of morbidity measured here is age dependent; and each age group shows a different relationship between illness and growth.

USE OF BEST DIAGNOSTIC CRITERIA FOR ESTABLISHING INTERPOPULATION DIFFERENCES IN GROWTH STANDARDS

The results of these analyses of mortality and morbidity are useful in several ways.

1. They provide objective criteria for selecting the best anthropometric indicators of PEM.
2. They validate the conventional cut-off values of Gomez, Waterlow, Jelliffe, Kanawati and McLaren, and others for weight and height indicators of PEM.

Table 12.3
Best Cut-Off Values for Three Anthropometric Indicators of Nutritional Status in Indonesian Male Preschool Children.

| Group | Number | Mild-to-Moderate | | Severe | |
		Cut-off % of Standard[1]	Sensitivity (Se) & Specificity (Sp)	Cut-off % of Standard[1]	Sensitivity (Se) & Specificity (Sp)
		Weight-for-Age Classification by Age Group (months) [2]			
7	901	90	1.44	75	1.85
6–13	836	87	1.35	72	1.77
12–25	896	84	1.44	72	1.78
24	739	77	1.51	67	1.73
		Height-for-Age Classification by Age Group (months) [2]			
7	896	95	1.34	95	1.67
6–13	831	95	1.25	95	1.56
12–25	887	95	1.32	92	1.58
24	736	89	1.35	86	1.42
		Weight-for-Height Classification by Height Group (cm)			
75	1,711	92.5	1.37	85.0	1.74
72–85	1,028	92.5	1.39	82.5	1.76
82	662	92.5	1.35	82.5	1.69

[1] Cut-off value based on the % of reference standard median for healthy Indonesian children.
[2] Age groups represent overlapping (nonexclusive) distributions.

3. They can serve as the basis for establishing local cut-off values for the international growth standards where criteria of risk of illness in a specific environment are used to evaluate severity of growth failure.

The last two issues are important to the understanding of growth in children who migrate to new environments as well as in children from different ethnic groups living in similar environments. The current debate over the applicability of local versus international growth reference standards is based on whether the *average* growth of healthy well-nourished children is different between populations. The general consensus is that these interpopulation differences are small relative to the differences in growth that are related to socioeconomic variation within populations (Habicht et al. 1974). If one takes the position of those who advocate a single international reference standard, then does one also accept that the conventional cut-off points for diagnosis of various types and grades of PEM are applied with these standards to all populations? Or, if one accepts that local standards are appropriate for specific populations, what then are the criteria for diagnosis that are to be used? For example, does one now apply the conventional Gomez cut-off values of 90, 75, and 60 percent of the new local reference weight-for-age or does one use the cut-off values established relative to the international reference but use the local standard to reflect mean growth only?

Table 12.4 demonstrates the complexity of various cut-off values that are possible for Indonesian children. The absolute cut-off values used in this table are those established by Gomez, Waterlow, and Kanawati and McLaren as computed from two reference populations: Indonesia and the United States (WHO/NCHS reference). These conventional cut-off values are compared to cut-off values for different grades of growth failure as computed from the sensitivity and specificity analysis described in Table 12.3. Male children at thirty months are the basis for these comparisons.

The 60 percent of reference weight is commonly used by nutritionists worldwide as a criterion for severe PEM or wasting. If the WHO/NCHS reference standard (WHO 1983) for male thirty-month-old children is a medium weight of 13.67 kg, then the 60 percent cut-off is 8.20 kg. However, if the Indonesian reference median for healthy well-nourished children is 12.41 kg then the 60 percent weight cut-off is 7.45 kg or 54 percent of the WHO/WCHS reference median. If one refers to Table 12.3, it is clear that the best cut-off point for diagnosing severe PEM based on sensitivity and specificity analysis of the Indonesian data is 69 percent of the Indonesia reference standard or 8.56 kg. This weight corresponds to 63 percent of the WHO/NCHS reference.

One can assume that the Gomez 60 percent cut-off is meant to screen the most severe cases who have a high risk of dying and not just a risk of hospitalization. Data on prospective mortality risk from a different subsample of the same Indonesian population (Jahari 1982) suggest a cut-off value of 9.16

Table 12.4
Comparison of Various Cut-Off Values for Assessing Nutritional Status in Thirty Month-Old Indonesian Male Children.

Criteria for Diagnosis	Conventional Cut-Off Points from Various Published Sources			Empirically Derived Cut-Off Points from Indonesian Morbidity/Mortality Study		
	% of Standard	Anthropometric Value NCHS	Indonesia	Anthropometric Value	%of Standard NCHS	Indonesia
Stunting or Height-for-Age (cm) (Kanawati & McLaren 1970)						
Median	100	92.3	87.8	87.8	95	100
Mild	95	87.7	83.4	78.1	85	89
Moderate	90	83.1	79.0	75.5	82	86
Severe	85	78.5	74.6	76.6	83	87
Underweight or Weight-for-Age (kg) (Gomez et al. 1956)						
Median	100	13.67	12.41	12.41	91	100
Mild	90	12.30	11.17	10.05	74	81
Moderate	75	10.25	9.31	8.56	63	69
Severe	60	8.20	7.45	9.16	67	74
Wasting or Weight-for-Height at 93 cm (kg) (Waterlow 1972)						
Median	100	13.65	13.71	13.71	100	100
Mild	90	12.29	12.34	12.75	93	93
Moderate	80	10.92	10.97	11.93	87	87
Severe	70	9.55	9.6	11.87	87	87

kg or 67 percent of the WHO/NCHS reference for the most severe grade of PEM. It appears as if the 60 percent level of the international standard is somewhat low but, nonetheless, a relatively efficient cut-off point for this population, and that 60 percent of the Indonesian standard would be too low and result in a considerable misclassification of false negative children.

Even though the most severe Gomez classification relative to WHO/NCHS reference standards may be valid in this case, the less severe levels of wasting and stunting are not so clearly related to functional outcomes. It is apparent that the best cut-off points of weight and height in this population do not correspond to the conventional published cut-off values, regardless of which reference population one chooses. In fact, some classifications, such as Waterlow's weight-for-height criteria for severe PEM, are totally inappropriate. The point to be made from this analysis is that the currently recognized criteria for assessing nutritional status from anthropometry suffers from considerable insensitivity to the functional consequences of PEM, at least in this Indonesian population. There is also evidence that some of these criteria for misclassification vary from population to population (Haas and Habicht 1990).

SUMMARY

It appears that the issue for individual assessment of nutritional status is not which growth reference standards are the "best" for a particular population but whether cut-off points and criteria for assessment of different grades of PEM differ among populations for which a particular reference is used. At this point, there is insufficient published evidence to evaluate this proposition. Clearly more research needs to be done with populations from diverse genetic backgrounds, living in widely differing environments, and possessing variable morbidity and mortality patterns. Populations in transition are good prospects for this type of study. An anthropological approach to the question will provide insights to the environmental and population-specific nature of these standards and cut-off values.

The adaptive significance of human morphological variation has long been a central theme in biological anthropology. For studies of the functional consequence of human biological variation, growth failure provides both a clinical and epidemiological basis for using growth assessment and a way of testing the adaptive significance of growth variation. The anthropological approach can be viewed in two ways. One approach applies the concept of adaptive domains as proposed by Mazess (1975). This approach emphasizes the current state of biological fitness or adaptedness of individuals, and with proper sampling procedures and careful interpretation some population level inference can be made. By focusing on adaptation of individuals, the approach does not presume to evaluate population adaptations in an evolutionary sense. Some inference regarding the population can be made from carefully selected samples. However, child growth has never been studied under the proper conditions to permit strong conclusions regarding the evolutionary forces that might have led to phenotypic variation in body size. It is important to remember that studies of growth and function in contemporary humans provide little direct documentation of the adaptive significance of certain phenotypic traits that may have been of benefit in historical or prehistorical environments. This is especially true for specific nutritional and disease factors that may have been important selective agents in the past but no longer function as such today (Haas 1983). The examples presented in this chapter all deal with short-term observation of complex biological characteristics in very changeable environments. This greatly limits our ability to address evolutionary questions from these data.

The second approach attempts to assess the intensity of natural selection in specific environments by examining the morphological variation of a presumed adaptive characteristic before and after selection. Previous research on the intensity of selection for birthweight at high and low altitudes in Peru (Beall 1981) provides some evidence for a lower optimal birthweight at high altitude. However, one must also be cautious in assuming adaptively significant selection in these kinds of studies without some knowledge of the genetic component of phenotypic variation in the characteristic being measured within the context of short-term observations and changeable environments.

NOTE

I am grateful to Hector Balcazar for permission to use unpublished data from his study of newborns in Mexico City. I am also grateful to Yayah Husaini and Abas Jahari for their help in collecting and analyzing the Indonesian data. Laura Caulfield provided considerable insight in the development of ideas presented here. I especially wish to thank fellow participants in the Wenner-Gren conference for their constructive criticisms of an earlier draft of this chapter. The National Science Foundation (Grant BNS 8407407) and the World Bank provided financial support for the research reported herein. This is a report of research from the Agricultural Experiment Station, Division of Nutritional Sciences, Cornell University.

REFERENCES

Balcazar, H. 1988. Birthweight-mortality relationships in an urban poor population of Mexico City: Implications for screening infants at risk. Ph.D. diss., Cornell University.

Balcazar, H., and J. D. Haas. In press. Retarded fetal growth patterns in relation to early neonatal mortality in an urban population of Mexico City. *Bulletin of the Pan American Health Organizaion.*

Baker, P. T. 1966. Human biological variation as an adaptive response to the environment. *Eugenics Quarterly* 13:81–91.

Beall, C. M. 1981. Optimal birthweights in Peruvian populations at high and low altitudes. *American Journal of Physical Anthropology* 56:209–16.

Brownie, C., and J.-P. Habicht. 1984. Selecting a screening cut-off point or diagnostic criteria for comparing prevalences of disease. *Biometrics* 40:675–84.

Brownie, C., J-P. Habicht and B. Cogill. 1986. Comparing indicators of health or nutritional status. *American Journal of Epidemiology* 124:1031–44.

Caulfield, L. E. 1989. An epidemiological study of the determinants and postnatal helath consequences of variation in ponderal index among intrauterine growth retarded infants. Ph.D. diss., Cornell University.

Chen, L. C., A. K. M. A. Chowdhury, and S. L. Huffman. 1980. Anthropometric assessment of energy-protein malnutrition and subsequent risk of mortality among preschool age children. *American Journal of Clinical Nutrition* 33:1836–45.

Chen, L. C., E. Hug, and S. L. Huffman. 1981. A prospective study of the risk of diarrheal diseases according to the nutritional status of children. *American Journal of Epidemiology* 114:284–92.

Cogill, B. 1982. Ranking anthropometric indicators using mortality in rural Bangladesh children. M.S. thesis. Cornell University.

Conlisk, E. A. 1987. The effect of high altitude on birthweight and mortality in Bolivia. M.S. thesis. Cornell University.

Fraccaro, M. 1956. A contribution to the study of birthweight based on an Italian sample. *Annals of Human Genetics* [London] 20:282–97.

Garrow, J. S., and M. C. Pike. 1967. The short-term prognosis of severe primary infantile malnutrition. *British Journal of Nutrition* 21:155–65.

Goldstein, H., and Peckham. 1976. Birthweight, gestation, neonatal mortality and child development. In *The Biology of Human Fetal Growth*. D. F. Roberts and A. M. Thomson, eds. London: Taylor & Francis.

Goldstein, H., and J. M. Tanner. 1980. Ecological considerations in the creation and the use of child growth standards. *Lancet* i: 582–85.

Gomez, F., R. Ramos-Galvan, S. Frenk, J. Craviato, R. Chavez, and J. Vazquez. 1956. Mortality in second and third degree malnutrition. *Journal of Tropical Paediatrics* 2:77–83.

Haas, J. D. 1983. Nutrition and high altitude adaptation: An example of human adaptability in a multistress environment. In *Rethinking Human Adaptation: Biological and Social Models*. R. Dyson-Hudson and M.A. Little, eds. Boulder, Colo: Westview.

———. 1981. Human adaptability approach to nutritional assessment: A Bolivian example. *Federation Proceedings*. 40:2577–82.

Haas, J. D., H. Balcazar, and L. Caulfield. 1987. Variation in early neonatal mortality for different types of fetal growth retardation. *American Journal of Physical Anthropology* 73:467–73.

Haas, J. D., E. Conlisk, and E. A. Frongillo. 1989. Fetal growth and neonatal mortality at high and low altitudes in Bolivia. *American Journal of Physical Anthropology* 78:233.

Haas, J. D. and J-P. Habicht. 1990. Growth and growth charts in the assessment of preschool nutritional status. In *Diet and Disease in Traditional and Developing Societies*. G. A. Harrison and J. C. Waterlow, eds. Cambridge: Cambridge University Press.

Habicht, J-P. 1980. Some characteristics of indicators of nutritional status for use in screening and surveillance. *American Journal of Clinical Nutrition* 33:531–35.

Habicht, J.-P., R. Martorell, C. Yarbrough, R. M. Malina, and R. E. Klein. 1974. Height and weight standards for preschool children. How relevant are ethnic differences in growth potential? *Lancet* i:611–15.

Habicht, J.-P., L. Meyers, and C. Brownie. 1982. Indicators for identifying and counting the improperly nourished. *American Journal of Clinical Nutrition* 35:1241–54.

Hamill, P. P. V., T. A. Drizd, C. L. Johnson, R. B. Reed, and A. F. Roche. 1977. NCHS *Growth Curves for Children from Birth to 18 Years: United States* Publ. No. PHS 78–1650: Vital Statistics Series 11, no. 165. US Department of Health, Education and Welfare, Hyattsville, Md.

Hellier, L. J., and H. Goldstein. 1979. The use of birthweight and gestational age to assess perinatal mortality risk. *Journal of Epidemiology and Community Health* 33:183–85.

Hoffman, H., and L. Bekketeig. 1984. Heterogeneity of intrauterine growth, retardation and recurrence risk. *Seminars in Perinatology* 8:15–24.

Hollingsworth, M. J. 1965. Observation on the birthweights and survival of African babies: Single births. *Annals of Human Genetics* [London] 28:291–300.

Jahari, A. B. 1982. Anthropometric measures for use in monitoring risk of death in under five years of age for the Nutritional Surveillance System in Indonesia. M.S. thesis. Cornell University.

Jayant, K. 1966. Birthweight and survival: A hospital survey repeated after 15 years. *Annals of Human Genetics* [London] 29:367–76.

———. 1964. Birthweight and some other factors in relation to infant survival: A study on an Indian sample. *Annals of Human Genetics* [London] 27:261–73.

Jelliffe, D. B. 1966. *The Assessment of the Nutritional Status of the Community. World Health Organization Monograph.* [Geneva] No. 53.

Kahn, E. 1959. Prognostic criteria of severe protein malnutrition. *American Journal of Clinical Nutrition* 7:161–65.

Kanawati, A. A., and D. S. McLaren. 1970. Assessment of marginal malnutrition. *Nature* 228:573.

Karn, M. M., and L. S. Penrose. 1951. Birthweight and gestation time in relation to maternal age, parity and infant survival. *Annals of Eugenics* 16:147–64.

Kielman, A. A., and C. McCord. 1978. Weight-for-age as an index of risk of death in children. *Lancet* ii:1247–50.

Lubchenco, L. O., C. Hansman, and E. Boyd. 1966. Intrauterine growth in length and head circumference as estimated from live births at gestational ages from 26–42 weeks. *Pediatrics* 37:403–8.

Lubchenco, L. O., D. T. Searls, and J. V. Brazie. 1972. Neonatal mortality rate: Relationship to birthweight and gestational age. *Journal of Pediatrics* 81:814–22.

Martorell, R., J.-P Habicht, C. Yarbrough, A. Lechtig, R. Klein, and K. A. Western. 1975. Acute morbidity and physical growth in rural Guatemalan children. *American Journal of Diseases of Childhood* 129:1296–1301.

Mazess, R. B. 1975. Human adaptation to high altitude. In *Physiological Anthropology.* A. Damon, ed. New York: Oxford University Press.

McDowell, I., and F. S. King. 1982. Interpretation of arm circumference as an indicator of nutritional status. *Archives of Diseases in Childhood* 57:292–96.

McLaren, D. S., E. Shirajian, H. Loshkajian, and S. Shadarevian. 1969. Short-term prognosis in protein-calorie malnutrition. *American Journal of Clinical Nutrition* 22:863–70.

O'Donald, P. 1970. Measuring the change of population fitness by natural selection. *Nature* 227:307–8.

———. 1968. Measuring the intensity of natural selection. *Nature* 220:197–98.

Rowland, M. G. M., T. J. Cole, and R. G. Whitehead. 1977. A quantitative study into the role of infection in determining nutritional status in Gambian children. *British Journal of Nutrition* 37:441–50.

Sansing, R. C., and J. P. Chinnici. 1976. Optimal and discriminating birthweights in human populations. *Annals of Human Genetics* [London] 40:123–31.

Sommer, A., and M. S. Lowenstein. 1975. Nutritional status and mortality: A prospective validation of the QUAC stick. *American Journal of Clinical Nutrition* 28:287–92.

Swets, J. A., R. M. Pickett, S. F. Whitehead, D. S. Getty, J. A. Schnur, and J. B. Swets. 1979. Assessment of diagnostic technologies. *Science* 205:753–59.

Thomson, A. M., and W. Z. Billewicz. 1963. Nutritional status, maternal physique and reproductive efficiency. *Proceedings of the Nutrition Society* 22:55–60.

Trowbridge, T. L., and A. Sommer. 1981. Nutritional anthropometry and mortality risk. *American Journal of Clinical Nutrition* 34:2591.

Van Valen, L., and G. W. Mellin. 1967. Selection in natural populations. 7 New York babies (Fetal Life Study). *Annals of Human Genetics* [London] 31:109–26.

Villar, J., and J. M. Belizan. 1982a. The relative contribution of prematurity and fetal growth retardation to low birthweight in developing and developed societies. *American Journal of Obstetrics and Gynecology* 143:793–98.

————. 1982b. The timing factor in the pathophysiology of the intrauterine growth retardation syndrome. *Obstetrical and Gynecological Survey* 37:499–506.

Waterlow, J. C. 1972. Classification and definition of protein-calorie malnutrition. *British Medical Journal* 3:566–69.

World Health Organization (WHO). 1983. *Measuring Change in Nutritional Status. Guidelines for Assessing the Nutritional Impact of Supplementary Feeding Programmes for Vulnerable Groups.* Geneva: World Health Organization.

Weinstein, M. C., and H. V. Fineberg. 1980. *Clinical Decision Analysis.* Philadelphia: W. B. Saunders.

III SOCIAL EPIDEMIOLOGY

13 CULTURAL EVOLUTION, PARENTAL CARE, AND MORTALITY

Henry C. Harpending, Patricia Draper, and Renee Pennington

In this chapter we will suggest that mortality among infants and toddlers in many societies of the world, especially those of intermediate complexity, may be usefully approached through a model of how natural selection would shape parental care in fitness-optimizing adults. In a multiparous species with prolonged dependence of offspring on parental care, there will be lots of "parent-offspring conflict" (Trivers 1974) about the allocation of that care among several offspring. If humans are disposed to allocate this care in ways that have maximized fitness in the course of their evolution, then we might observe patterns of investment and care that result in levels of morbidity and mortality that are higher than public health workers and other professionals consider to be necessary and appropriate in a given environment.

Our ethics about health include the idea that suffering and death must be minimized. But natural selection has instead maximized the number of surviving offspring of two parents whose interests may not always (or even often) have coincided. We wish to discuss the hypothetical nature and consequences of this unappealing residue of human evolution in this chapter.

Infant and childhood mortality among the prosperous segments of Western industrial society may approach the lower limit imposed by the vulnerability of our genetic code and by the inevitability of some accidents. The cultural assumptions that accompany this low mortality include the idea that children are to be essentially saturated with physical care and the investment of parental time and energy.

We will cite examples in this chapter from European history and from ethnographies of other societies, especially from low-energy agricultural societies and from prosperous hunter-gatherers, of much lower levels of physical care and of parental investment in children. It seems clear from the comparative perspective of the cultural anthropologist that "modern" Western ideas about the value of children are special, not universal.

Our approach to this issue is to acknowledge the universality of cultural transmission of values and of much of parental behavior, at the same time acknowledging that the capacities and the propensities for cultural transmission shared by our species are the product of Darwinian evolution. We assume that in order to understand what we are willing to learn and to believe, we must understand the ultimate biological forces that shape the mechanisms maintaining culture.

Evolution favors the genetic code that causes the production of more copies of itself than does any competing genetic code. Organisms bearing a genetic code favoring intense saturating parental care, in the context of preindustrial human society as well as in the context of most mammalian evolution, would generally have lost in competition with organisms with more measured allocation of resources. When we speak of a genetic code "favoring" something, we mean "favoring" as a correlated character with the underlying chemistry of the genetic material in question. A code favoring intense parental care might work, for example, by increasing parental vulnerability to the demands of children. The nature of these links is generally unknown.

The ethnographic record describes a great diversity of human cultures in space and in time. This probably means that any set of human genetic material has passed through a variety of cultural ecologies in the last, say, ten thousand years and that there is little reason to suspect any direct genetic adaptation in our species to local social environments. Rather, we are looking for innate potentials and predispositions, "phylogenic constraints" in Wilson's (1974) terminology, shared by all humans. Patterns of child care are learned, we believe, but we do not understand how a given environment, or a given perception of an environment, determines goals and standards of the learning process. Boyd and Richerson (1985) speak of "direct bias" as a force conditioning cultural transmission, wherein an organism chooses among alternatives or modifies acquired traits in the direction of some (perhaps unconscious) goal. These direct biases seem to us to be the crucial characteristics of our species that anthropology must understand and make explicit.

At issue, then, is the old question of what we are really like, down deep. How do members of our species respond to environmental perceptions and adjust allocation of effort? We cannot get at these questions through introspection, since social psychologists tell us that we are notoriously poor at describing and predicting our own behavior. The ethnographic record is too complex for correlational studies to be very informative. Here, we wish to approach the problem by developing some models of optimal parental behavior, then to confront various sources of data to see whether our models account for much of what has been observed.

THEORY AND PREDICTIONS

In this section we try to sketch a graphic framework for developing a theory of how parental investment patterns in humans may have been shaped by natural selection. Figure 13.1 shows the probability that an average child survives to adulthood as a function of the age of the child. The left end point may be taken from standard life tables—it is the probability that a newborn survives to the (somewhat arbitrary) age of 20. The right end point is 1.0, that is, a living twenty-year-old has survived to twenty. The solid curve we have sketched is typical of those found in life tables from moderately high mortality populations.

Neglecting population growth, this curve is an analogue of R. A. Fisher's reproductive value. We take it as a proxy for a graph of the value of the average child for the fitness of the parent under prevailing (that is, average) conditions of nurturing. The evolutionary problem, then, is how this curve is perturbed by alternative patterns of nurturing. More generally, the problem is to specify the optimum allocation of nurturing among a variable number of offspring.

Our goal now is to generate a simple model of the fitness effects of parental care that will provide us with qualitative insight. Our initial simplifying

Figure 13.1
Probability of Survival to Adulthood.

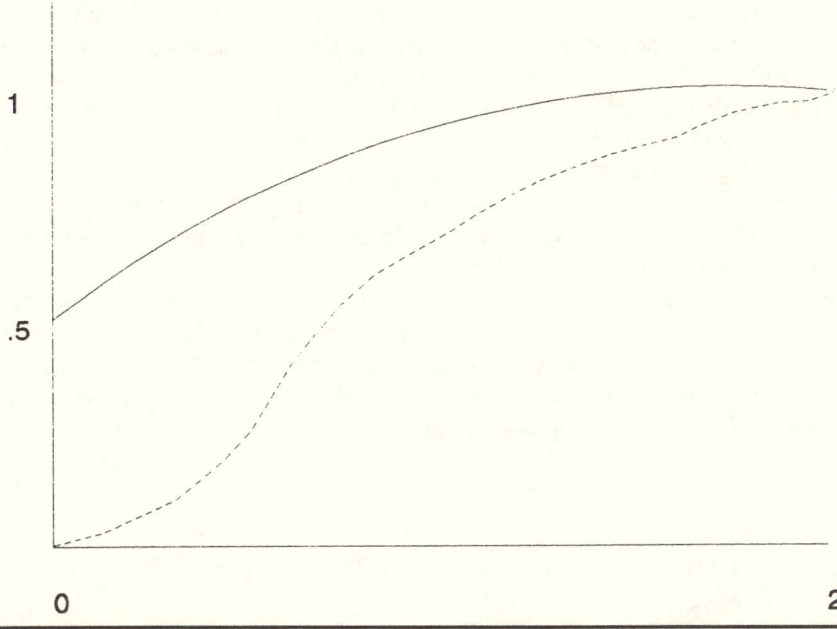

Key: — = Survivorship under prevailing conditions
     --- = Survivorship of child abandoned to the social group

assumptions are that a single parent (usually the mother) nurtures offspring and that there is no grading of nurturing. That is to say, a mother has only the options of provisioning the child at some average level or abandoning the child completely. Assume further that decisions are made only once per year, so that mothers annually make a discrete decision about continued investment versus termination of investment and starting a new offspring. We will try to relax these constraints later.

The dotted line on the same graph represents the (entirely hypothetical) probability that the same child survives to adulthood in the absence of any parental care from the parent. It starts in infancy very close to zero, since a child abandoned from birth will hardly ever survive, but it converges with the curve showing survivorship with parental care at age 20 at the value of 1.0. Note our assumption that there is no fitness payoff to parental care after age 20. This may be reasonable for many horticultural societies of intermediate complexity and for some hunter-gatherers, but it is certainly not reasonable if there is heritable wealth.

As we have drawn these curves, the probability of the abandoned child surviving increases sharply at around age two to four, that is, the ordinary age of weaning. Especially in societies where village children forage cooperatively in peer groups, such a child may survive even if effectively abandoned (but in the context of a social group) by the parents.

This simplest of all possible models already provides useful qualitative insight. Consider a parent with a toddler. In the metric of fitness the benefit of continued nurturing for another year is the probability that the child survives to adulthood as a function of its age and prevailing mortality schedules less the probability that same child survives if it is abandoned to the care of the larger social unit. The cost of continued nurturing is the loss of a year of her finite childbearing years that could instead have been spent on a new offspring. This cost is approximately twice the net reproduction rate (that is, the total number of live births) divided by the reproductive span. In this simplest model, for example, the cost may be 2 / 20 or .1 offspring per year.

It may be easier to grasp the implications of a model like this if an algebraic expression is presented. If P_c is the probability that the child survives with continued care, P_a is the probability that the child survives if abandoned, R_0 the net reproduction rate, and I the length of the fertile interval, then continued care will be favored (by evolution) whenever

$$P_c - P_a > 2 R_0 / I$$

This implies that nurturing will be favored by:

1. High P_c. Other things being equal, lower mortality rates will favor the evolution of longer parental care if the lower mortality is a payoff to parental care (e.g., nutrition of the child). On the other hand, higher

mortality rates from care-independent causes like infectious diseases will favor briefer parental care and higher fertility.

2. Low P_a. It seems obvious that the lower the likelihood of survival without parental care the more parental care is favored. P_a will be higher if there are alternate caretakers available and willing to provision the child. Peer groups among many sedentary horticulturalists function as a rearing agent for many toddlers. Accessible kin of the mother who will undertake care of the offspring will also, sensibly, favor abandonment to foster parents. Other obvious factors are settlement pattern and climate. Isolated nuclear families in northern Europe, for example, face a much lower P_a than do Samoan villagers.

3. A low R_0 will favor extended parental care. Other things being equal, population growth will favor briefer parental care even with survival probabilities held constant.

An important determinant of the distance between P_c and P_a for children is simply the availability of energy. Energy-stressed subsistence systems will not favor the survival of children who do not enjoy parental care for at least two reasons. First, a child represents a bundle of reproductive energy. In an economy limited in energy, it therefore represents a larger proportion of total energy than in an economy where energy is more plentiful. Thus the child is equivalent to a higher reproductive energy value in which a little investment has a big payoff. Conversely, if the risk is high that the child will die without parental care, the mother faces a reproductive loss of greater magnitude and it probably would not pay her to redirect reproductive energy into a new offspring until the first one has a good chance of making it on its own. Second, mothers in energy-stressed environments probably cannot care for two youngsters at once or may need to recoup, or save up, energy to reproduce again.

This model is stark and simple, but it provides predictions that were not intuitively obvious, at least to us. But what use are they? We do not believe for a moment that natural selection operating on genetic material directly could have led in our species to any of the effects we describe. But it is certainly plausible that humans are engineered to sense the state of the environment and to favor (read "learn more easily") certain behaviors over others depending on their perception of the environment. If these learning rules evolve, then our model may tell us what kind of learning rules to look for.

ETHNOGRAPHIC EVIDENCE

Anthropology, with the most interesting species and the richest set of models, is cursed with the worst data of any biological science. Here we can only muster a motley collection of anecdote, poor data, and corrupt information to examine our surmise that humans do under certain circumstances terminate parental care or, at least, reduce it well below levels that seem "natural" to westerners.

The most dramatic description of the strategy of high fertility/low parental care that we have read is William Langer's famous essay (1972) describing infant and childhood mortality in European cities of the late seventeenth and eighteenth centuries. He cites reports of city dumps scattered with corpses of dogs and babies. The situation apparently reflected finite agricultural land and a shortage of property-holding males for many young women to marry. These women migrated to the cities and engaged in low-level employment as domestics. They bore many illegitimate offspring (Langer calls this the "age of seduction") but were unable to provide useful nurturing. They abandoned them to orphanages and elsewhere, and many or most of them died. In terms of our model, the survivorship-with-care probability, P_c, was very low, so the distance between P_c and P_a became equal to R_0 / I at a very low age of offspring.

Much the same portrait of urban migration of young women who exhibit high fertility followed by abandonment is described by Schuster (1979) in *New Women of Lusaka*. In Lusaka the ecological details are quite different. In Europe we hypothesize that the women were migrating in response to a shortage of land-holding rural males. In Lusaka the women are coming from rural areas where female farming was the predominant subsistence activity (Boserup 1970). Men did not provide much help with subsistence even under traditional circumstances. The Lusakan women are also abandoning their children, but to the care of relatives in rural areas rather than to deadly orphanages, so the children are not receiving any worse care than they would have had they been born to rural women. Schuster describes child care in much the same terms as Draper and Harpending (1987) have described it for "peer-rearing societies": the children are intensely nurtured until weaning, then left to the almost exclusive care of others.

Other descriptions of societies where mothers have little to do with children after weaning and where most of the care of toddlers is in the hands of peers are not difficult to find (LeVine and LeVine 1981; Murphy and Murphy 1974; DuBois 1944). One of the most detailed descriptions we have found is for Polynesia (Ritchie and Ritchie 1979). There the infant is intensely cared for by the mother prior to weaning, but after weaning it is actively discouraged from returning to the parents for care. It is denied parental attention and even kept away from the mother.

Here is a description of parental separation from the toddler in Hawaii:

An infant that cries and fusses until picked up, fed, changed, and so on, is acceptable: a whining, clinging, demanding toddler is not. While babies live in the midst of an adult world, indeed, often at its very center, children are expected to function in a separate sphere that overlaps with that of adults at the peripheries. To a large extent, they are not to intrude into adult activities except on invitation, or if they must have adult assistance, they should request it in a subtle and unobtrusive fashion, marking the presence of a need without making demands to which an adult must respond.

[O]ther instances of reaction to intrusiveness include: scolding toddlers for approaching and responding to a field worker, pushing children away from groups of grown-ups, spanking a toddler for crying, and so on. (Gallimore, Boggs, and Jordan 1974:119–20)

A toddler is sometimes seen wandering from one sibling to another seeking some kind of assistance, sometimes approaching the parent. With experience, most learn to signal their needs unobtrusively, to which mothers may respond with the desired assistance, by ignoring, or by pointing out the problem to a sibling. At times ... there may be little satisfaction from any source. (Ibid.: 124–25)

Descriptions of child-rearing in much of rural Africa reveal similar patterns (Weisner 1982; LeVine and LeVine 1981). Here mothers provide intense care for the first year of life, but after weaning the toddler is turned over to older children and maternal provisioning terminates. Toddlers are discouraged from seeking adult attention, especially from the mother, and from drawing unnecessary attention to themselves in any way.

Among the West African Kpelle studied by Bledsoe and Murphy (n.d.) children are turned over to a group of peers, usually children of the polygynous compound, after weaning. Typically one meal a day is prepared, and toddlers and children are fed together, separately from adults. A common pot is prepared, from which they are expected to share. Adult supervision is not routine, and older children eat faster and elbow aside younger children. Outright malnutrition is not rare, and mortality is high. Many of these children are fostered out to kin and even nonkin, and these foster children suffer even higher mortality. Much of the food intake of children is foraged wild food, and parents report resenting the season when wild fruits are available since, at that time, adult threats of food denial are less effective in disciplining the children.

Children born to prosperous western parents are most vulnerable to death immediately after birth, and their vulnerability declines relatively smoothly to reach a minimum immediately before the onset of puberty. Children in other groups like those we have described may show different patterns, with mortality remaining high or even increasing toward the end of the first year of life. They may remain quite vulnerable through the first three to five years of life. A familiar example is the "weaning diarrhea" and other correlated diseases that kill many children throughout the world during the second and third years of life.

We try in Figure 13.2 to assess these ideas by assuming that infant mortality rates reflect the underlying biology and environmental conditions of a group while toddler mortality rates are more culture specific and sensitive to parental

Figure 13.2
Survivorship to Age 1 (x-Axis) and Age 20 (y-Axis).

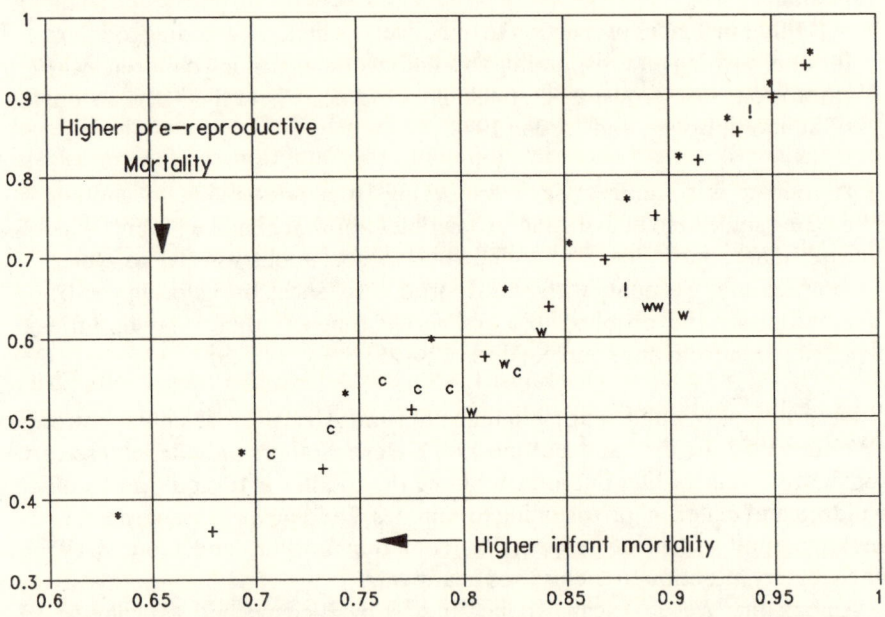

Key: *, + = European
      w, c = West African
        !   = Kung Bushmen

care. (Wills and Waterlow [1958]) propose a similar hypothesis, i.e., that childhood mortality is more sensitive to nutritional adequacy than early infant mortality.) The figure is a scatter-plot of probability that a newborn survives the first year (horizontal axis) and the probability that a newborn survives to age twenty (vertical axis). The points marked by "*" and by " + ", which form more or less smooth lines, are representative of the mortality experience and history of European populations. These are taken from the model life tables in Coale and Demeny (1966).

These tables are a kind of standard set of null hypotheses for demography. The populations marked with the symbol "w" are a series of populations from West Africa reported in Brass et al. (1968). Notice that they are all well to the right of the Coale-Demeny line; they show lower survivorship to age twenty than they "should," given their levels of infant mortality.

Ethnographies of many (but not all) West African societies reveal a pattern of family organization and parental care that Draper and Harpending (1987) call "peer rearing" societies, as for example the Kpelle described above. Pair bonds are neither durable nor accompanied by male provisioning of their own

Figure 13.3
Milk Production (Calories/Day) by Month Postpartum.

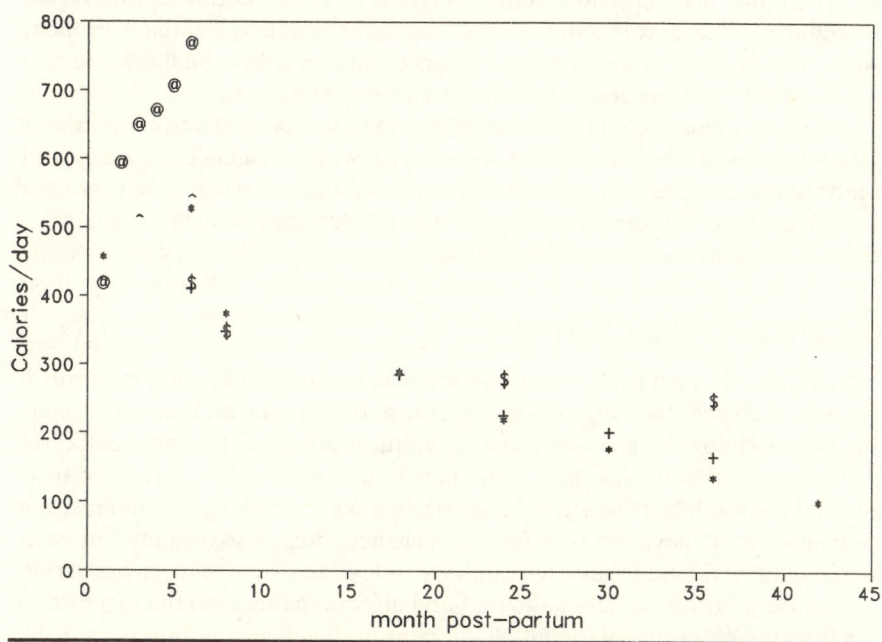

Key: * = Summary of Rattigan, Ghisalberti, and Hartmann (1981) (Australia);
        Whitehead and Paul (1981) (England); Prentice et al. (1981) (Gambia);
        Van Steenbergen et al. (1981) (Kenya); Goplan (1958), and Rao et al.
        (1959) (India); Martinez and Chavez (1971) (Mexico); Becroft (1967)
        (New Guinea)

  @ = Widdowson (1976) (Western)

  ^ = Jelliffe (1976) (Western)
  $ = Casey and Hambidge (1983) (Western)
  + = Chavez and Martinez (1980) (Indonesia, India, Mexico)

offspring. Children are nursed through infancy, then parental care is sharply
reduced. Many children are fostered to kinsmen or to others, and even those
who remain at home are not exclusively fed by their parents. Children forage in
groups of other children only occasionally supervised by adults (Bledsoe 1980;
Verdun 1983).

We went to these sources after we had formulated our hypothesis that
childhood mortality should be higher here, relative to infant mortality, than the
European norms would predict. We are the first to admit that there is no clear
confirmation of our hypothesis in the West African pattern because of the
multitude of confounding agents. For example, malaria is a major cause of

seasonal childhood mortality, and its age pattern may be the cause of this West African pattern. Further, the data may not be good. The points indicated by "c" on the figure are the same data "corrected" by orthodox demographic procedures. These corrections, however, are derived from the European experience, so there is good reason to expect that they should be shifted, as they are, to resemble more closely the known European pattern.

In an interesting monograph, Garenne (1981) shows on the basis of intense data collection in a restricted West African population that childhood mortality is indeed much higher, relative to infant mortality, than what would be predicted on the basis of the European experience. He also provides examples of a number of other populations showing this pattern.

THE COURSE OF LACTATION

Another approach from which to infer variation in human parental effort is to examine the characteristic temporal course of lactation and the variation in this course among women and among cultural groups. This is potentially a fruitful area in which to work because there is no way for culture to escape from the fundamental laws of physics; if energy is at issue, then energetic commitment to lactation must inevitably be reflected in changes in energy consumption, body weight, and work and leisure activities.

Data from various societies show a fairly uniform pattern of milk production as a function of the age of the infant.

As Figure 13.3 shows, milk production in a variety of groups reaches a maximum at about six months postpartum and then declines. By one year or so after birth, production is only on the order of 300 calories per day in the groups which have been studied. In order to maintain activity levels characteristic of the nonpregnant nonlactating state, a woman would have to consume almost 400 extra calories per day. This is about 20 to 25 percent of the ordinary daily caloric intake and represents a substantial demand upon the mother's subsistence system.

Why should production achieve its maximum at six months of age? It may be that in the past several tens of thousands of years our physiology has adapted to environments where substantial supplementation has been commonplace at and after six months of age. This perspective is somewhat different from that derived from studies of !Kung and other hunter-gatherers where lactation persists at high levels for several years and where supplemental food is difficult to generate (Howell 1979).

There is usually deposition of extra fat stores in women during pregnancy. This fat, laid down within the first thirty weeks of pregnancy (Hytten 1980), is thought to serve either as a subsidy for postpartum lactation or as a buffer against energy shortage in later pregnancy. Ironically, these fat stores are greatest in populations where they are most inappropriate. Studies on pregnant Western women report weight gains ranging from 10.3 kg in a group of Swedish women (English and Hitchcock 1968) to 14.7 kg in a group of American women (Blackburn and Calloway 1976). Hytten (1980), who reports an average pregnancy weight gain of 12.5 kg for healthy western women, estimates that 3.5 kg of this gain composes the fat store. These weight gains are significantly higher than those reported for women elsewhere. Pregnant women gain as little as 6.0 kg in parts of Ethiopia (Gebre-Medhin 1980) and 7.9 kg in Nigeria (Edozien 1980). Rajalakshmi (1980) reports that poor Indian women gain as little as 7.0 kg but still manage to give birth to infants weighing 2.6 to 3.0 kg and to provide 700 to 750 ml per day of breast milk. !Kung women gain only 7 to 9 kg during pregnancy, yet they typically breastfeed their offspring for four to five years (Howell 1979). Since these low weight gains allow for little fat storage, compared to those noted for Western women, the role of the fat store in pregnancy is unclear at this time.

THE KALAHARI BUSHMEN

Two points are shown as exclamation marks (!) on Figure 13.2. These two points represent samples collected by Harpending of Kalahari !Kung Bushmen. One (the leftmost !) is from people whose reproductive years were spent predominantly hunting and gathering, the other is from a population of !Kung which has been sedentary for approximately seventy-five years. We discuss the !Kung because there is a great deal known about them, they are an interesting group of people, and we have been asked about them.

The hunting and gathering !Kung have durable pair bonds, strong nuclear family organization, low fertility, and child-nurturing and intense mother-father-infant interaction well into toddlerhood and beyond. This kind of cultural pattern is characteristic of parent-rearing societies, according to the Draper and Harpending (1987) typology. It is the hypothesis of this chapter that such rearing will result in a low ratio of childhood to infant mortality, that is, that the foraging !Kung mortality rates will conform to the European pattern.

The sedentary !Kung of Ghanzi, on the other hand, live in more settled villages, and they may exhibit some of the indicators which we believe to be associated with weaker pair bonds, low male parental investment, and peer group rearing. Hence it seemed of interest to compare mortality rates between the two !Kung groups and between them and the European norm.

The hunting and gathering !Kung of Ngamiland have been thoroughly described in the anthropological literature. For our purposes here the relevant facts are that children are fed predominantly by their own parents and that this parental provisioning extends without apparent discontinuity throughout childhood (and often beyond). Fertility is low, and this is thought by some to be related to long lactation by mothers. To the naive observer and to pediatricians the health of children seems excellent (Trusswell and Hansen 1976). Children are active, noisy, and full of boisterous play.

The !Kung of Ghanzi contrast with their relatives in Ngamiland in interesting ways. They have been associated with European farmers for approximately seventy-five to one hundred years in a relatively stable sedentary adaptation. Patterns of interaction between the sexes are very different from those in Ngamiland — men and women seem to occupy more separate social spheres, and women respect and fear men in a way unfamiliar in the bush. Detailed observational data on the behavior of children like those collected by Draper in Ngamiland (1976) are not available for these sedentary people (Draper and Cashdan 1988). We hypothesized, on the basis of field impressions, that peer groups of children would be more important here and that this would be reflected in mortality patterns. The Ghanzi !Kung are noticeably fatter than the lean !Kung foraging in Ngamiland (Harpending and Wandsnider 1982).

Given this, we expected that examination of mortality levels during infancy and during childhood would reveal different patterns. We expected the mobile !Kung to show patterns like those in European populations, while we expected that the sedentary !Kung might be below the European line on Figure 13.2, that is, to show higher prereproductive mortality for a given level of infant mortality than would be characteristic of the European past. A glance at Figure 13.2 shows that the foraging !Kung do indeed look very European in this context, while the sedentary !Kung are also completely like Europeans. Our only (weak) conclusion is that !Kung in general show mortality schedules that are consistent with the European norm and not like the high childhood mortality schedules described by Garenne (1981) and others. The sedentary people differ drastically from the mobile people in levels of mortality, but they are also firmly on the European line.

CONCLUSIONS

It is important for many academic and nonacademic disciplines to understand what universal human predilections for caring for children are. There is much cross-cultural variation, and this variation is in some sense learned. Human biology must comprehend cultural variation and try to incorporate it into its Darwinian paradigm. It is not useful to ascribe variation to culture regarded as a random or inexplicable black box: rather, learned variation must be subject to evolutionary pressures analogous in some way to evolutionary pressures on genetic code (Boyd and Richerson 1985).

We have taken the strategy of modeling how selection has acted on human learning propensities to allocate effort among competing demands, and we have sketched a theory that makes plausible predictions about relationships among mortality, fertility, and family structure across cultures.

We were able to cite ethnographic and historical cases which accorded well with our theory, but a test using demographic data from mobile and sedentary !Kung Bushmen showed no effect.

The comparative ethnography of lactation is the natural area in which to pursue our models, since lactation is influenced by learning and the cultural milieu, yet the allocation of energy during lactation is directly measurable and the system is clearly constrained by basic bioenergetics. Milk production is the allocation of calories, while ethological measures like mother-child and adult-child proximity and interpersonal interactions, costing little or nothing, are much further from the basic biology.

REFERENCES

Becroft, T. C. 1967. Child-rearing practices in the highlands of New Guinea: A longitudinal study of breast feeding. *Medical Journal of Australia* 2: 598–601.

Blackburn, M. W., and D. H. Calloway. 1976. Energy expenditure and composition of mature, pregnant and lactating women. *Journal of the American Dietetic Association* 69:29–37.

Bledsoe, C. 1980. *Women and Marriage in Kpelle Society.* Stanford: Stanford University Press.

Bledsoe, C., and W. Murphy. n.d. personal communication.

Boserup, E. 1970. *The Role of Women in Economic Development.* London: Allen and Unwin, Ltd.

Boyd, R., and P. J. Richerson. 1985. *Culture and the Evolutionary Process.* Chicago: University of Chicago Press.

Brass, W., A. J. Coale, P. Demeny, D. F. Heisel, F. Lorimer, A. Romaniuk, and E. Van de Walle. 1968. *The Demography of Tropical Africa.* Princeton: Princeton University Press.

Casey, C. E., and K. M. Hambidge. 1983. Nutritional aspects of human lactation. In *Lactation, Physiology, Nutrition and Breast-Feeding.* M. C. Neville and M. R. Neifert, eds. New York: Plenum Press.

Chavez, A., and C. Martinez. 1980. Effects of maternal undernutrition and dietary supplementation on milk production. In *Maternal Nutrition During Pregnancy and Lactation.* H. Aebi and R. Whitehead, eds. Nestlé Foundation Publication Series No. 1. Bern: Hans Huber.

Coale, A., and P. Demeny. 1966. *Regional Model Life Tables and Stable Populations.* Princeton: Princeton University Press.

Draper, P. 1976. Social and economic constraints on !Kung childhood. In *Kalahari Hunter-Gatherers.* R. B. Lee and I. DeVore, eds. Cambridge: Harvard University Press.

Draper, P., and E. Cashdan. 1988. Technological change and child behavior among the !Kung. *Ethnology* 24(4): 339–65.

Draper, P., and H. Harpending. 1987. Parent investment and the child's environment. In *Parenting Across the Lifespan.* J. Lancaster, A. Rossi, and J. Altmann, eds. Chicago: Aldine.

Dubois, C. 1944. *The People of Alor.* Minneapolis: University of Minnesota Press.

Edozien, J. C. 1980. Dietary influences on human lactation performance. In *Maternal Nutrition During Pregnancy and Lactation.* H. Aebi and R. Whitehead, eds. Nestle Foundation Publication Series No. 1. Bern: Hans Huber.

English, R. M., and N. E. Hitchcock. 1968. Nutrient intakes during pregnancy, lactation and after the cessation of lactation in a group of Australian women. *British Journal of Nutrition* 22:615–24.

Gallimore, R., J. Boggs, and C. Jordan. 1974. *Culture, Behavior, and Education: A Study of Hawaiian-Americans.* Beverly Hills: Sage.

Garenne, M. 1981. The age pattern of infant and child mortality in Ngayokheme (Rural West Africa). Working Paper 9, Population Studies Center, University of Pennsylvania.

Gebre-Medhin, M. 1980. A comparison of nutrient intake during pregnancy and lactation in Sweden and Ethiopia. In *Maternal Nutrition During Pregnancy and Lactation.* H. Aebi and R. Whitehead, eds. Nestle Foundation Publication Series No. 1. Bern: Hans Huber.

Goplan, C. 1958. Studies in lactation in poor Indian communities. *Journal of Tropical Pediatrics* 4:87–92.

Harpending, H., and L. Wandsnider. 1982. Population structures of Ghanzi and Ngamiland !Kung. In *Current Developments in Anthropological Genetics* vol. 2. M. Crawford and J. Mielke, eds. New York: Plenum.

Howell, N. 1979. *Demography of the Dobe !Kung.* New York: Academic.

Hytten, F. E. 1980. Nutritional aspects of human pregnancy. In *Maternal Nutrition During Pregnancy and Lactation.* H. Aebi and R. Whitehead, eds. Nestlé Foundation Publication Series No.1. Bern: Hans Huber.

Jelliffe, E. P. 1976. Maternal nutrition and lactation. In *Ciba Foundation Symposium* 45 (n.s.). *Breast-feeding and the Mother.* New York: Elsevier North-Holland.

Langer, W. 1972. Checks on population growth: 1750–1850. *Scientific American* 226:92–99.

LeVine, S., and R. LeVine. 1981. Child abuse and neglect in sub-Saharan Africa. In *Child Abuse and Neglect: Cross-Cultural Perspectives.* J. Korbin, ed. Berkeley: University of California Press.

Martinez, C., and A. Chavez. 1971. Nutrition and development in infants of poor rural areas. I. Consumption of mother's milk by infants. *Nutrition Reports International* 4: 139–49.

Murphy, Y., and R. Murphy. 1974. *Women of the Forest.* New York: Columbia University Press.

Prentice, A. M., R. G. Whitehead, S. B. Roberts, and A. A. Paul. 1981. Long-term energy balance in child-bearing Gambian women. *American Journal of Clinical Nutrition* 34:2790–99.

Rajalakshmi, R. 1980. Gestation and lactation performance in relation to the plane of maternal nutrition. In *Maternal Nutrition During Pregnancy and Lactation.* H. Aebi and R. Whitehead, eds. Nestle Foundation Publication Series No. 1. Bern: Hans Huber.

Rao, K. S., M. C. Swaminathan, S. Swarup, and V. N. Patwardhan. 1959. Protein malnutrition in South India. *Bulletin of the WHO* 20:603–39.

Rattigan, S., A. V. Ghisalberti, and P. E. Hartmann. 1981. Breast-milk production in Australian women. *British Journal of Nutrition* 45:243–49.

Ritchie, J., and J. Ritchie. 1979. *Growing Up in Polynesia.* Sydney: Allen & Unwin.

Schuster, I. M. G. 1979. *New Women of Lusaka.* Palo Alto: Mayfield.

Scrimshaw, S. C. M. 1978. Infant mortality and behavior in the regulation of family size. *Population and Development Review* 4: 383–403.

Trivers, R. 1974. Parent-offspring conflict. *American Zoologist* 14:249–64.

Trusswell, S., and J. Hanson.1976. Medical research among the !Kung. In *Kalahari Hunter-Gatherers.* R. Lee and I. DeVore, eds. Cambridge: Harvard University Press.

Van Steenbergen, Wil M. , J. A. Kusin, and M. Van Rens. 1981. Lactation performance of Akamba mothers, Kenya. Breast feeding behavior, breast milk yield and composition. *Journal of Tropical Pediatrics.* 27:155–61.

Verdun, M. 1983. *The Abutia Ewe of West Africa: A Chiefdom That Never Was*. New York: Mouton.

Weisner, T. 1982. Sibling interdependence and child caretaking: A cross-cultural view. In *Sibling Relationships*. M. Lamb and B. Sutton-Smith, eds. Hillsdale, N. J.: Erlbaum.

Whitehead, R. G., and A. A. Paul. 1981. Infant growth and human milk requirements. *Lancet* 2:161–63.

Widdowson, E. M. 1976. Changes in the body and its organs during lactation: Nutritional implications. In *Ciba Foundation Symposium* 45 (n.s.). *Breast-Feeding and the Mother*. New York: Elsevier North-Holland.

Wills, V. G., and J. C. Waterlow. 1958. The death-rate in the age-group 1–4 years as an index of malnutrition. *Journal of Tropical Pediatrics* 3: 167–70.

Wilson, E. O. 1974. *Sociobiology: The New Synthesis*. Cambridge: Harvard University Press.

14 ASSESSING THE IMPACT OF ENVIRONMENTAL CHANGE, WITH SPECIAL REFERENCE TO THE ROLE OF URINARY HORMONES

G. A. Harrison and D. A. Jenner

Organisms tend to be genetically adapted to their environment. A rapid change of environment, particularly to a state never previously experienced, might well be expected to lead to a loss of Darwinian fitness. The forms of transition that have occurred and are occurring in most human societies as they move from traditional hunter-gatherers to modern urban conditions represent such rapid environmental change when seen from an evolutionary point of view. Even when seen from an individual's position the amount of environmental change experienced in a lifetime can be formidable. S. V. Boyden (1970, 1972) has analyzed these premises in great detail and has concluded that most human populations should be showing signs of what he terms "phylogenetic maladjustment." One can take issue with specifics, including the terminology. Not all environmental change need be bad. The eradication of infectious disease — an enormous change — can hardly be viewed in any sense as responsible for loss in fitness. But, notwithstanding such points, the general proposition is worth examination in considering the health and disease of populations in transition.

How may the Boyden hypothesis be tested? A number of population comparisons might prove revealing. Perhaps most directly relevant are comparisons of people in modern developed societies to those still living a hunter-gatherer, or at least a highly traditional, life. There are, however, difficulties in interpreting such comparisons. Present-day hunter-gatherers only survive in rather special and in general inhospitable environments: their lifestyles do not properly represent the ancestral condition of all human behavior. More practically, some comparisons are biologically meaningless because environments are qualitatively as well as quantitatively different. Thus for example there is little point comparing fertility in a contracepting versus a noncontracepting society, at least from the position of testing the Boyden hypothesis.

A more rigorous, if less contrasting, comparison is to examine the differences between urban and rural groups in the same society. In many of the features which Boyden finds distinguish traditional from developed societies, rural groups show quantitatively less development than urban ones. This is perhaps most evident in nutritional factors but also tends to be true of others such as crowding, levels of infections with many diseases, and social cohesiveness. Care needs to be taken in the documentation of the environmental variety, and it certainly cannot be assumed that in all features rural people will be exposed to less change. For instance a farmer endlessly driving a tractor may experience much more noise than any city dweller. Nevertheless, the approach might be rewarding.

A final method is to compare the effect of the diversity of lifestyles which occur within a single population. No two people are exposed, or expose themselves, to exactly the same environmental circumstances, and the variety can reflect many of the differences that are of interest here. Fundamentally this is the epidemiological approach and is the most rigorous of all. However, within-population variety tends only to embrace a small proportion of the full range of environmental experience one is attempting to investigate.

Various components of fitness can be measured in these three approaches. With Darwinian fitness as the focus, the critical measures, of course, are demographic: such fitness is composed solely of variance in fertility and mortality. As already mentioned, there are major problems in interpreting fertility variation, particularly in between-population comparison. And measures of biological fecundity are hard to obtain. So far as mortality is concerned, the evidence from hunter-gatherers/traditional versus modern comparison unequivocally "falsifies" the Boyden hypothesis. People have shorter life expectancies in the former societies, and this is as evident in the archaeological record as among living groups. On the other hand, when one has made allowance for the provision of systems of modern hygiene and health care, as in the urban/rural and within-group analysis, it would appear that many of the features of modern living are associated with higher mortality.

While genetically determined, or associated, variations in Darwinian fitness are the vehicle of evolution, there are other elements to the fitness concept. Some of these are quite closely related to Darwinian fitness, others less so. One that is related, through its clear connection to mortality, is morbidity. Morbidity, of course, is also fundamentally related to the concept of health. The evidence from studies of morbidity, both physical and psychological, have been reviewed elsewhere (Harrison 1980). It will not be considered in detail here, but it can be said that urban/rural and within-population analyses tend to favor Boyden's position. Even so, the fact that the diseases present in hunter-gatherer and modern societies are so different makes this comparison essentially useless.

Another important element is "well-being." By this, one means an individual's own perception of his homeostatic condition. Well-being may have little to do with fertility or mortality, but it is a crucial component of health. It is widely recognized now that absence of medically diagnosable disease is not the same as having "good health." The difference lies in the ill-explored in-between area of varying well-being. This area is of great importance in both practical and academic terms and plays an important part in the etiology of many physical as well as psychological diseases (Sterling and Eyre 1981; McQueen and Siegrist 1982). Unlike many diseases, particularly the noninfectious ones, well-being tends to relate to the environments prevailing when subjects are actually being studied. Environmental contributions to cardiovascular or neoplastic diseases will have occurred long before there is any morbidity manifestation. This should make well-being more amenable to analysis.

It does, however, also suffer from an extreme disadvantage: its fundamental subjectivity. Various questionnaires have been devised and employed in attempts to measure it, but many authors feel it can only be established by intensive psychological interviews and then only within a single society. Certainly no one would feel confident in any results pertaining to comparison between hunter-gatherers and modern urbanites! A few studies do suggest that rural inhabitants complain less about their lifestyles than neighboring townfolk (Millar 1979), and in general the happy tend to be healthy, though which is cause and which is effect are far from clear. Evidently it would be of enormous value if there were objective and accurate physiological correlates of well-being.

It is well known that acute psychosocial stress is associated with increased heart rate, and sympathetic sweating is evidenced in changed skin conductance. Measuring these changes as people go about their daily lives is not of much value for various reasons. However, it is widely held that certain hormones, the catecholamines and the corticosteroids, do also reflect stress (Levi 1982; Selye 1976), and these can be assayed in urine which slowly accumulates in the bladder over a period of many experiences and feelings. Implicit in thinking about these relationships are the suppositions that low psychosocial stress and high well-being amount to the same thing and that being stressed is a pejorative state (Cox 1978).

Most of the early stress hormone studies were undertaken on subjects in experimental or semiexperimental conditions. They certainly showed that experiences such as hospital admission and academic examinations and risky jobs such as motor racing and battle were associated with high excretion (with presumed high secretion) of catecholamines and corticosteroids.

Following these observations we decided some years ago to attempt to monitor in a similar way normal daily activity in a group of local Oxfordshire populations — the Otmoor villages — focusing mainly on levels of excretion of the catecholamines adrenalin (epinephrine) and noradrenalin (norepinephrine) in relation to a number of aspects of varying life-style, health, and reported feelings.

Analyses were based on timed urine samples collected first thing in the morning, around midday, and in the early evening on both a workday and a rest day. The results of these analyses for both men and women have been mainly

Table 14.1
Adrenalin Excretion Rates in Otmoor Men Born or Working Locally and Nonlocally.[1]

Mean (s.e.)

Workday	Born Local (N = 145)			Born Nonlocal (N = 223)		
	Work Local (N = 55)		Work Nonlocal (N = 90)	Work Local (N = 59)		Work Nonlocal (N = 164)
Overnight		.383 (.016)			.411 (.013)	
	.389 (.031)		.379 (.018)	.405 (.023)		.413 (.015)
Morning		.924 (.020)			.951 (.014)	
	.935 (.033)		.917 (.029)	.903 (.030)		.968 (.016)
Afternoon		.866 (.019)			.880 (.015)	
	.845 (.028)		.878 (.025)	.850 (.026)		.892 (.018)
Rest Day						
Overnight		.394 (.017)			.428 (.015)	
	.408 (.029)		.386 (.020)	.411 (.028)		.434 (.017)
Morning		.865 (.024)			.854 (.017)	
	.883 (.039)		.854 (.030)	.854 (.031)		.854 (.020)
Afternoon		.750 (.021)			.757 (.017)	
	.764 (.041)		.742 (.024)	.734 (.033)		.766 (.019)

[1] Log ng/min corrected for urine volume, time of urination, and bodyweight.

published (Jenner, Reynolds, and Harrison 1980; Reynolds et al. 1981; Harrison et al. 1981), and there is no need to repeat them in detail here. In summary, they show the well-known marked circadian rhythm in catecholamine excretion, with highest rates of output being around midday, and a number of significant associations with life-style features, especially for adrenalin. The latter include, in men, greater adrenalin excretion on a workday than on a rest day, greater excretion in nonmanual workers than in manual workers on the workday but not on the rest day, and higher outputs associated with coffee drinking, cigarette smoking, feeling mentally tired and time pressured, and wanting to change one's job as established by questionnaire interview. Interestingly, those who find their work "boring" tend to have low adrenalin excretion rates on a workday; those who report that the day on which they gave urine samples was "more stressful than usual" gave significantly higher outputs than those who reported a less stressful day than usual.

In women, workday/rest day and occupational differences are less clear, though housewives tend to have low outputs. Furthermore, there is a marked association in married women with their husbands' occupation, even on rest days! Various reported feelings as well as the pharmacological effects are detectable. Women, for example, who report frequent frustration tended to have high rates of adrenalin output.

An analysis not previously reported was to examine catecholamine output according to the migratory status of individuals and whether they work in the Otmoor area or not (Harrison 1982). In principle this might be of particular relevance to transitional societies since it affords a possible indication of comparative social stability. Table 14.1 presents the data for adrenalin excretion for men according to whether they were born or work locally or nonlocally. Although over each time period on the workday those who were born locally tend to have lower mean rates of excretion than those who were born nonlocally, none of the differences is statistically significant. However, if one takes some account of the length of time which has elapsed since nonlocally born men migrated into Otmoor, significant linear analyses of variance are found; the shorter the time in Otmoor, the higher the adrenalin excretion rate (Table 14.2). To some extent the same phenomenon is evidenced in women, particularly housewives. This relationship is not due to subjects' age, which is little related to adrenalin excretion in this population. It might, at first sight, be thought to arise from an inverse relationship between "stress" and the extent of integration of immigrants into the Otmoor community. However, analysis of the occupation of the immigrants shows that there has been an ever-rising proportion of people in nonmanual work and particularly professional people. The relationship is thus essentially another expression of the effect of occupational variation on adrenalin excretion, which explains why it is only evident on the workday.

Notwithstanding this negative result and considering the room for technical errors and the many deficiencies of a questionnaire approach, a surprisingly high proportion of population adrenalin variance can be explained by multiple

Table 14.2
Adrenalin Excretion Rates in Otmoor Men in Relation to Length of Time Resident in the Area (Radius 10 Miles).

		Born Local	Length of Time Resident in the Area				
			> 10 Years	5–10 Years	3–5 Years	< 3 Years	
		(N = 138) (39.1)[1]	(N = 114) (44.3)	(N = 36) (38.7)	(N = 36) (38.2)	(N = 40) (33.3)	ANOVA (Linear Trend)
Workday							
Overnight	mean	.377	.396	.423	.446	.425	p < .05
	s.e.	.016	.020	.024	.029	.025	
Morning	mean	.921	.931	.951	.974	.992	p < .05
	s.e.	.022	.021	.036	.029	.029	
Afternoon	mean	.858	.839	.913	.888	.990	p < .05
	s.e.	.019	.020	.039	.036	.033	
Rest Day							
Overnight	mean	.391	.428	.411	.447	.428	nonsig.
	s.e.	.017	.018	.048	.024	.042	
Morning	mean	.860	.838	.874	.872	.887	nonsig.
	s.e.	.024	.025	.035	.033	.044	
Afternoon	mean	.742	.760	.762	.762	.768	nonsig.
	s.e.	.022	.023	.046	.031	.043	

[1] Mean age.

regression analysis of the Otmoor data. In males on a working day, for example, something of the order of 25 percent of the adrenalin variance is explicable. The proportion of female variance "explained" is rather smaller (Harrison et al. 1981), but the questionnaire was poorly equipped to examine the life-styles of those who were not in employment. Factor analysis allowed the identification of statistically independent contributions, and the elements summarized earlier are of this form. It was, however, impossible on these data to determine whether coffee drinking is associated with high or tea drinking with low adrenalin excretion! They are so strongly inversely correlated. More experimental studies have, however, shown a direct coffee effect.

On the bases of these results it was adjudged that population approaches to urinary hormone analysis are worthwhile and deserving of further development. In particular, it was felt that the extension of the work to other kinds of society, including traditional and transitional ones, might be revealing, not only from the perspective of identifying determinants of hormone excretion but also for monitoring stress and health.

One early extension was undertaken in collaboration with G. D. James and P. T. Baker of Pennsylvania State University, who were examining health changes under acculturation in Samoa. They were able to send overnight and morning timed samples from groups of men who could be classified into traditional villagers, physically active urban dwellers, sedentary urban dwellers, and students. These groups are considered to show increasing acculturation. Analyses of these data (James et al. 1985) again show significant adrenalin association with life-style characteristics such as coffee drinking and social status, but, more particularly, there is a relationship between the output of this hormone (at least judged by excretion rate) and the level of acculturation. One problem with the interpretation of these results is that the acculturation association becomes much less marked if the analysis is based on hormone/creatinine ratios rather than in terms of absolute excretion rates (nanograms per minute). This might arise through the less acculturated being also less time conscious and systematically overestimating the time elapsed since the previous urination. The analysis certainly highlights the potential problems of using timed samples in non-time-conscious societies and for between-population comparisons they are totally inappropriate. Different societies schedule their daily routines in quite different ways: to compare afternoon samples in societies with a siesta with those without one is clearly quite meaningless in terms of measuring overall stress.

At this stage we turned from timed samples to twenty-four-hour collections. These have the advantage that subjects do not need to be able to record time, that circadian rhythms in hormone secretion and urine flow are immaterial (such rhythms need to be allowed for statistically in timed samples), and the timing of daily events is inconsequential. But they suffer not only from the potential problem of missed samples but also from the greater pooling of the effects of a variety of different experiences over the day. Under such circumstances it will clearly be more difficult to detect single associations, but if there is a relationship between hormone and stress then the cumulative excretion rate is the best daily measure of the latter one has.

So far, the main study we have undertaken of a traditional society using twenty-four-hour collections has been that of the Pacific Polynesian Islands of the Tokelau group. These have been done at Wellington Hospital, New Zealand, in collaboration with Dr. I. A. M. Prior and his colleagues who have been analyzing Tokelauan epidemiology for many years (Prior et al. 1977). To provide a basis for comparison in a Western society, twenty-four-hour collections have been obtained from two groups of Oxford City inhabitants. Results from the latter, by comparison with the Otmoor studies, do indeed indicate that it is more difficult to detect certain kinds of association on twenty-four-hour samples than on limited time samples, though the relationships between adrenalin and coffee drinking and tobacco consumption are endorsed.

A disturbing feature of the Tokelau samples is that in them there is a positive correlation between catecholamine hormone output (and creatinine output) and twenty-four-hour urine volume. This particularly affects noradrenalin and men. It could arise from varying loss of hormone in sweat in this tropical environment, but perhaps most likely is a failure of some subjects to collect all urinations. The effect can be minimized by analyzing hormone/creatine ratios rather than absolute hormone excretion, though the results are basically similar whichever approach one uses.

As in Western societies, there are detectable associations between catecholamine excretion and lifestyle, in particular with educational, occupational, and social status factors and, for reasons not at all clear, with the particular island inhabited. There are also suggestions of positive relationships between noradrenalin excretion and blood pressure in both men and women. But the striking finding is that the excreted amounts of both catecholamines are very significantly lower than in the Oxford City samples. That missed urinations have contributed something to this is probable, but the contrast is as evident in creatinine ratios as in absolute quantities, and preliminary findings on other traditional societies (e.g., Australian aborigines) also support the conclusion that in them catecholamine excretion is low.

By the time Tokelau and Oxford City samples were collected, we were also in a position to analyze urinary cortisol and cortisone by HPLC. Unfortunately, the best conditions for preserving catecholamines involve collecting over sodium metabisulphite, and this causes a gradual breakdown of cortisol and cortisone. The absolute amounts of these hormones have therefore not been established in the populations studied so far, but lifestyle associations with them do occur. It is also worth mentioning that in every population examined there is a marked positive correlation between output of these steroids and diuresis.

What do these various findings mean concerning comparative levels of stress and well-being? Stress is widely regarded as a determinant or an element of well-being and is known to play an important role in the etiology of a number of diseases. One might therefore be tempted to conclude from these results that the elements of health and well-being which are due to stress, and particularly psychological state, would favor traditional and stable societies and physical rather than mental occupations. These results rest, however, on the categorization of adrenalin as a "stress hormone." There is no doubt that many pejorative states are associated with increased adrenalin secretion—anxiety, frustration, rushedness and mental overload—and the hormone was first identified as part of the fight-or-flight response. High levels of catecholamine have also been involved in models of the etiology of coronary heart disease (Carruthers 1969; Friedman and Rosenman 1974). But other states that are viewed pejoratively, like boredom, are associated with low levels of adrenalin, and circadian rhythms in catecholamine output can hardly be explained in terms of stress. It seems to us that the patterns of association described here are much more readily explained on the basis that adrenalin output is providing insight into comparative levels of psychosocial arousal. In a study of associations between hormone output and response to a mood questionnaire in Oxford City, only weak relationships were detectable; these, however, were mainly with moods containing components of arousal (Jenner, Anderson, and Harrison 1985).

The hormone has indeed for long been considered as an arousal hormone, involved in the anticipation of a potential need for physical activity. On this view, the results described here would mean no more than that levels of psychological arousal tend to be lower in traditional than developed societies and in physical rather than mental occupations. Such a conclusion carries no value judgment with respect to health or anything else. Whether or not prolonged high output of adrenalin has an adverse effect in the short or the long term is another question. The answer may very well depend on whether or not it is accompanied by high levels of physical activity.

It may turn out that corticosteroids are a better measure of the well-being of populations, but preliminary results are not encouraging (Summers et al. 1983). However, from other studies of the Otmoor populations we consider that objective correlates of well-being are evidenced in certain characteristics of sleep (Palmer, Harrison, and Hiorns 1980; Palmer and Harrison 1983). Little is known of the natural history of sleep, but in Otmoor reported habitual sleep latency (the length of time it takes for an individual to fall asleep) associates quite strongly with almost all reported states of comparative well-being. Long latency is, for example, associated with general lassitude and discontent as well as with many minor "morbidities" which can only be diagnosed through report. Sleep quality (a subjective perception of an element of well-being) is also very strongly correlated with, if not primarily determined by, sleep latency.

The problem with sleep characteristics is that they are very difficult to determine in traditional societies, especially those with little time consciousness. Only observation can here provide accurate data, and this itself poses many problems. We therefore know almost nothing of individual sleep patterns among hunter-gatherers. However, the Otmoor analysis does support the view that

Table 14.3
Summary Evaluation of Evidence Relating to Boyden's Hypothesis of "Phylogenetic Maladjustment" in Modern Societies.

Comparison	Mortality	Physical Morbidity	Mental Morbidity	Subjective Well-Being	"Stress" Hormones	Sleep
Hunter-gatherer and traditional versus modern	X	—	X?	—	√?	?
Rural versus urban	√	√	√	√	√?	?
Varying life-style within populations	√	√	√	?	√?	√

Key: √ = Evidence in favor of hypothesis
     X = Evidence against hypothesis
     ? = Data insufficient or equivocal
     — = Comparison not possible or meaningful

country life, that is, those in the villages who are engaged in agricultural and similar physical and outdoor occupations, has short sleep latency and long sleep duration.

In Table 14.3 the evidence for the Boyden hypothesis, as presented here and in the previous review (Harrison 1980) is summarized. Overall, it would seem that most of the analyses which can or have been made offer some support. The one outstanding exception is comparative longevity in modern and traditional societies, and length of life is by no means an inconsequential element of quality. It would also be misleading to maintain that the comparisons which support the hypothesis do so in an overwhelming way. Perhaps the most impressive support comes from the etiology of coronary heart disease if, as many believe, psychological stress/arousal play a significant role in this. The fight/flight response is clearly an important element of individual adaptability in hunter-gatherer life: a response which must have been favored throughout most of human evolution. During this time it would inevitably be associated with the physical activity implied in fight or flight. The triggering of this response in modern societies is often not associated with such activity, and under such circumstances the lipid released by catecholamine secretion will not be catabolized for the provision of energy and may, as Carruthers (1969) suggested, play a part in atheromatus plaque formation. Further, the increased coagulability of blood accompanying adrenalin secretion, which is advantageous in wounding in fights, can also facilitate thrombus formation in coronary arteries. Under these circumstances the fight/flight response might well be regarded as a once adaptive strategy which is now overall maladaptive.

REFERENCES

Boyden, S. V., ed. 1970. *The Impact of Civilization on the Biology of Man.* Toronto: University of Toronto.

Boyden, S. V. 1972. Ecology in relation to urban population structure. In *The Structure of Human Populations.* G. A. Harrison and A. J. Boyce, eds. Oxford: Oxford University Press.

Carruthers, M. E. 1969. Aggression and atheroma. *Lancet* 2:1170–71.

Cox, T. 1978. *Stress.* London: Macmillan.

Friedman, M., and R. H. Rosenman. 1974. *Type A Behavior and Your Heart.* New York: Knopf.

Harrison, G. A. 1980. Urbanization and stress. In *Disease and Urbanization.* E. J. Clegg and J. P. Garlick, eds. London: Taylor and Francis.

———. 1982. Dissecting populations. *Perspectives in Biology and Medicine* 25:649–61.

Harrison, G. A., C. D. Palmer, D. A. Jenner and V. Reynolds. 1981. Associations between rates of urinary catecholamine excretion and aspects of lifestyle among adult women in some Oxfordshire villages. *Human Biology* 53:617–33.

James, G. D., D. A. Jenner, G. A. Harrison, and P. T. Baker. 1985. Differences in catecholamine excretion rates, blood pressure and lifestyle among young Western Samoan men. *Human Biology* 57:635–47.

Jenner, D. A., A. W. Anderson, and G. A. Harrison. 1985. Endocrine associations with mood and sleep. *Stress Medicine* 1:101–107

Jenner, D. A., V. Reynolds, and G. A. Harrison. 1980. Catecholamine excretion rates and occupation. *Ergonomics* 23:237–46.

Levi, L., ed. 1982. *Stress and Distress in Response to Psychosocial Stimuli.* Oxford: Pergamon Press.

McQueen, D. V., and J. Siegrist, eds. 1982. Sociocultural factors in chronic disease. *Social Science and Medicine.* Symposium Issue. 16, no. 4.

Millar, S. 1979. *The Biosocial Survey in Hong Kong.* Australian National University Press for UNESCO/UNEP.

Palmer, C. D., and G. A. Harrison. 1983. Sleep latency and lifestyle in Oxfordshire villages. *Annals of Human Biology* 10:417–28.

Palmer, C. D., G. A. Harrison, and R. W. Hiorns. 1980. Sleep patterns and lifestyle in Oxfordshire villages. *Journal of Biological Science* 12:437–67.

Prior, I. A. M., A. Hooper, J. W. Huntsman, J. M. Stanhope and P. E. Salmond. 1977. The Tokelau Island migrant study. In *Population Structure and Human Variation.* G. A. Harrison, ed. Cambridge: Cambridge University Press.

Reynolds, V., D. A. Jenner, C. D. Palmer and G. A. Harrison. 1981. Catecholamine excretion rates in relation to lifestyles in the male population of Otmoor, Oxfordshire. *Annals of Human Biology* 8:197–209.

Selye, H. 1976. *Stress in Health and Disease.* Boston: Butterworths.

Sterling, P., and J. Eyre. 1981. The biological basis of stress-related mortality. *Social Science and Medicine* 15:3–42.

Summers, K. M., G. A. Harrison, D. A. Hume and D. A. Palmer. 1983. Urinary hormone levels: A population study of associations between steroid and catecholamine excretion rates. *Annals of Human Biology* 10:99–110.

15 SOCIAL SUPPORT AND MORTALITY IN POST-TRANSITION POPULATIONS

Stephen J. Kunitz

The transition from infectious to noninfectious diseases is thought to have made host factors of a psychosocial nature of relatively more etiological significance than in past times. Among these, social support has been considered to be of particular importance. In this chapter I shall review the results of a number of prospective cohort studies of the relationship between social support and mortality. My points shall be:

1. Most studies do show an association between some measure of contact with other people and mortality, though the causal mechanism is unknown.

2. The studies showing no association have been done in kin-based societies in which social isolation is sufficiently uncommon as to be an inadequate predictor of mortality—which is to say, in societies with a low variance in social isolation, it is not possible to detect an association with mortality.

3. The reason epidemiologists have considered social isolation to be a generally important variable has to do with the way Western social scientists typically have understood the transition from "traditional" to "modern" life.

That transition has not been the same everywhere, however, and "modernization" in northwest Europe and its overseas extensions seems to have been very different from what has occurred elsewhere. Such differences may help to account for the anomalous findings.

John Cassel was perhaps the first epidemiologist to attempt to develop a theory of the relationship of psychosocial processes to health (Cassel, Patrick, and Jenkins 1960). He suggested that, as epidemics of infectious diseases declined, host factors of a psychosocial nature became increasingly significant as determinants of health status (Cassel 1970). Among the factors that enhanced susceptibility to disease, he believed, were situations in which "the actor is not receiving adequate evidence [feedback] that his actions are leading to anticipated consequences" (Cassel 1976:478). The protective factors he thought most important, "Might be envisioned as . . . buffering or cushioning the individual from the physiologic or psychologic consequences of exposure to the stressor situation. It is suggested that the property common to these processes is the strength of the social supports provided by the primary groups of most importance to the individual" (Cassell 1976:478).

As defined by Sidney Cobb (1976), social support includes information leading the subject to believe that he or she is cared for and loved; is esteemed and valued; and belongs to a network of communication and mutual obligation. This definition includes nothing about the sources of such support, whether from within the household, from nonresident kin and friends, or from community organizations. It also blends together several dimensions of support, most significantly the instrumental and the affective. Presumably both are important, but their relative importance is unspecified, and perhaps unspecifiable.

Sources of social support may be found within the household and/or the extended family, among friends and neighbors, and in formal social institutions. It is by no means necessary that neolocalism and nuclear family organization, for instance, be associated with increasing isolation, as Segalen (1984) has shown. On the other hand, in a society with a high proportion of solitary individuals living alone, the chances are increased that social isolation will be more prevalent than where the proportion of solitaires is low; a high proportion of single-person households does seem to be characteristic of societies in which nuclear families are the norm.

I have used the terms "social isolation" and "lack of social support" interchangeably, blurring an important distinction. Contact with other people does not necessarily imply that one is receiving any of the kinds of support listed by Cobb. As I shall indicate below, most studies assume that social support is present when individuals report that they have some sort of contact with other people or with social institutions, but this is to assume in advance the presence of that which is to be demonstrated. "In order to study the conditions under which individuals do get support, we must allow for the possibility that many of their ties are not necessarily supportive" (Wellman 1981:172). Nonetheless, even assuming that these studies measure isolation rather than the lack of support, the results do show an association with mortality in most instances. My task will be to attempt to explain the seemingly anomalous results in which no association is observed.

MORTALITY AND SOCIAL SUPPORT/ISOLATION

As already noted, Cassel's work stimulated a number of empirical studies of the relationship between social support and mortality. Of those, I shall review only the cohort studies.[1] The first to be published was the Alameda County (California) Study, in which a large sample of county residents was interviewed and then followed for up to nine years (Berkman and Syme 1979). It was observed that even when pre-existing self-reported health status, health related practices and habits, social class, and age were controlled, the number of social ties people reported was inversely related to the risk of death from a wide variety of diseases. This was true of both men and women.

Perhaps because this was a very large study, in which the survey instrument covered an enormous range of topics, or perhaps because the significance of social support was only appreciated after the data were collected, the variables used cannot really be said to measure support. They included marital status (married or unmarried); contacts with friends and relatives (high, medium, and low); church membership (member or nonmember); and member or nonmember of other formal or informal associations. While it may be inferred that group membership and marriage provide support of some sort, it is by no means clear of what kind — financial? other instrumental help such as house cleaning? companionship? It is perhaps safer to use these variables as measures of social contact or its absence.

A very similar study in Tecumseh, Michigan, reported roughly comparable results (House, Robbins, and Metzner 1982). A large sample of community residents between thirty-five and sixty-nine years of age in the period 1967–1969 was interviewed, examined, and then followed for up to twelve years. Again controlling for age, health status as determined on physical examination, and a variety of risk factors, it was observed that, among men, those who reported the most social relationships were at lowest risk of death in the follow-up period. The results were in the same direction for women but did not reach statistical significance.

The measures of social relationships fell into four major categories:

1. Intimate social relationships (marital status, visits with friends and relatives, going on pleasure drives and picnics);
2. Formal organizational involvements outside of work (going to church or meetings of voluntary associations);
3. Active and relatively social leisure (going to classes or lectures, movies, plays, fairs, museums, etc.); and
4. Passive and relatively solitary leisure (watching television, listening to the radio, reading). (House, Robbins, and Metzner 1982:126)

It was observed that, unlike Alameda County, in Tecumseh membership in formal organizations or attendance at formally scheduled events seemed to be especially significant, whereas visiting with friends, relatives, and neighbors was not. The authors speculated that these patterns

> reflect the differing processes of social integration and activity which characterized a small city in a rural area such as Tecumseh vis-à-vis a metropolitan area such as Alameda County, California. It is possible that meaningful social relationships and activities are more likely to occur as part of the normal fabric of daily life in places like Tecumseh. Thus, for example, friends and relatives may be seen and "visited with" more often at work or while shopping and performing other routines of daily life. (The term "visit" in Tecumseh is used to mean merely talking with another person, as well as physically going to see him.) This may be especially true for women. The result is that these specific measures may be less differentiating among persons in a small city than among residents of a metropolitan area where such interactions are more frequently special events. Generally, the measures in the Tecumseh data may more accurately index the actual level of social integration and activity of men than women, since men more often have to make special efforts to foster social relationships through formal organizations and activities. (House, Robbins, and Metzner 1982:139).

Two studies of the association between social support and mortality have been reported among elderly populations. The first, in Durham County, North Carolina, followed a sample of 331 people aged sixty-five years and older for thirty months after they had been interviewed (Blazer 1982). Three parameters of social support from the Older American Resources and Services (OARS) Social Support Scale were used: roles and available attachments; frequency of social interactions; and perceived social support. Controlling for a variety of risk factors, it was observed that the relative risk of dying was greatest among those who had least interaction and perceived themselves to be most isolated. Moreover, in contrast to the Alameda County study, "No consistent pattern of increased mortality rates was associated with a progressive decrease in social interaction or perceived social support. Rather, a threshold effect appears to be operational with only those subjects with the least perceived support and social interaction exhibiting an increased mortality rate" (Blazer 1982:691).

The second study of elderly people was done in several Connecticut cities and found that, among the 400 people followed for two years, excess risk of mortality was associated with "religiousness," happiness, and the presence of living offspring (Zuckerman, Kasl, and Ostfield 1984). In relation to social support, nine questions addressed contacts with friends and relatives. Several dealt with the presence or absence and frequency of interaction with a confidant. Several others were concerned with friendship and visiting patterns. Two questions dealt with the number of living children and the number of children living nearby (scored as none, one, and two or more). Only two of these questions "were significantly related to mortality, when gender and health status were controlled: respondents who have more living children and more children living nearby are more likely to survive" (Zuckerman, Kasl, and Ostfield 1984:417). As in the previous studies, support may be inferred from these variables, but what sort is not known. It is perhaps more accurate to label this, as the authors do, social contact rather than support.

Despite the differences in measures of social support, social isolation, and social contact, these studies all find associations between involvement with other people and reduced risk of mortality in the follow-up period. There are, however, two anomalous studies so far that show no association. The first is of a large sample of Japanese-American men living in Hawaii and followed for up to seven years after interview and examination (Reed, McGee, and Yano 1984). The incidence of death was unrelated to what was termed "sociocultural inconsistency" (changes in religion, occupation, and diet) and to "social networks" (marital status, household size, number of living children, and geographic proximity of parents.) Clearly, the variables used to measure "social networks" do not measure networks at all but rather are related to the organization and size of the domestic group. Analyses using "A scale which included interactions with co-workers, social groups, and religious organizations" were also done but added nothing and were not included in the published results (Reed, McGee, and Yano 1984:359). The authors commented: "While we have used measures similar to the ones that have been associated with disease in other studies, it may be that this group of men perceive things differently or have some other attributes that neutralized the effects of what are usually considered adverse circumstances. If this should be true, then the general susceptibility hypothesis is weakened to the extent that it operates only in certain cultures or social subgroups" (Reed, McGee, and Yano 1984:368).

The second study with anomalous results is of a sample of 270 elderly Navajo Indians followed for only two years as yet (Kunitz and Levy, unpublished data). Preliminary analyses of family organization patterns (household and camp size and composition, marital status), and visiting and support patterns, indicate no differences between the people who have died and controls, matched for age and sex, who are still alive.

It has sometimes been suggested that social isolation and morbidity and/or mortality are the results of a common cause, perhaps depression or mental illness. Depressed people become isolated and are also more likely to die from a variety of unexplained causes. This suggestion is plausible, but why should it not be the case among the Japanese and Navajos as well?

The authors of the study of Japanese men in Hawaii observed: "If psychosocial processes are associated with an increased rate of disease in one city and not another, or in one ethnic group but not others, then the accumulating body of information will grow more confusing and beliefs will become more controversial" (Reed, McGee, and Yano 1984:368). Their suggestions for future research were for the most part aimed at the individual level of analysis. This criticism is surely appropriate, but there is another level that might usefully be considered as well.

It is striking that the two populations in which no associations between social support and mortality have so far been observed are in fact kin-based societies. Though Japan may not be kin-based in the usual sense of the term, since there is no clan system and since stem rather than extended families are the usual form of family organization, family solidarity and loyalty are a dominant feature of Japanese life (Lebra 1976). Indeed, a survey of elderly Issei (Japanese-born immigrants to the United States) found that 14 percent lived entirely alone, although many of the solitaires belonged to various formal and informal associations (Montero 1979). This result contrasts with 25 percent of a sample of elderly American Indians and 38 percent of a sample of elderly residents of Cleveland, Ohio, who lived alone (National Indian Council on Aging 1981).

It seems likely, then, that the explanation of the anomalous findings has to do with patterns of social organization that characterize different societies. In those with a high proportion of solitaires, the chances are that a substantial enough number will be socially isolated that social isolation will be predictive of mortality. In those in which solitaires are uncommon or unknown, social isolation will not occur frequently enough to be predictive of mortality. We may then consider briefly the settings in which future studies might be expected to show an association between mortality and social isolation.

MORTALITY AND SOCIAL ISOLATION

I began by suggesting that the relationship between mortality and host factors of a psychosocial nature has become important only recently, occurring after the decline in infectious disease epidemics. It is unlikely that social support would provide any protection in the face of a pandemic. Indeed, to the degree that isolated individuals were not brought in contact with the etiological agent, isolation may have reduced the risks of mortality. No studies have examined the association of social isolation and mortality in epidemic circumstances as rigorously as the studies cited above have examined it in nonepidemic situations, but there is some tenuous evidence that there is no relationship. For example, Schofield has described a plague epidemic in Colyton, Devon in 1645–1646, even then not a kin-based society, and has shown that "For every family size, the number of families with extreme experiences (no one dying; everyone or almost everyone dying) was greater than expected, and the number of families with some dying and others surviving was correspondingly fewer than expected" (1977:107). Had social support made a difference, we might expect mortality in large households to be disproportionately lower than in small households. One must, of course, be careful about inferring lack of support from the fact that England was not a kin-based society for, as Schofield has pointed out (personal communication), support may well have come from kin elsewhere in the neighborhood, from nonkin neighbors, or even from social institutions such as the church. Thus, when a household became infected, others may have felt it too dangerous to maintain contact and would have discontinued support, such as nursing care, that would have been provided with more benign diseases. This is a reasonable explanation, but it is not clear just how important nursing care would be in the face of a plague epidemic in which everyone was susceptible,[2] especially in the absence of antibiotics. In either case, the result is the same; in the face of a pandemic, either social support was irrelevant to begin with in a non-kin-based society, or existing support structures collapsed and became irrelevant.

In an entirely different, kin-based society, Neel and his colleagues described a measles epidemic in a virgin soil population of Brazilian Indians during which everyone fell ill at about the same time, leaving no one available to provide nursing care (Neel et al. 1970). In such a situation, social support became irrelevant in the wake of the rending of the social fabric. It seems reasonable to suggest, therefore, that no matter what the pattern of social organization of a society, the presence of pandemic and severe epidemic diseases to which virtually everyone is susceptible will render social isolation and social contact insignificant as predictors of mortality.

What kinds of societies, then, have a high proportion of solitaires and low mortality? Low mortality characterizes all the industrial nations and many of the less-developed ones. Social isolation is another matter, however. We usually assume that as industrialization and urbanization proceed, families become nuclear in organization and the proportion of socially isolated people increases. There is some reason to think that this is not inevitably the case. Table 15.1 displays characteristics of household and work organization in four regions of premodern Europe (Laslett 1984:359).

Although the explanation of these patterns is speculative as yet (Goody 1983), it is clear that societies with a high proportion of solitaires also had a high proportion of small, simple-family households in which the institution of life-cycle service was common. That is, it was common for children to leave home to work for a few years on the farm of someone other than their family of origin before themselves marrying and establishing an independent home of their own. Hajnal (1982) suggests that this pattern may have been associated with the definitions of individualism and economic rationality that characterize much of Western thought and are very different from notions of rational behavior found in "joint household populations." Significantly, such patterns of organization and thought seem to have antedated the development of the market economy, capitalism, and industrialization. This is important for our topic because it calls into question the notion that nuclear family organization, small household size, and social isolation emerge only as an inevitable consequence of industrial development and "modernization." Laslett observes that, "It is already apparent that various types of social structure can exist alongside established industrialization, even if it may also be true that only one particular social structure could give rise to industrialization in the first place" (1983:559–60).

TABLE 15.1
Sets of Tendencies in Domestic Organization in Traditional Europe.

Overall criteria	Sets 1 and 2 Northern and western		Sets 3 and 4 Southern and eastern	
	1 West	2 West/central or middle	3 Mediterranean	4 East
Occasion and method of group formation				
a 1 Formed at marriage of household head	Always	Usually	Seldom	Never
a 2 Formed by fission or fusion of existent household(s)	Never	Sometimes	Frequently	Always
a 3 Marriage important to household formation	Always	Usually	(Seldom)[a]	Never
a 4 Takeover of existent houshold by new head	Occasionally	Frequent	Frequent	Usual
Procreational and demographic criteria				
b 1 Age at marriage, female	High	High	Low	Low
b 2 Age at marriage, male	High	High	High	Low
b 3 Proportions marrying	Low	Low	High	High
b 4 Age gap between spouses at first marriage	Narrow	Narrow	Wide	Narrow
b 5 Proportion of wives older than husbands	High	Very high	Low	High
b 6 Proportion of widows remarrying	High	Very high	Very low	Very low
Criteria of kin composiiton of groups				
c 1 Proportion of resident kin	Very low	Low	High	High
c 2 Proportion of multigenerational households	Low	Low	High	Very high
c 3 Proportion of households headed by never-married women	High	High	(Low)[a]	High
c 4 Proportion of solitaries	Very high	High	Low	Absent
c 5 Proportion of no-family households	High	High	Low	Absent
c 6 Proportion of simple-family households	High	High	Low	Low
c 7 Proportion of extended family households	Quite high	High	Low	Low
c 8 Proportion of multiple-family households	Very low	Low	High	Very high
c 9 Proportion of complex-family households (c7 + c8)	Very low	Low	High	Very high
c 10 Proporiton of frereches	Absent	Low	High	Very high
c 11 Proportion of stem-family households	Very low	High	Low	Low
c 12 Proportion of joint-family households	Absent	Low	Very high	Very high

Criteria of organization of work and welfare

d	1	Addition to household of kin as workers	Rare	Common	Very common	Universal
d	2	Added working kin called servants	Rare	Common	?	Irrelevant
d	3	Addition to household of life-cycle servants	Very common	Very common	Not uncommon	Irrelevant
d	4	Married servants	Uncommon	Common	?	Irrelevant
d	5	Attachment to household of inmates as workers	Very rare	Common	?	Occasional
d	6	Mean number of adults per household	Low	High	Very high	Maximal
d	7	Mean number of households of ≤3 persons	Very high	High	Very low	Very low
d	8	Mean number of persons of working age (15–65) per household	Low	Medium	Very high	Very high
d	9	Household head described as laborer, journeyman, out-servant, cottager	Often	Sometimes	Never	Never
d	10	Household head described as pauper	Often	Sometimes	?	?
d	11	Attachment of secondary household to houseful	Absent	Common	Absent	Absent

Table 15.2 displays data from several European nations and one non-European nation concerning the proportions of people sixty years of age and above who live with four or more other people. Though not perfect, it is clear that people in northwestern and central Europe are much less likely than people in southern and eastern Europe and the Balkans to live with four or more other people. There may be a variety of reasons for this pattern, including the lack of available housing for young families, something that is clearly the case in Belgrade and Zagreb. Nonetheless, the pattern is too similar to what would have been predicted on the basis of the premodern pattern to believe that traditional forms of social organization are entirely irrelevant. Note, moreover, that I am not asserting that co-residence necessarily implies support. That may or may not be the case. At the very least, however, it implies contact with other people.

Thus, it is not self-evident that social isolation will be observed frequently enough to be predictive of mortality in all low mortality, industrialized nations. Indeed, we might reasonably predict that it will be significant only in northwest European nations and in their overseas extensions, such as North America, Australia, and New Zealand. In such industrial nations as are found in eastern Europe, the Balkans, and the Far East, for instance, it is by no means clear that social isolation is a relevant variable. That depends upon patterns of social organization developed in the course of their recent industrialization. If indeed family organization retains many of its traditional features, then even in the face of urbanization and industrialization social isolation will not be common enough to be significantly associated with mortality.

The Ideological and Intellectual Response to Transitions

If the conventional wisdom is wrong, and industrialization and urbanization are not invariably associated with increasing social isolation, we may ask why it has usually been assumed by Western social scientists that they will be? I have already cited John Hajnal's observation that "Adam Smith, Ricardo, and their successors based their theories on the social system they knew, namely that of Northwest Europe" (1982:475). That system transformed the world, perhaps especially rapidly since the dual revolutions of the 1780s — the Industrial Revolution in Britain and the democratic revolution in France (Hobsbawm 1962). And it is to the reaction to those events and what followed in their train that the assumptions of much Western social science may be traced (Nisbet 1966). The perceived destruction of *gemeinschaft* by *gesellschaft*, status by contract, and the traditional by the modern, all are part of the intellectual legacy left by nineteenth-century social philosophers to twentieth-century social scientists, along with such concepts as alienation, anomie, and mass society.

These are European ideas, but like so much else in the world, they have been Americanized in the course of the past century (Bramson 1961). It has often been pointed out that Europeans are concerned with The Social Problem of

TABLE 15.2
Percentages of People 60 Years of Age and Above Living With Four or More People, by Age, Sex, and Region.

Region	Sample Area	Men 60–4	65–9	70–4	75–9	80–4	85–9	Women 60–4	65–9	70–4	75–9	80–4	85–9
N.W. Europe	Brussels (urban)	0	0	4	4	0	0	3	0	4	0	4	7
	Leuven (mixed urban and rural)	16	14	5	2	6	12	3	8	7	12	18	9
	Tempere, Finland (mainly urban)	5	4	1	1	3	5	3	2	1	3	4	0
	Upper Normandy (both urban and rural)	1	5	5	0	5	0	3	1	1	4	3	13
Central Europe	West Berlin (urban)	2	1	0	0	2	3	2	2	0	1	3	2
Southern Europe	Midi-Pyrenees (mainly rural, with Toulouse)	13	8	8	13	21	18	7	7	7	11	11	15
	Florence (urban)	16	10	15	16	18	25	13	22	25	20	18	12
	Low Ombrone (mixed rural-urban)	23	32	33	40	47	46	26	34	44	37	42	43
	West Amiata (rural)	9	7	13	11	12	11	9	6	11	17	16	12
Eastern Europe	Bialystak (urban)	36	31	23	20	27	—	27	25	16	6	24	—
	Kiev (urban)	19	20	17	22	20	11	19	20	15	14	16	18
Balkans	Belgrade (urban)	23	20	14	14	18	11	14	20	13	13	16	18
	Zagreb (urban)	20	24	11	24	12	13	13	14	18	12	13	20
	Rural Greece	22	22	24	33	31	35	27	10	32	27	27	33
	Bucharest (urban)	8	2	11	7	22	20	10	11	11	9	18	13
Persian Gulf	Kuwait (entire country)	84	89	89	92	87	84	81	84	86	95	94	94

class, whereas Americans are concerned with social problems resulting from the necessity to assimilate wave upon wave of immigrants from many different societies. C. Wright Mills observed that the response of early sociologists to the growth of cities peopled by newly arrived immigrants was conditioned by their origins in the small towns of America. "Most of the 'problems' considered arise because of the urban deterioration of certain values that can live genuinely only in a relatively homogeneous and primarily rural milieu. The 'problems' discussed typically concern urban behavior. When 'rural problems' are discussed, they are considered due to encroaching urbanization" (1943:136).

Immigration was thought to be disruptive both for the rural communities whose citizens felt threatened by alien, urban forces and for the immigrants themselves, who displayed all sorts of problematic behavior until they "adapted" — another favorite notion of the social pathologists, according to Mills. But the sociologists' fundamentally conservative idealization of the "primary-group community," a "Christian-democratic version of the rural village," was combined with a liberal belief in progress and upward mobility. Therefore, failure to adapt was often seen as an example of "cultural lag," the inability or unwillingness to shed beliefs and behaviors inappropriate in the new situation.

Thus sociologists in the United States Americanized many of the notions of their European predecessors and teachers by focusing increasingly upon social problems and the significance of primary groups in retarding or encouraging the adaptation of individuals to industrial civilization, rather than by attending to the social problem of class conflict and the emergence of bourgeois society (Shils 1951). Indeed, the belief in progress and the adaptive function of primary groups was an important source of insights regarding industrial management, as the seminal work of Elton Mayo at the Harvard Business School suggests. Summing up twenty years of research, including the classic studies at the Hawthorn Western Electric plant, Mayo (1945) made the by-then-familiar distinction between "established" and "adaptive" societies. The former were characterized by face-to-face relationships and training in apprenticeships in which technical and social skills were learned simultaneously. Adaptive societies were characterized by rapid change, high degrees of mobility, and, at the individual level, increased breakdown and psychoneurosis. Primary groups could retard or promote adaptation. It was the task of administrators to foster adaptation — often utilizing primary work groups — to the changes produced by industrial civilization.

Many of these notions of adaptation, change, and the role of primary groups were drawn upon explicitly by Cassel and his colleagues (Cassel, Patrick, and Jenkins 1960) and have had a profound impact upon social epidemiology. But there is a curiously related tradition that has also been influential. I refer to the importance of concepts taken over from physiology into the social sciences.

Physiology had developed as a flourishing science when it was submerged by the bacteriological revolution in the last quarter of the nineteenth century and the first two decades of the present century. The germ theory provided an explanation for the most significant causes of morbidity and mortality and had a profound impact upon public health, medical practice, and research. But by the 1920s it was clear that infectious diseases had declined in significance and new conditions were becoming prevalent, what Peyton Rous (1929) called "The Modern Dance of Death" — heart disease, nephritis, apoplexy (stroke), and cancer — and what Alfred Cohn (1931:133) called "physiological disharmony."

L. J. Henderson, physiologist and social philosopher at Harvard, wrote in his 1927 introduction to the English translation of Claude Bernard's *Introduction to the Study of Experimental Medicine*:

> Today, looking backward, we see how it was that bacteriological researchers for a long time took the first place which Claude Bernard believed to be already assured to those of his own science. When Pasteur began the study of micro-organisms a great gap existed in our knowledge of the organic cycle and of natural history. His work and that of his successors filled this gap, completed our present theory of the cycle of life and established the natural history of infectious diseases, of fermentation and of the soil. This was perhaps the most rapid advance of descriptive knowledge in the history of science. For the moment the researches of physiologists were overshadowed and the work of the young men diverted to new fields. In time bacteriology grew into a fully developed science, perfected its methods, exploited its domain, and then, the most pressing work well done, resigned its leadership of the medical sciences. (Henderson 1948:ix-x)

It was in this context that physiology re-emerged in the 1920s and 1930s. Its central concern is perhaps best captured by the term "homeostasis," coined by Henderson's colleague Walter Cannon to describe the ability of organisms to maintain "dynamic equilibrium" in the face of a continually changing environment (Cannon 1939). He even proposed that failure to maintain homeostasis of the sympathico-adrenal system might be the mechanism explaining "voodoo death" (Cannon 1942), and also applied it to the functioning of the welfare state (Cannon 1939).

Moreover, like Rous, Cohn, and many others, Cannon believed that "Since the turn of the century an important change in the phenomena of disease has occurred — the seriousness of infection has undergone a remarkable decline, and strains and stresses, especially affecting the nervous system, have been on the increase" (Cannon 1936:1454). Indeed, stress research began to increase appreciably in the 1930s, notably with the work of Hans Selye (1956) on the general adaptation syndrome and with the growth of psychosomatic medicine.

Even ideas about infectious diseases began to change. Lecturing in 1934 toward the end of a distinguished career as a microbiologist and pathologist at the Rockefeller Institute, Theobald Smith observed that predation led "by gradual evolutionary steps" to parasitism – "the finding of lodgement and food by one organism on or in another." And "parasitism may be regarded, not as a pathological manifestation, but as a normal condition having its roots in the interdependence of all living organisms."

> Parasitism is in a sense a compromise or truce between two living things, accompanied by predatory processes whenever opportunity is offered one or the other party. The universality of parasitism as an offshoot of the predatory habit negates the position taken by man that it is a pathological phenomenon or a deviation from the normal processes of nature. The pathological manifestations are only incidents in a developing parasitism. (Smith 1934:3–4)

By the 1930s, then, shifting morbidity and mortality patterns and growing knowledge of carrier states (Winslow 1943) led some observers to conclude that it was an oversimplification to say that infectious diseases were synonymous with "disease agents." They were the result of incomplete evolutionary mutual adaptation of parasites and hosts and could follow from a disturbance in the precarious equilibrium between them (e.g., Dubos 1965:164).

This reconceptualization of infectious and noninfectious diseases as the result of failures of adaptation, and of the inability to maintain equilibrium, was resonant with broader themes in social philosophy and the emerging social sciences (Russett 1966; Kunitz 1970). Rapid change overwhelmed the ability of individuals and societies to adapt and resulted in personal and social disequilibrium and various forms of breakdown. The connection between physiology and social science was made explicit in the work of L. J. Henderson, a colleague of both Mayo and Cannon, who, in addition to his physiological research, taught sociology at Harvard, including a famous seminar on the sociology of Pareto attended by such budding luminaries of American social science as Clyde Kluckhohn, George Homans, Talcott Parsons, and William F. Whyte (Heyl 1968). Henderson made explicit the relationship between social and personal health: "The conclusion of Hippocrates was that the state of health is similar to that state defined by Pareto in his treatise on *General Sociology, The Mind and Society*, as equilibrium" (Henderson 1970:73; see also Henderson 1935). Personnel management and patient management were thus similar, both requiring the special talent of the therapist to help the worker or patient adapt to change and restore equilibrium.

It was this complex of ideas from social philosophy and physiology that formed the basis for Cassel's earliest formulations of a new kind of epidemiology. In an early statement on the health implications of culture change, he and his co-authors wrote:

> Dating from the discovery of bacteria, medical thinking has until recently favored a closed-system mechanistic model of illness and health. This

model ascribed a single specific cause to each disease which, if present, would ideally always cause the disease. Conversely any disease would always be due to a specific cause . . . .

This concept, while useful in the study of communicable disease, posed difficulties where micro-organisms were not involved . . . .

In order . . . to gain understanding of other diseases, particularly the diseases of contemporary industrialized society, a more useful model would appear to be the open-system model suggested as applying to both physics and biology by von Bertalanffy. (Cassel, Patrick, and Jenkins 1960:939)

They went on to say that within this framework, health represented successful adjustment (homeostasis) and disease a failure of adjustment. Such a conception, they believed, would prove fruitful for epidemiology as it would provide a means of showing "the relationship between strain in the various systems [biochemical, physiological, psychological, social, and cultural—S. J. K.] and alterations in the state of health under study" (Cassel, Patrick, and Jenkins 1960:940).

They drew upon the work of a number of anthropologists and sociologists to begin developing a model of the kinds of sociocultural changes that would influence the health of individuals by challenging their adaptive capacities. In this context, they leaned heavily upon Robert Redfield's notion of the folk-urban continuum, characterizing rural folk cultures as found in relatively homogeneous communities where relationships are based upon long-continued personal interaction; which are self-contained and self-supporting; where traditions are stable and the pace of change slow; and where values are implicitly held, taken for granted, and sacred inasmuch as they are not subject to challenge or criticism (Cassel, Patrick, and Jenkins 1960:945).

They hypothesized:

1. That the process of culture change, as manifested by rural migration to an industrial area, will be associated with changes in health status. The group experiencing culture change will have higher indices of poor health and adjustment than the group that has not experienced the change or the group that experienced the change more than a generation ago.
2. (a) The association between culture change and poor health and adjustment will be maximal in those families in which there has been least sharing of the process of change and in which there is least solidarity.
   (b) Upward social mobility will accentuate the association between culture change and poor health and adjustment. (Cassel, Patrick, and Jenkins 1960:944)

Cassel and his co-authors were careful to say that the urban dweller was not necessarily cut off from all meaningful contacts, but rather that "the culture of the city is organized on different principles" (Cassel, Patrick, and Jenkins 1960:946). The urbanite is a member of many groups rather than one all-encompassing group and has not lost commitment to values but develops values appropriate to the urban setting. Likewise, family structure changes: "The isolated nuclear family, centering its functions on sex, companionship, and the socialization of the young, may be of crucial importance for the members of an industrial society as a buffer against the impersonal, competitive, occupational world" (Cassel, Patrick, and Jenkins 1960:947). This sort of family organization was adaptive to urban life. The maintenance of "extended folk-type kinship relations" might thus be useful "as a temporary buffer" for new migrants to the city, but "the long continuation of extended forms of the family may be regarded as dysfunctional in urban-industrial society."

Some of the health and adjustment problems of lower-class people in industrial cities, who tend not completely to have made the transition to the nuclear family, may be subject to interpretation in the light of the "social lag" hypothesis. It is possible that the very form of these lower-class families tends to unfit their members for adequate functioning in the new type of social reality. (Cassel, Patrick, and Jenkins 1960:948)

Cassel's theoretical position contained some of the same ambiguities as those of the social pathologists before him. On one hand, stable communities are conducive to health; on the other, progress is inevitable, and pathology results from cultural and social lags which impede adaptation to change. He did not take the position that rural life was necessarily happier and healthier than urban life and that the transformation from the former to the latter implied the inevitable degradation of the population. Rather, it was during the transition that morbidity would be expected to increase, and it would remain high so long as adjustment was incomplete. Nonetheless, it is clear that woven into the very fabric of social epidemiology is the view that urbanization and industrialization — modernization — are disruptive and bad for one's health, at least until such time as one becomes successfully modern.

Thus, like the Fore described by Shirley Lindenbaum in Chapter 16 of this volume, social epidemiologists have produced explanations of disease based upon perceptions of the past and of the consequences of major social and epidemiological transformations. In this case the perception is of a past characterized by extended family organization in stable, slowly changing communities. Modernization was understood to mean unilinear change to societies based upon nuclear families, in which the alienated individual is both psychologically and socially isolated. We have seen that this does not seem to be an accurate picture of family organization in premodern or early modern Europe and instead represents a romantic idea of a past that may never have existed and against which the present may be judged and found wanting. Similarly, modernization of kin-based societies may not necessarily mean either that extended families are rendered obsolete or that social isolation increases. The perceptions of social philosophers and social scientists that individualism can have some harmful consequences may thus be accurate but perhaps only for the societies that gave birth to the insight.

NOTES

Theodore M. Brown, Jerrold E. Levy, Robert McC. Netting, and Roger Schofield commented on an early version of this chapter.

1. A useful review of a very large number of recent studies on the association between social support and health is Campbell (1985).
2. Unlike measles and smallpox, plague does not cause immunity, though resistance to a repeat infection does seem to be enhanced.

REFERENCES

Berkman, L. F., and S. L. Syme. 1979. Social networks, host resistance, and mortality: A nine-year follow-up study of Alameda County residents. *American Journal of Epidemiology* 109:186–204.

Blazer, D. G. 1982. Social support and mortality in an elderly community population. *American Journal of Epidemiology* 115:684–94.

Bramson, L. 1961. *The Political Context of American Sociology.* Princeton: Princeton University Press.

Campbell, T. L. 1985. *Family's Impact on Health: A Critical Review and Annotated Bibliography.* NIMH Contract Report No. 84M0267612. Rochester, N. Y.: Department of Preventive, Family, and Rehabilitation Medicine, University of Rochester Medical Center.

Cannon, W. B. 1942. "Voodoo" death. *American Anthropologist* 44:169–81.

———. 1939. *The Wisdom of the Body.* New York: W. W. Norton.

———. 1936. The role of emotion in disease. *Annals of Internal Medicine.* 9:1453–65.

Cassel, J. 1970. Physical illness in response to stress. In *Social Stress.* S. Levine and N. A. Scotch, eds. Chicago: Aldine.

———. 1974. Psychosocial processes and stress: Theoretical formulation. *International Journal of Health Services* 4:471–482.

———. 1976. The contribution of the social environment to host resistance. *American Journal of Epidemiology* 104:107–23.

Cassel, J., R. Patrick, and D. Jenkins. 1960. Epidemiological analysis of the health implications of culture change: A conceptual model. *Annals of the New York Academy of Sciences* 84:938–49.

Cobb, S. 1976. Social support as a moderator of life stress. *Psychosomatic Medicine.* 38:300–14.

Cohn, A. 1931. *Medicine, Science and Art.* Chicago: University of Chicago Press.

Dubos, R. 1965. *Man Adapting.* New Haven: Yale University Press.

Goody, J. R. 1983. *The Development of the Family and Marriage in Europe.* Cambridge: Cambridge University Press.

Hajnal, J. 1982. Two kinds of preindustrial household formation systems. *Population and Development Review.* 8:449–94.

Henderson, L. J. 1970. Sociology 23 Lectures. In *Henderson on the Social System.* B. Barber, ed. Chicago: University of Chicago Press.

————. 1948. Introduction. In *An Introduction to the Study of Experimental Medicine.* C. Bernard, ed. New York: Henry Schuman.

————. 1935. *Pareto's General Sociology.* Cambridge: Harvard University Press.

Heyl, B. 1968. The Harvard "Pareto Circle." *Journal on the History of the Behavioral Sciences.* 4:316–334.

Hobsbawm, E. J. 1962. *The Age of Revolution.* London: Weidenfeld & Nicolson.

House, J. S., C. Robbins, and H. L. Metzner. 1982. The association of social relationships and activities with mortality: Prospective evidence from the Tecumseh community health study. *American Journal of Epidemiology* 116:123–40.

Kunitz, S. J. 1970. Equilibrium theory in social psychiatry. *Psychiatry.* 33:312–28.

Laslett, P. 1984. The family as a knot of individual interests. In *Households: Comparative and Historical Studies of the Domestic Group.* R. M. Netting, R. R. Wilk, and E. J. Arnould, eds. Los Angeles: University of California Press.

————. 1983. Family and household as work group and kin group: Areas of traditional Europe compared. In *Family Forms in Historic Europe.* R. Wall, ed. Cambridge: Cambridge University Press.

Lebra, T. 1976. *Japanese Patterns of Behavior.* Honolulu: University of Hawaii Press.

Mayo, E. 1945. *The Social Problems of an Industrial Civilization.* Boston: Graduate School of Business Administration, Harvard University.

Mills, C. W. 1943. The professional ideology of the social pathologists. *American Journal of Sociology.* 49:165–80. Reprinted in *The Sociology of Sociology.* L. T. Reynolds and J. M. Reynolds eds. New York: David McKay. 1970.

Montero, D. 1979. Disengagement and aging among the Issei. In *Ethnicity and Aging.* D. E. Gelfand and A. J. Kutzick, eds. New York: Springer-Verlag.

National Indian Council on Aging. 1981. *American Indian Elderly: A National Profile.* Albuquerque: National Indian Council on Aging.

Neel, J. V., W. R. Centerwall, N. A. Chagnon, and H. L. Casey. 1970. Notes on the effect of measles and measles vaccine in a virgin-soil population of South American Indians. *American Journal of Epidemiology* 91:418–29.

Nisbet, R. 1966. *The Sociological Tradition.* New York: Basic.

Reed, D., D. McGee, and K. Yano. 1984. Psychosocial processes and general susceptibility to chronic disease. *American Journal of Epidemiology* 119:356–70.

Rous, P. 1929. *The Modern Dance of Death.* Cambridge: Cambridge University Press.

Russett, C. E. 1966. *The Concept of Equilibrium in American Social Thought.* New Haven: Yale University Press.

Schofield, R. 1977. An anatomy of an epidemic. In *The Plague Reconsidered.* Matlock, Derbyshire: *Local Population Studies Supplement.*

Segalen, M. 1984. Nuclear is not independent: Organization of the household in the Pays Bigouden Sud in the nineteenth and twentieth centuries. In *Households: Comparative and Historical Studies of the Domestic Group.* R. M. Netting, R. R. Wilk, and E. J. Arnould, eds. Los Angeles: University of California Press.

Selye, H. 1956. *The Stress of Life.* New York: McGraw-Hill.

Shils, E. 1951. The study of the primary group. In *The Policy Sciences.* D. Lerner and H. D. Lasswell, eds. Stanford: Stanford University Press.

Smith, T. 1934. *Parasitism and Disease.* Princeton: Princeton University Press.

Wellman, B. 1981. Applying network analysis to the study of support. In *Social Networks and Social Support*. B. H. Gottlieb, ed. Beverly Hills: Sage.

Winslow, C. E.-A. 1943. *The Conquest of Epidemic Disease*. Princeton: Princeton University Press.

World Health Organization (WHO). 1983. *The Elderly in Eleven Countries*. Copenhagen: Regional Office for Europe.

Zuckerman, D. M., S. V. Kasl, and A. M. Ostfeld. 1984. Psychosocial predictors of mortality among the elderly poor: The role of religion, well-being, and social contacts. *American Journal of Epidemiology* 119:410–23.

16 THE ECOLOGY OF KURU

Shirley Lindenbaum

The anthropological perspective on health and disease encompasses interactions among the culture, biology, and demography of human hosts and the environmental associations between host-factors and pathogens/insults in space and time. Assuming that illness beliefs and behaviors, as much as host-pathogen associations, are part of the ecology of disease, an anthropological approach further attempts to provide an account of these connections from the natives' as well as from the observers' point of view. In the account that follows, I discuss the beliefs and behaviors of the Fore of the Eastern Highlands of Papua New Guinea, widening the discussion to include kuru as well as other diseases and ailments. The Fore concern with the pathogenesis of disease is seen to convey a particular, if changing, world view.

Following a short account of Fore beliefs about the etiology of illness in the early 1960s, I show how these beliefs change over time, point to social changes that accompanied these cognitive shifts, and indicate the merits of reflecting upon the intellectual history of a region. By viewing the contexts in which Fore models of disease and danger shift, we learn something of the ways paradigms and behaviors change in other times and places. Moreover, just as an appreciation of the genesis of our own contemporary illness beliefs and behaviors stems from social and intellectual changes that had their beginning in the "scientific revolution" of the sixteenth and seventeenth centuries, an account of Fore currents of thought and the contexts in which they change is relevant to an understanding of the present-day health status of the Fore.

FORE ILLNESS BELIEFS AND BEHAVIORS

In the lower montane forests of the Eastern Highlands of Papua New Guinea, the Fore, a population of some 14,000 horticulturalists, tend gardens of sweet potato, taro, yam, corn, and other vegetables. They also grow sugarcane and bananas, keep pigs, and in the sparsely populated southern regions, still hunt for birds, mammals, reptiles, and cassowaries. Coffee, introduced in 1957, became an important cash crop by the late 1960s as the coffee trees matured.

In the early 1960s, the Fore classified illness in a systematic way, defined by beliefs about causation. Within the overall class of illness, there were two significant categories: maladies resulting from actions of men against men, or acts of sorcery (*kio'ena* "the hidden thing"), and second, conditions attributed not to the machinations of sorcerers but to assault by various less malign forces — by nature spirits inhabiting spirit places associated with one's parish of residence, by ghosts of the recently dead, and by punishment for violation of social rules and expectations among co-residents. (In the 1960s there were thirty-nine parishes in the South Fore, their populations ranging from 41 to 525, with a mean of 150.) Calamities ascribed to sorcery involved life-threatening disorders such as kuru, liver disease, or respiratory illness, conditions that endangered the survival of important members of the society, the women who ensured its continuity and the men who protected it. Ailments ascribed to other causes involved minor afflictions and temporary illness among adults and sickness and death among children.

Spirit-induced ailments were believed to result from human intrusion into spirit places, the forest reserves associated with every parish. Gardening was permitted at the edge of a spirit place but not within, and certain timbers, vines, animals, and wild foods that could be collected elsewhere were not to be touched in one's own spirit place. In some, to speak or to make a loud noise was considered dangerous. Not all products were absolutely forbidden, however, and limited use was made of these sacred groves. Minor illness in adults or the birth of a slightly impaired child indicated the spirit's anger at the removal of a particular item.

Diagnosis is retrospective. A child born deaf was called a "spirit child" because the pregnant mother was thought to have touched a certain tree, vine, or other spirit-inhabited object in the forest reserve. Relief was gained by bringing the offended tree spirit a gift of wealth or food. Shells were hung temporarily on the tree's branches, and its trunk was rubbed with pig fat, while the victim ate a medicinal meal of pork with *ni* (cyanotis), a red-leafed vine found growing in forest reserves and believed to contain the power of the place.

Spirit place beliefs, then, operated as zoning regulations for the protection of small areas of wilderness — an important concern for the Fore who, in the 1960s, still depended on the forest for wild foods and for the game they were obliged to give to their affines. People with physical impairments were a living reminder of past offenses against this group resource.

Ghost-caused ailments were said to occur if a person removed food from the gardens of a man recently deceased. To remove the growing plants was to sever the head decorations of the man lying buried in his garden and, if committed during the period of mourning, was an offense. This was a period when death payments were to be distributed to kin and agemates of the deceased, not a time to plunder his property and disturb his ghostly identity. Offenders were said to be punished by the angered ghost, suffering nausea, weakness, and fainting spells. Those who had poor relationships with living parents similarly succumbed to ghost attack when the parents died.

Ghosts, then, monitored considerate attention toward close kin and the correct modes of property exchange. They also ensured a period of fallow for parish gardens. Curers blew the angered ghost from the victim's body, but the insulted ghost was placated only by the sacrifice of pork and the libation of pig blood poured into the head of the grave.

Infringements of social rules among the living produced the simplest ailments and the most direct remedies. A man cut down a tree belonging to another, and the offender's son or daughter immediately fell ill. Recovery was assured when the guilty party offered the tree owner a compensatory payment and the latter provided for the sick child a reviving meal of pork and medicines.

These three subcategories of non-sorcery-caused ailments have several things in common. Encroachments against nature spirits, ghosts of the dead, or injured neighbors must all be made good by some kind of indemnity; spirits and ghosts receive "symbolic" food, the angry person, material payment. The victim is restored to health. The therapy has a conceptual basis that seems characteristically Melanesian: the notion of compensation for injury, with its emphasis on equality and a return to the status quo. (Indigenous court fines, for instance, are set equal to estimates of the damage incurred, and wartime allies were bribed or persuaded by gifts to join one side of a contest.)

A few conditions, such as war fatalities, epidemic illness (dysentery), and mild conditions that at times affect everyone (colds, headaches) fell outside theories of causation that depended on the selective malevolence of spirits, ghosts, or perverted humans and were said to be forms of "illness." All other maladies required judgment as to cause, which involved some kind of socially disapproved act. Sorcery resulted from the deliberate activities of hostile outsiders, enemies in another parish or local parish section, who were to be exposed by divination or threat. Responsibility for lesser ailments fell within the local parish section, the minimal political unit. (Wanitabe parish, the central fieldwork location, had 350 residents in three sections of 170, 139, and 42 members.) Within this small residential unit, the offense was patent and required no detection. These minor illnesses stemmed from some wrongdoing by the victim or close kinsperson and involved the relationship of a person to his or her group's land, to people who had until recently been members of the group, or to present residents. In sum, sorcery allegations appeared to be statements about contemporary political relations with other groups, whereas interpretations of other ailments referred to personal relations, rules of behavior, property rights, and common responsibilities within the group itself. These involved issues common to legal systems everywhere: the proper definition of murder, manslaughter, negligence, accident, and theft.

At one level, then, Fore analyses of the etiology of disease can be viewed as assertions about the structure of their society, the dangers to which its composite units are exposed, and the measures that can be taken to protect them. In the early 1960s, lesser dangers were thought to originate from within the community, great dangers from without. Most sorcery accusations thus occurred between men residing in different parishes, but as the discussion that follows indicates, this was in the process of change, reflecting the epidemiological and existential concerns of the decade. The Fore medicinal idiom exhibits a fit between environmental, cognitive, and historical experience.

CHANGING TAXONOMIES

The literature on the topic frequently depicts two kinds of sorcery said to occur in the Papua New Guinea region. Glick describes "the more usual form," which he calls "projective sorcery" (1972:1029). Here, the sorcerer is said to be a single individual acting on his own initiative or on behalf of others. Sorcerer and victim do not come into contact; the sorcerer works at a distance, propelling harmful objects into his victim or cooking bits of bodily refuse or food scraps with poison. Illnesses attributed to projective sorcery are usually those of gradual onset, and the victim and his or her kin often attempt to find a cure. The second type, "assault sorcery," is almost a reverse of the first. Here, several assailants ambush their victim and carry out an "uncompromisingly vicious" attack. Overpowering the victim, the assailants jab poisons into his body, twist and rip out organs, and are "not satisfied until he is thoroughly befuddled, unable to remember who or what has afflicted him" (Glick 1972:1029) The victim staggers home and dies without identifying his attacker. There is little emphasis on a cure, for it is apparent to everyone except the victim, who has no memory of the attack, that he is beyond the range of ordinary curative powers.

If we adopt Glick's useful schema for the Fore as well as for other contemporary societies in Papua New Guinea, it is evident that both kinds of sorcery are on the increase, and both are changing in significant ways. The most striking change is a shift from what might be called exosorcery to endosorcery (Lindenbaum 1981:119). Sorcery attacks formerly directed against "outsiders" are now said to occur within the phratry (the Agarabi of the Eastern Highlands, Westermark 1981:94) or the village (the Kilenge of West New Britain, Zelenietz 1981:115), within the larger villages (Ambrym of Vanuatu, Tonkinson 1981:83), or between former allies and "brothers" (the Mendi of the Southern Highlands, Lederman 1981:16). Fore data confirm the trend. Whereas Berndt reported that in 1951–1953 North Fore sorcerers were apparently not feared within the district (1958: 6), in the early 1960s the South Fore indicated that this was no longer the case. By late 1962, South Fore were speculating on the changing locus of disease origin:

> During wartime, we men of Wanikanto [parish] fought against Amora [a neighboring parish] and they fought back. But since kuru has come amongst us, we don't think it is our enemies who are killing us. We think it is people in our own community who are finishing off our women.

As later discussion illustrates, current endosorcery accusations in Papua New Guinea resemble witchcraft complaints in sixteenth and seventeenth century Europe, as well as nineteenth century Africa, reflecting in part the contradictory claims of kin-based communities and the new worlds of wage labor, business, and trade. The income from coffee and other small ventures has created tension between ceremonial exchange obligations, on the one hand, and market-based activities on the other, between an ethic of generosity to kin and neighbors and one of competitive individualism.

The changed locus of projective sorcery indictments in the 1960s, as well as the escalating number of sorceries identified,[1] shows the Fore rearranging their taxonomic system to account for the new pathogens and experiences they were confronting. The transformed idioms of assault sorcery, however, provide a more striking commentary on contemporary social conditions. Since Codrington's first account of assault sorcery (called *vele*) in the Solomons in 1891, various permutations of this form of sorcery have been recorded. Known as *sangguma* or *shut'im nil* in Melanesian pidgin, or by the indigenous term in each location, the geography of the phenomenon covers island, coastal and highland Papua New Guinea, as well as some parts of Northern Australia.[2] Its recent presence in the Eastern Highland is documented by several anthropologists who note its increasing incidence, as well as the fact that it is said to be "perhaps the most feared sorcery technique" (Westermark 1981, writing about the Agarabi) or "the form of sorcery most dreaded" (Johannes and Keil 1974, on the Nekematigi). Glick observes that Gimi assault sorcerers, called "violent men," a name Gimi gives also to Papua New Guinea policemen, are considered bold, aggressive, and virile.

While the broad outlines of assault remain constant—the vicious attack by multiple assailants, the victim's loss of consciousness and subsequent revival with no memory of what has taken place, and his final demise—the imagery of assault transmutes as it travels through time and moves from the coast to the highlands. The apparently solitary Solomon Island sorcerer, who bites his victim's neck, stuffs magical leaves down his throat, and stuns him with the blow of an axe (Codrington 1891:206), has his counterpart in Wogeo where the weaponry includes needlelike slivers of black palm wood or lengths of sharp stingray spines and medicines (Hogbin 1970: 149, based on fieldwork in 1934). The documented spread of recent assault sorcery in the Eastern Highlands, however, begins to tell of sorcerers whose paraphernalia includes an updated technology of knives, razor blades, bicycle spokes, and battery acid. Moreover, some assault sorcerers are now reported to be available as assassins for hire beyond their own linguistic region.

Assault sorcery, called *tokabu* by the Fore, is not a category in the Western sense. Part murder, part hypnosis, part sudden death, part magic, it seems to us to "confuse" a number of separate concepts. Since corpses are occasionally discovered providing evidence of dramatic mutilation — the victim's Adam's apple is severed and a three-inch nail driven into his skull — the tendency is to assume that assault sorcery is merely a kind of murder. A historical glance at Fore attributions of *tokabu* deaths provides us with a more precise picture.

Berndt's North Fore genealogies recorded between 1951 and 1953 show sangguma (*tokabu*) accounting for 199 of 1,863 North Fore deaths, more than twice the number of deaths from kuru during the same period. My own South Fore genealogies from a decade later, representing four generations of remembered deaths in Wanitabe parish, shows *tokabu* second only to kuru in this more highly kuru-affected southern region. The South Fore attribution of *tokabu* as a cause of death, however, registers an interesting change. In the great-grandparental generation, *tokabu* is an equal danger to both men and women; in the following two generations, *tokabu* is said to kill twice as many men as women. In this more contemporary period, nineteen of the fifty-eight male victims were unmarried at the time of death, while only three of the thiry-one female victims were single women. In some cases the Fore also indicated a "Western" cause of death, not regarded as a primary cause. (*Tokabu* killers may enlist agents to do their bidding.) A number of men are thus said to have died of arrow wounds received during wartime, and three women (two married and one widowed) are said to have been suicides. In this latter case, the victims are thought to have been told what to do to bring about their own deaths. *Tokabu* thus accounts for the demise of those who have suffered a loss of volition, placing them in dangerous or destructive environments, seen increasingly as the fate of young unmarried men. From day to day in the South Fore during the 1960s, cries of "*Tokabu*" issued also from the women's seclusion hut or from young women gardening alone in locations distant from the hamlet, alerting those within earshot of suspected sexual intruders.

Classical *tokabu* ideology, as well as the ethnographic record, thus portrays the *tokabu* victim as a lone individual, separated from his or her community, set upon by an ill-defined party of antagonistic forces. (The Fore term *tokabu* indicates assault, *kabu*, by strangers, *to-gina*). In contrast to projective sorcery, the assailants are not merely unknown, they are unknowable. Various Fore accounts describe the victims as mute: "He can't tell his wife or father or brother what happened." "The rope in his neck is cut." "His larynx is eaten away." "They tightened a net bag around his neck, severed part of his throat, and blood came out of his mouth." Assault sorcery deaths are also sudden and unexpected: "On the first day he was sick, unable to eat, and on the fifth day he died." As Mathews observes (1971:47), *tokabu* represents a residual nosological entity to account for any death unexplained by more specific types of sorcery, reflecting in part the impact of a new viral strain on a virgin population.[3] *Tokabu* diagnosis thus precludes lengthy divination or curative procedures, suggesting the assumed impotence and uselessness of such public social therapies.

A central image of this form of sorcery is loss of consciousness by a victim caught in an isolated place. Fore men fear *tokabu* most on sunny days when traveling alone on roads beyond their own parish territory. For protection, they move rapidly from the shade of one roadside tree to the next or carry a large umbrella. One's shadow, one's "soul," one's psychic self is exposed in an encounter with strangers beyond the security of the home parish. The Eastern Highlands Agarabi say they recover from the trance of assault sorcery when they recognize the familiar smells of their parish hearth fires and the feces of their dogs and pigs (Westermark 1981:93), the very odor and idea, one might say, of their own moral community. Glick was thus correct, I think, to emphasize that "the victim is permitted to stagger home but only as a shell, a mocking sign to kinsmen and neighbors that in this man's person they have all in a sense been assaulted and are now helpless to resist" (1972:1029). For many Papua New Guineans, the experiences of the past few decades have disassembled the old physical and mental barricades that kept out enemies and strangers. Gone, too, is the degree of mutual trust and support which magnetized the communities from within, as the growing allegations of endosorcery indicate.

The epidemic of assault sorcery in the Eastern Highlands and elsewhere in Papua New Guinea thus provides a moving account of the experience of individuals and communities stripped of their former autonomy, confronting new kinds of physical and mental assault. Young men, predominantly, pulled out of context by wage labor and the newfound mobility occasioned by the end of warfare and the construction of public trunk roads, encounter new kinds of diseases and new forms of random and sudden death. It is not by chance that many of the new instruments of attack—battery acid, bicycle spokes, and sometimes umbrella ribs—come from the "high tech" of Western transport and life on the road. Young men leave their communities to reside temporarily in a world of strangers, with no well-defined etiquette for the exchange of food, friendship, and mutual support and little moral basis for affirmation of "common substance." As the social geography of assault sorceries in Papua New Guinea indicates, these island and coastal communities were experiencing in the late nineteenth and early twentieth centuries the dislocations which only began to disturb highland communities during the last few decades.

In larger perspective, however, the increasing concern with sorcery in Papua New Guinea, especially the identification of assault sorcery as the most threatening visitation, suggests that Papua New Guineans are reaching a kind of intellectual and experiential turning point, as did Europeans during the "witch crazes" of the sixteenth and seventeenth centuries, and Africans in the nineteenth. Like other Papua New Guinea populations, the Fore are confronting new pathogens/insults, many of which we would classify as medical—kuru, syphilis, viral disorders, and perhaps an increase in liver disease. As the Fore *tokabu* category indicates, however, many of the new experiences are of another order. Assault sorcery accounts for mortality from conditions we consider to be varied and discrete: disease, rape, assassination, and accidents on the road and in the air. The image of assault fuses political, economic, biological, and existential ailments in a single diagnosis; it is a quick gauge of multiple disturbances. Moreover, this indigenous explanatory subset expands to account for a ballooning of sudden, unexpected, uncontrollable, and otherwise unnameable forms of dislocation and death. Just as the European witch craze settled upon demonic illnesses that were "strange," not easily accommodated within any regularly constituted nosology (Estes 1984), Fore *tokabu* killers inhabit a similar category of cognitive space.[4]

During the great antisorcery campaigns of the late 1950s and early 1960s, the Fore publicly tested their taxonomic categories. One recurrent theme, as noted above, concerned the locus of disease origin. Another was whether kuru (and sometimes other conditions) should be regarded as sorcery or as a form of "illness." This latter theme was often debated at length in light of recognition that Europeans did not share Fore theories of causation. By the end of the decade,[5] the Fore still retained their conviction that kuru was a form of sorcery and that *tokabu* killers were a major threat to the unwary.

THE CONTEXT OF CHANGING TAXONOMIES

The Fore tested their taxonomic categories during the 1950s and 1960s to accommodate the monumental expansion of knowledge and transformations of daily life. They had recently confronted a new political order in which they were at first subjects rather than autonomous actors. They adjusted to a new sense of themselves as "the Fore" (having previously had no concept of themselves as a single "people"), in contest now with neighboring and distant populations whose wealth, power, and skills differed from their own. The end of warfare during colonial times (during the early 1950s in the South Fore) altered the political relations within and between small residential groups, unsettled the hegemony of the senior male in local power arrangements, and "freed" young men to travel to distant parts for adventure and wage labor. Gender relations, too, were modified by a new legal system that protected wives from the harsh treatment of husbands,[6] and new cash crops added to the gardening labors of women. Taxes were imposed (in 1967), trade stores entered the area (from none in the Okapa Subdistrict in 1960, there were over twenty by 1971), and by 1971 newly planted coffee trees provided the area with a cash income of $400,000, an average of $30 to $40 per annum per adult male (Mathews 1971:63). During the same period, missions and then the government opened primary schools for Fore children.

The burgeoning of sorceries (projective and assault) occurs in this time of rapid metamorphosis of the known world. The paradigms that explain perceived experience are tested in the great sorcery debates and antisorcery campaigns, as well as in daily interaction. "Revision" of the taxonomic system was not, however, a novel process. The Fore, like other Papua New Guineans, had other explanations for disease and danger before a density of sorcerers came to occupy the landscape. Until recently, the Fore had considered the forest to be a location of some peril. It was a rule that one should not hunt or travel bush paths except in the company of others, and the failure to return from forest expeditions was proof that the travelers had been set upon by bush spirits. Yet these cultural precursors of the *tokabu* killers were ambiguously evil, less malicious than their human ancestors. Nokoti, the best-known bush spirit in the Wanitabe region, might cause the death of infants or illness among adults, but his characteristic mark was that of a trickster. During the 1940s, however, Nokoti's behavior is said to have begun to change. At that time he began stealing into people's houses to spirit away old time wealth—men's and women's skirts, shells, and *kinta*, a decorative black seed bead grown locally and exchanged among matri-kin. For a time the forests retained their strong image as the home of bush spirits, places of danger, and sources of medicinal power. But as forests were trimmed and depleted of wildlife, as men turned their energies from hunting and horticulture to coffee and cash, and as a foreign colonial power established towns and markets in new locations, the bush/power/sorcery metaphor lost much of its force. With the arrival of a government administrative post in the North Fore in 1954 and the construction of a jeep road into the South Fore during the next few years, Nokoti the trickster disappeared from sight and almost from consciousness. His last appearance, said to have been in the mid-1950s in the Wanitabe region, signals the end of an era. By then, a new political and economic order had provided a reoriented geography of danger and another meaning to the fearsome experience of being out of context.

The construction of the trunk road through the South Fore lands in the mid-1950s was a momentous event. Until that time, the Fore had traveled along bush and grassland paths cleared, owned, and sustained by small localities. The occasional journey beyond the home parish followed trails through the lands of current friends and allies. The construction of a public road in peacetime thus facilitated the new flow of traffic; it led also to a flood of ideas, information, novel cultigens, and diseases that precipitated a new set of attitudes and a new metaphysic.

The gradual passing of Nokoti and his world was a process of ecological transition that Fore had been negotiating apparently without great anxiety. The poignant stories told by old men of waning encounters with the spirit were backward glances at less paradoxical times. With Nokoti's demise, the Fore moved from the narrow horizons of subsistence horticulture, hunting, and parish "nationalism" to a colonial and postcolonial world of increased mobility, competition, a partly monetized economy, and an experience of new ways to die beyond the comforting support of community and kin. Moreover, the community now appeared to harbor the enemy within the gates.

By the 1970s, the Fore sorcery beliefs remained intact, perhaps strengthened by a decade of inquisition and self-reflection. An etiology that placed responsibility for death in the hands of Fore sorcerers was an assertion of Fore authority over their own affairs during an era of waning autonomy, particularly in face of an alternate paradigm proposed by foreign kuru investigators and a colonial administration. As indicated, however, Fore paradigms were not unchanging. During the 1950s and 1960s the projective sorcery count had risen even as the zones of safety contracted. Endocausation, once the mark of capricious spirits, now accounted for major afflictions which were the work of malevolent enemies, possibly located within the parish. The identification of close-range sorcery fears contributed to and also registered the disintegration of former kin communities.

The taxonomic shift whereby *tokabu* killers (not projective sorcerers) began to account for a larger burden of sudden illness and death provides evidence of an explanatory system increasingly distanced from a theory in which the Fore assert their own sense of control. *Tokabu* killers are the "unknowable." As killers for hire, they operate now at distances beyond the social epidemiology of political and personal contest. In contrast to the symptoms of projective sorcery which can be "read" (with some slippage) for their clinical and diagnostic social contents, *tokabu* is a grab-bag category rather than a uniquely perceived condition. The symptoms of the victims of *tokabu* are notably vague.[7] Beyond control or therapeutic intervention, *tokabu* killers appear more demonic, more superhuman, than detectable, enemy sorcerers. If the identification of projective sorcery shows the Fore analyzing changing social, political, and epidemiological conditions with some authority, the designation of *tokabu* deaths tells a less confident story.

FORE "MEDICINE" AND WESTERN "MEDICINE"

A comparison of some aspects of recent Fore intellectual history reveals that similar changes of metaphysics have occurred in our own systems of belief and currents of thought. Western beliefs reached a similar watershed in the sixteenth and seventeenth centuries, when the "new sciences" brought a body of knowledge, a method, an attitude of mind, and a metaphysic that became the directive force of Western civilization, displacing theology and antique letters (Van Baumer 1952: 249). The relevance of this shift in Western thought to the discussion of Fore notions of ultimate causation lies in the fact that the sixteenth and seventeenth century witch hunts (like Fore antisorcery campaigns) appear to have been instrumental in helping to formulate, publicize, and reframe the assumptions of an influential segment of the populations—the university-trained physicians, the church, and the investigators in the courts of law. Diseases with regular symptomatology were increasingly naturalized, even as the witch hunts were climbing to a peak. The classical ailments attributed to witches in the Middle Ages—impotence, madness and the incubus/nightmare complex—were regarded by sixteenth and seventeenth century physicians as forms of sickness stemming from natural causes. That is, in Europe after 1500 ailments that could be named unambiguously were no longer attributed to witchcraft; on the other hand, illnesses that were viewed as inconstant, variable, and irregular were judged to be "strange" and thus demonic (Estes 1984). Much as the changes in Fore society led to the demise of Nokoti, to an efflorescence of sorcerers and the rise of the *tokabu* killers, social changes in sixteenth and seventeenth century Europe led to the "evaporation" of medieval cognitive schemes and to the notion of witch-caused illness dissociated from earlier cosmological arrangements.

I am not suggesting here that the Fore are on the brink of abandoning current sorcery beliefs about the etiology of illness.[8] The theories of sixteenth and seventeenth century physicians, concerned with what was reducible under regular laws and categories, were similarly not in conflict with a belief in the power of witches. Instead of treating a devil-inspired illness, they would inform the secular and religious authorities (Estes 1984:18). The Fore are similarly engaged in refining and shaping the content and profile of their mental categories, heightened by a new historical sense of the sharp divide in life before and after the arrival of Europeans.

Just as the European physicians took a prominent place in defining what was treatable or nontreatable illness, Fore specialists have emerged to deal with certain newly named conditions. In the 1950s and 1960s a number of specialist-curers appeared.[9] Technicians of the new order, they received payment for their work (in cash, pigs, and consumer goods), treated and defined the cause of the ailment, and in some cases acquired a political prominence that would have been unavailable in the past. Somewhat like sixteenth and seventeenth century physicians who refused to treat demonic disease, the new curers focused on projective sorcery (kuru, in particular) and made no claim to holding power to counteract assault sorcery.

The rise of the specialist-curer was to some degree triggered by the high profile of physicians in the colonial administration and by the creation of a class of Fore trainees, "Dr. Boys," whose job it was to monitor the health and epidemiological status of the population. At the same time, in some places Fore abandoned or trimmed the divination tests that determined guilt for particular deaths. Various tests using the opossum as an oracle are no longer performed.[10] Missions have appealed to their followers to forego the custom,[11] the kin of the deceased now buy rice and canned meat rather than hunt for opossums in the forest, and the mortuary ceremonies in which divination occurred now take place before many sick and elderly people expire. That is, the explanatory schemes and behaviors associated with illness and death show signs of transferring the powers of investigation and therapy from social groups to individuals who are paid for service.

In their discussion of sorcery and witchcraft the Fore and seventeenth century Europeans tested and reevaluated their experimental procedures and assumptions and altered their conception of the sorts of entities the universe contained and those it did not (cf. Kuhn 1970). Conceptual shifts in both places proceeded by making marginal what was perceived as anomalous, strange, and untreatable. The ailments attributed to European witches, like those caused by *tokabu* assailants, are a public recognition of anomalies that cannot be assigned to existing theories of "reasonable" causation. Both the Fore and the European example illustrate also the importance of listening to the apparently innocent language of the victim. By chronicling the natives' as well as the observers' point of view, we learn something of paradigm shifts from within and some notion of what is really troubling the patient.

NOTES

1. In the early 1950s, Ronald Berndt and Charles Julius recorded seven and six types of sorcery respectively. My own records a decade later show sixteen kinds of sorcery (Lindenbaum 1979:74).

2. For early and late examples, see Spencer and Gillen (1899) and Reid (1983).

3. One *tokabu* victim taken to Okapa hospital in 1966 had bowel obstruction and died shortly after operation (Mathews 1971:45).

4. Nicolas Remy, a famous judge and demonologist from Lorraine, described the case of Bernard Bloquat, who fell from his cart and was killed, "yet no part of his body was injured, there was no wound or bruise or swelling, no limb was dislocated or twisted, nor was there any lesion in any part" (quoted in Estes 1984:22). The similarities with *tokabu* diagnosis are apparent.

5. And to the present (Robert Klitzman, personal communication).

6. Fore began to acknowledge that their attention was deflected from the care of sisters to the care of wives.

7. Witchcraft "illnesses" in the sixteenth and seventeenth centuries are also diverse and vague. The symptoms were not only diverse, but the illnesses were rarely named. Indeed, it was a mark of a witch-caused ailment that it could not be named (see Estes 1984:10, 50).

8. Several hundred years would pass in the western world before the theoretical discussion of contagion would lead to an acceptance of the germ theory of disease.

9. Robert Klitzman interviewed a contemporary curer on the North Fore borderlands in 1984 (personal communication). The trend thus continues.

10. A guilty person is thought to become ill, for example, after eating the opossum meat distributed at the mortuary gathering for the deceased person.

11. Many seventeenth century churchmen were also opposed to the divination tests of peasants (cf. Estes 1984:41).

REFERENCES

Berndt, R. M. 1958. A "devastating disease syndrome": Kuru sorcery in the Eastern Highlands of New Guinea. *Sociologus* 8:4.

Codrington, R. H. 1891. *The Melanesians.* Oxford: Clarendon Press of Oxford University Press.

Estes, L. L. 1984. The structure of medicine in early modern Europe and the rise of the witch-craze. Paper given at American Anthropological Association meeting, Denver, Colorado.

Glick, Leonard B. 1972. Sangguma. In *Encyclopedia of Papua and New Guinea.* vol. 2. P. Ryan, ed. Melbourne: Melbourne University Press.

Hogbin, H. I. 1970. *The Island of Menstruating Men: Religion in Wogeo, New Guinea.* Scranton: Chandler.

Johannes, A., and D. Keil. 1974. Fighting with illness: Sorcery in the Eastern Highlands of New Guinea. Paper prepared for American Anthropological Association meeting, Mexico City.

Kuhn, Thomas S. 1970. *The Structure of Scientific Revolutions.* Chicago: University of Chicago Press.

Lederman, R. 1981. Sorcery and social change in Mendi. In *Sorcery and Social Change in Melanesia.* M. Zelenietz and S. Lindenbaum, eds. *Social Analysis* 8.

Lindenbaum, S. 1981. Images of the sorcerer in Papua New Guinea. In *Sorcery and Social Change in Melanesia.* M. Zelenietz and S. Lindenbaum, eds. *Social Analysis* 8.

————. 1979. *Kuru Sorcery. Disease and Danger in the New Guinea Highlands.* Palo Alto: Mayfield.

Mathews, J. D. 1971. Kuru: A puzzle in culture and environmental medicine. Ph.D. diss., University of Melbourne.

Reid, J. 1983. *Sorcery and Healing Spirits: Continuity and Change in an Aboriginal Medical System.* Canberra: Australian National University Press.

Spencer, Sir W. B., and F. J. Gillen. 1899. *The Native Tribes of Central Australia.* London: MacMillan

Tonkinson, R. 1981. Sorcery and social change in southeast Ambrym, Vanautu. In *Sorcery and Social Change in Melanesia.* M. Zelenietz and S. Lindenbaum, eds. *Social Analysis* 8.

Van Baumer, Franklin Le. 1952. *Main Currents of Western Thought.* New York: Alfred A. Knopf.

Westermark, G. D. 1981. Society and economic change in Agarabi. In *Sorcery and Social Change in Melanesia.* M. Zelenietz and S. Lindenbaum, eds. *Social Analysis* 8.

Zelenietz, M. 1981. One step too far: Sorcery and social change in Kilenge, West New Britain. In *Sorcery and Social Change in Melanesia.* M. Zelenietz and S. Lindenbaum, eds. *Social Analysis* 8.

17 CHANGING PATTERNS OF DISEASE IN INDIA WITH SPECIAL REFERENCE TO CHILDHOOD MORTALITY

Kailash C. Malhotra

The purpose of this chapter is threefold: (1) to provide an overview of the changing pattern of health and disease in India from the beginning of the twentieth century to the present time; (2) to identify major causes — socio-economic, cultural, environmental — that have been responsible for the disappearance/reduction/increase in select major diseases in the country; and (3) to highlight problems and strategies that need to be adopted in the future.

At the outset, it may be pointed out that about 40 percent of the Indian population consists of children below fifteen years; and 35 percent of these are below four years and account for nearly 35 percent of all the deaths. It is, therefore, appropriate that due emphasis be given to the health status of infants and children.

SOURCES AND QUALITY OF DATA

The data used in this chapter have been drawn from various sources such as decennial government census reports, Sample Registration Surveys (SRS), and health statistics reports.

Unfortunately the health statistics for India suffer from various shortcomings, and one of the most deficient aspects of mortality statistics relates to cause-of-death data (Bose, Gupta, and Premi 1982).

DEMOGRAPHIC PROFILE 1901–1981

Table 17.1 and Figures 17.1 and 17.2 present demographic characteristics of the population of India during the period 1901–1981. At the beginning of this century the population of India was about 240 million; in 1981 it was around 700 million. Thus, in eight decades the population nearly tripled. The history of Indian population growth can broadly be divided in two parts, with a separation date of 1921. From 1901 to 1921 the total growth was about 5 percent, with the net addition of 13 million people. However, during the last six decades (1921–1981) the population shows an alarming increase – a new addition of 433 million. In other words, the decennial variation in 1901 was 5.75, and in 1981 it was 24.78. The average density of population has also shown alarming increase, from 77 per square kilometer in 1901 to 220 in 1981.

The crude birth rate has shown progressive decline all along since 1901: in 1901 it was 48.8; in 1951, 1961, 1971, and 1981 it was 39.9, 40.0, 36.9, and 33.3, respectively. The death rate also shows steady decline, from 44.4 in 1901 to 27.4 in 1951, to 22.8 in 1961, to 12.4 in 1981. The life expectancy at birth has shown substantial increase, from 23.6 years in 1901 to 32.5 in 1951, to 41.9 in 1961, and 52.6 in 1981.

The literacy rates have shown a steady increase all along; from 5.35 percent in 1901 it reached 16.67 percent in 1951 and 36.17 percent in 1981. Another interesting aspect of literacy is the substantial increase in the female literacy rates; in 1901 it was barely 0.6 percent, in 1961 it was 12.9 percent, and in 1981 it was 24.9 percent.

Table 17.1
Crude Birth, Death, Life Expectancy, and Literacy Rates in India, 1901–1981.

Year	Crude Birth Rate	Crude Death Rate	Life Expectancy at Birth		Literacy Rates (%)
			Male	*Female*	
1901	48.8	44.4	23.6	24.0	5.35
1911	48.1	42.6	22.6	23.3	5.92
1921	49.2	48.6	19.4	20.9	7.16
1931	46.4	36.3	26.9	26.6	9.50
1941	45.2	31.2	32.1	31.4	16.10
1951	39.9	27.4	32.5	31.7	16.67
1961	40.0	22.8	41.9	40.6	24.02
1971	36.9	XX	XX	XX	29.45
1981	33.3	12.4	52.6	51.6	36.17

Key: XX = missing data

Sources: Misra (1970); Saxena (1971); Government of India (1982).

Figure 17.1
Growth of the Indian Population, 1901–1981

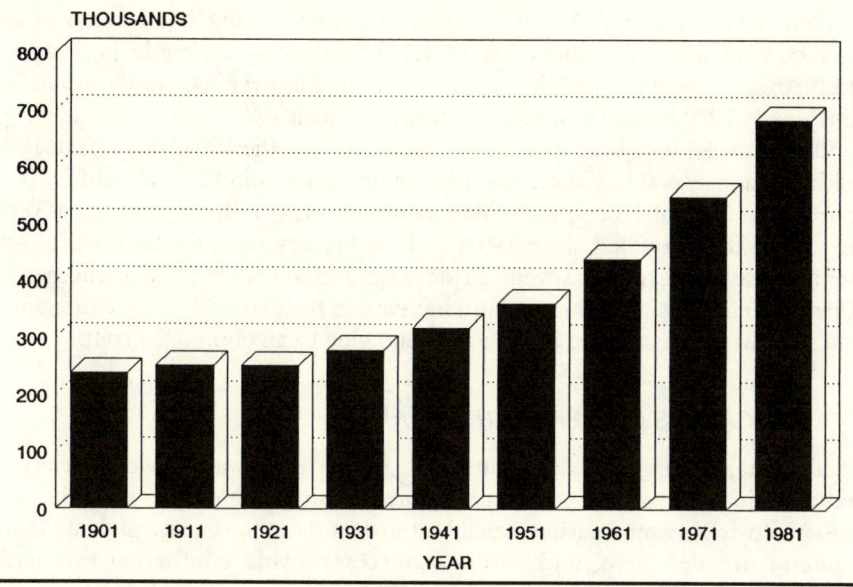

Figure 17.2
Population Density of the Indian Population, 1901–1981.

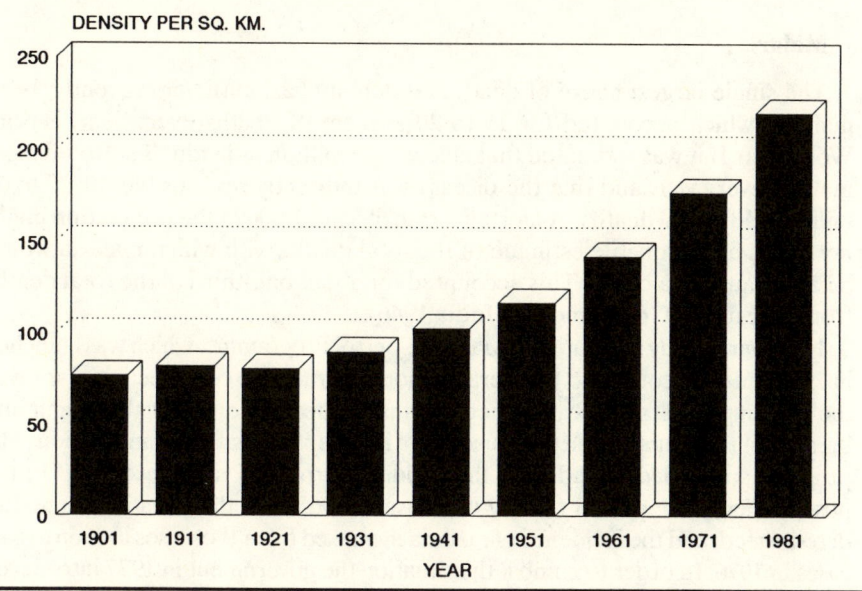

Sources (Both Figures): Registrar General of India (1983); Saxena (1971).

Although a more detailed treatment of infant and child mortality will be presented below, it is appropriate to mention here a few salient features. It is evident from Figure 17.3 that considerable progress has been made in the reduction of infant mortality rates (IMR) in the country during the period 1911 to 1980; at the beginning of the century the IMR was over 200 per thousand live births — by 1980 it had been reduced to 114 (Ghosh 1985).

It is thus evident from the above data that: (1) the birth rates have been reduced considerably since 1901; (2) the death rates in general, and IMR in particular, have also been contained substantially; (3) life expectancy at birth has more than doubled since 1901; and (4) literacy rates for both males and females have registered a sevenfold increase. Among other consequences of all these changes has been a mammoth increase in the country's population and a substantial increase in the population belonging to an older age group.

MAJOR CAUSES OF DEATH IN INDIA

The major cause of death in India in the past was a wide variety of communicable diseases such as plague, smallpox, cholera, malaria, and tuberculosis. As noted earlier, reliable statistics about the causes of death in the country are defective, and various sources provide conflicting estimates. Although it is thus impossible to ascertain the actual number of deaths caused by a particular disease, nevertheless we can appreciate the relative importance of these diseases in causing deaths.

Malaria

The single largest cause of death and debility has, until very recently, been malaria, which accounted for 15 to 20 percent of deaths every year. Before World War II it was estimated that at least 100 million individuals suffered from malaria every year and that the disease was indirectly responsible for 25 to 65 million additional deaths. A mortality rate of 8 per 1,000 of the population might not be an unreasonable estimate of the total deaths with which malaria would be associated as a cause. This accounted for about one-third of the total deaths from all causes (Government of India 1946).

However, during the National Malaria Control Programme, which was launched in 1953 and later converted to an eradication program in 1958, insecticidal spray in the dwelling houses and cattle sheds was introduced throughout the length and breadth of the country with the objective of interrupting malaria transmission. The program succeeded in reducing the incidence from 7.5 cases per 1,000 in the postindependence period to only one case in 1965. But the situation thereafter deteriorated, and the incidence of malaria increased from 1.48 cases in 1966 to 64.7 cases in 1976. In order to combat the situation the government in 1977 introduced a revised plan of operation. This program has slightly contained the incidence; in 1981 there were only 2.5 cases.

It appears that, among others, one major cause for the emergence of malaria has been the increased canal irrigation which leads to water clogging and thus provides good opportunities for mosquitoes to breed.

Smallpox

Smallpox was another major killer, and its incidence in India was the highest among all the countries of the world. However, due to sustained efforts such as the National Smallpox Eradication Campaign, started as late as 1962, the incidence of this dreaded disease was brought down to zero in July 1975. The country was declared to have eradicated smallpox by the International Assessment Commission on 23 April 1977. The decline of smallpox has occurred in three phases in the current century:

1. 1900–1920. Death rate varied from 0.19 to 0.80, with mean annual death rate of 0.37 per 1,000 population.
2. 1921–1946. Death rate varied from 0.09 to 0.70, with mean annual rate of 0.29 per 1,000 population.
3. 1947–1967. Death rate varied from 0.02 to 0.44, with mean annual death rate of 0.15 per 1,000 population.

Cholera

Cholera also took a heavy toll of Indian lives until recently. In 1900 it killed 805,698 persons; in 1906, 682,649; and in 1919 it took 556,533 lives. As late as 1943 it killed 459,930 persons; in 1957, 46,442 persons; in 1961, 26,947 persons; and in 1962, 11,404 persons. However, since 1966 the deaths caused by cholera have shown progressive decline; in 1966 it killed 2,788 persons and in 1983 only 309.

Plague

Until very recently, the plague was one of the major killers in the country. From 1898 to 1908 it killed 548,427 persons. Since then there has been a steady decline; the deaths due to this disease totaled 166 during 1961–1962, and in 1966 only eight deaths.

Dysentery and Diarrhea

The diseases grouped under this heading occupy the third place of importance among the diseases of India, the first being fevers and the second, respiratory diseases. It is estimated that at least 5 percent of the total deaths in India result from gastrointestinal diseases.

The other major diseases in the country are tuberculosis, leprosy, filariasis, and poliomyelitis. It is thus seen that India has been able to contain to a very

Figure 17.3
Infant Mortality Rates in India, 1911–1980.

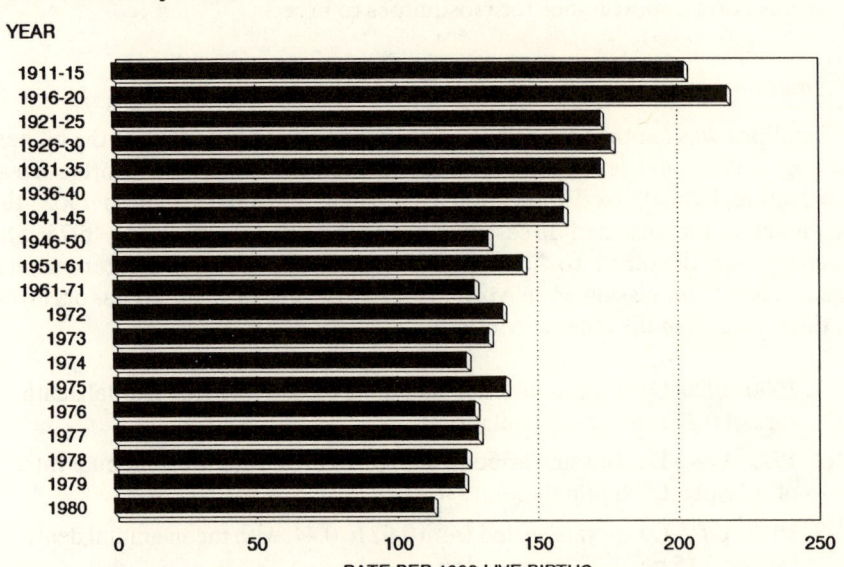

YEAR

RATE PER 1000 LIVE BIRTHS

Sources: The rates for 1911–1945 are from Davis (1951);1946–1950 from Chandrashekhar (1959); 1951–1971 from the Indian Census; 1970–1977 from Sample Registraion Survey; and 1978 from the Registrar General of India (1983).

large extent several of the major diseases, especially communicable diseases, during the current century. It may, however, be emphasized that although deaths due to various communicable diseases have been drastically reduced, the morbidity caused by these diseases is still alarming.

Some other diseases have shown dramatic rise in the country. For example, in 1955 sporadic cases of Japanese encephalitis were first detected in southern India. By 1973 it had spread to several districts in West Bengal, and by 1978 it was reported not only from Karnataka, Tamilnadu, Bihar, West Bengal, and Uttar Pradesh, but also from Assam, Pondicherry, and Boa. Similarly, dengue, a viral fever spread by the white-striped mosquito *Aedes aegypti*, found mainly in urban and semiurban areas and breeding in clear water sources, has assumed alarming proportions. The first known outbreak occurred in Calcutta in 1963.

Since then numerous epidemics have been reported from several towns in the country: Delhi, Hardoi, Kanpur, Asansol, Calcutta, Gwalior, Saugar, Jabalpur, Jaipur, Pune, and Surat among others. It is clear now that dengue is the result of improper urban planning, inadequate control over construction activity which blocks drainage and creates puddles, inadequate drinking water supply which forces people to store water, overhead water tanks which are seldom cleaned, discarded cans and plastic bags in which water can collect, and a lack of public hygiene and health education. A survey in Delhi carried out by the Medical Research Council in November 1982 showed that overhead tanks were major sources for the breeding of the dengue mosquito throughout urban Delhi, including rich and middle-class colonies (Argarwal and Narain 1985).

INFANT AND CHILD MORTALITY

Until recently, only estimates of mortality were available. In 1979, the Registrar General of India undertook a nationwide sample survey to provide mortality rates and their differentials (Registrar General of India 1983). The materials presented in this section have been primarily drawn from this source.

DEMOGRAPHIC AND SOCIAL CHARACTERISTICS

About 40 percent of the rural and 36 percent of urban population is below fifteen years of age. Thus, two out of five persons in India are below fifteen years. The proportion of population below fifteen years is more in the rural areas than in the urban areas; this is true for both sexes. A comparison of figures between 1951 and 1978 shows a declining trend in the proportion of children below fifteen years in both rural and urban areas; in 1971 there were 41.9 percent males and 42.2 percent females compared to 38.8 percent for males and 38.4 percent for females in 1978.

The percent distribution of children below fifteen years by quinquennial age groups shows that 35 percent of the children below fifteen years belong to the age group 0–4 years. One-third of the total children are in each of the age groups 5–9 and 10–14 years. The sex ratio of children below fifteen years shows that there is a preponderance of males (rural 1,085; urban 1,055). There is an appreciable increase in the literacy rate both for males and females. Among male children 41.65 percent are literate against 28 percent in 1971; among female children the rate is 29.4 percent against 17.8 percent in 1971. The rural-urban differentials are also noteworthy. In rural areas, literacy among female children is lagging behind.

LEVEL OF INFANT MORTALITY

The level of infant mortality is often considered as an index of health conditions and level of living of a society. The trend in the level of infant mortality from the turn of the century is given in Figure 17.3. It is evident that the infant mortality that was prevailing at the beginning of the century was over 200 per 1,000 live births, which was frightfully high. The country has marched progressively in reducing this rate to 114 by 1980.

As expected, infant mortality in rural areas is higher than that in urban areas, where health facilities are more readily available. It is noteworthy that until 1970 infant mortality rates in both rural and urban areas decreased overall. However,

Figure 17.4
Rural-Urban Comparisons in Infant Mortality in India, 1970–1978.

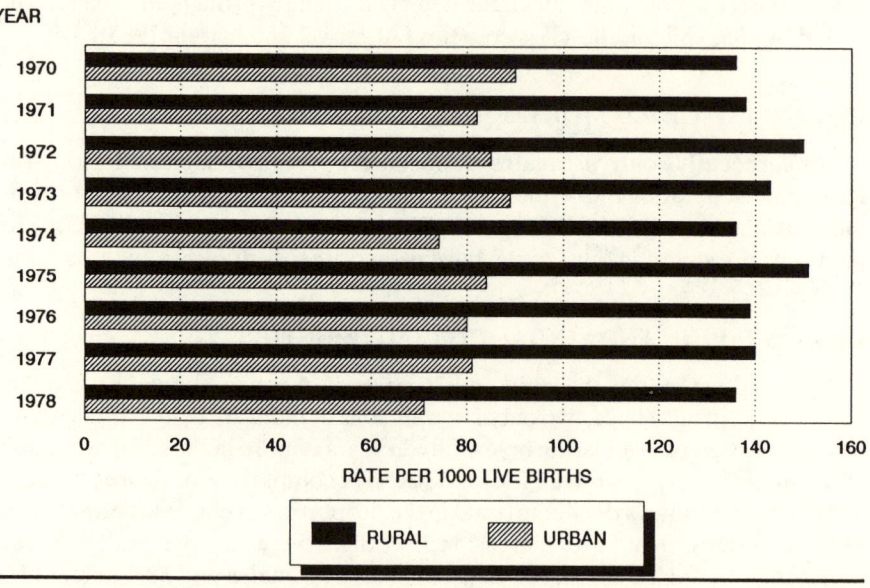

YEAR

RATE PER 1000 LIVE BIRTHS

RURAL   URBAN

from 1970 to 1978 urban infant mortality declined by about 20 percent while the rural rate actually increased for several years during the same period. (Figure 17.4).

Infant mortality by sex is a key factor indicating the social customs and prenatal care given to infants of each sex. It is seen that mortality among female infants is more than that among male infants, especially in rural areas (Table 17.2). In the case of urban areas, the sex differential is not significant.

It is often useful to consider infant mortality in two components, neonatal mortality and postnatal mortality. The former relates to deaths within the first four weeks after birth. In rural areas the neonatal mortality exceeds the postnatal mortality by nearly double (Table 17.3). The absence of proper medical care for expectant mothers, especially in the antenatal period, and the inadequate maternal and child care in the rural areas might be major contributory factors for this high neonatal mortality.

India is a vast country; its regions differ in ecosystems, cultural practices, level of economic growth, and literacy. It would, therefore, be of interest to see the magnitude of variation depicted by major states in India. Such data were readily available for 1972 and 1978, and the same are set out in Table 17.4. Several aspects are apparent from this table:

1. The interstate variability is enormous; it ranges from 39 in Kerala to 167 in Uttar Pradesh, the Indian average being 126.

Table 17.2
Infant Mortality by Sex per 1,000 Live Births in India, 1972–1978.

Year	Rural			Urban			Total		
	M	F	Total	M	F	Total	M	F	Total
1972	141	161	150	85	85	85	132	148	139
1973	141	144	143	88	90	89	132	135	134
1976	133	146	139	78	82	80	124	134	129
1977	136	146	140	80	82	81	126	135	130
1978	130	143	136	71	71	71	120	131	126

Source: Registrar General of India (1983).

Table 17.3
Neonatal and Postnatal Mortality Rates in India, 1970–1978.

Year	Rural			Urban		
	Neonatal	Postnatal	Infant Mortality	Neonatal	Postnatal	Infant Mortality
1970	72	64	136	46	44	90
1971	81	57	138	45	37	82
1973	77	73	150	45	40	85
1976	83	56	139	49	31	80
1977	88	52	140	42	39	81
1978	80	56	136	41	30	71

Source: Registrar General of India (1983).

Table 17.4
Infant Mortality Rates for Major Indian States, 1972, 1978.

State	Rural		Urban		Total	
	1972	*1978*	*1972*	*1978*	*1972*	*1978*
Andhra Pradesh	128	120	65	62	116	112
Assam	140	120	95	86	136	118
Bihar	—	98	—	44	—	—
Gujarat	139	127	94	88	128	118
Hariyana	98	116	72	59	94	109
Himachal Pradesh	120	99	38	52	116	97
Jammu & Kashmir	76	76	43	28	71	70
Karnataka	102	81	68	55	95	75
Kerala	66	42	43	26	63	39
Madhya Pradesh	165	141	102	86	156	135
Maharashtra	114	84	70	56	101	75
North Eastern Region	115	85	83	48	114	84
Orissa	136	137	73	80	131	133
Punjab	129	111	78	65	119	103
Rajasthan	132	139	76	65	123	129
Tamil Nadu	133	120	85	63	121	103
Uttar Pradesh	213	172	120	110	202	167
West Bengal	—	79	—	75	—	—
All India	150	136	85	71	139	126

Source: Registrar General of India (1983).

2. Infant mortality in the rural areas in all the states exceeds that in the urban areas.

3. The states of Madhya Pradesh, Orissa, Rajasthan, and Uttar Pradesh form one belt where infant mortality is above the national average.

4. Between 1972 and 1978 there has been appreciable reduction in the level of mortality in the states of Assam, Kerala, Madhya Pradesh, Maharashtra, and Uttar Pradesh.

The age-specific death rates in the age group 0–4 are a key indicator of general mortality (Figures 17.5, 17.6, 17.7). The child mortality among females is more (55.1 percent) than among males (51.7 percent). Child mortality in rural areas is higher than that in urban areas. Again, different states reveal different mortality data. The lowest, as expected, are observed in Kerala and in the northeastern region, and the highest are noted in Assam, Rajasthan, and Uttar Pradesh.

INFANT MORTALITY DIFFERENTIALS

The relationship between some socioeconomic variables and infant mortality rates is shown in Table 17.5. The literacy level of women appears to have a strong influence on the infant mortality rates; among the rural illiterates the rate was 145 while among women with education the rate was only 71.

The infant mortality rate is higher (150) among women engaged in production than among women working in agriculture (143). Again, among working women the rate is higher (142) than for non-working women (134); this is true in both rural and urban areas.

The age of women at marriage seems to have a profound influence on the infant mortality rates. In rural areas, for women married at or below eighteen years, the mortality is 159 as against 90 recorded for women married at the age of twenty-one years and above; the same pattern is observed in urban areas also.

The source of drinking water is an important variable which influences infant mortality (Figure 17.8). In rural areas infant mortality is lowest among that section of the population that uses tap water as the main source of drinking water. In comparsion, infant mortality is very high among that section of population using wells as their main source of drinking water. In urban areas also (among the population using well/pond/tank/river as the main source of drinking water), infant mortality is very high.

It is also observed that the easy accessibility of social amenities is an index of the development of the area and is reflected in the level of infant mortality. With the availability of facilities such as motorable roads, bus stands, railway stations, schools, and medical care, the infant mortality gets reduced substantially.

BIRTHWEIGHT

Birthweight to a great extent reflects the level of maternal nutrition. Dietary surveys in low economic groups have shown a daily deficit of 500–600 calories in women and 1,000–1,100 calories in pregnant and lactating mothers (ICMR 1974, 1981). This maternal malnutrition leads to low birthweight babies. The average birthweight of newborns in the lower socioeconomic groups is 2.7 kg

Figure 17.5
Age Specific Death Rates for Rural Children 0–4 Years, 1970–1978.

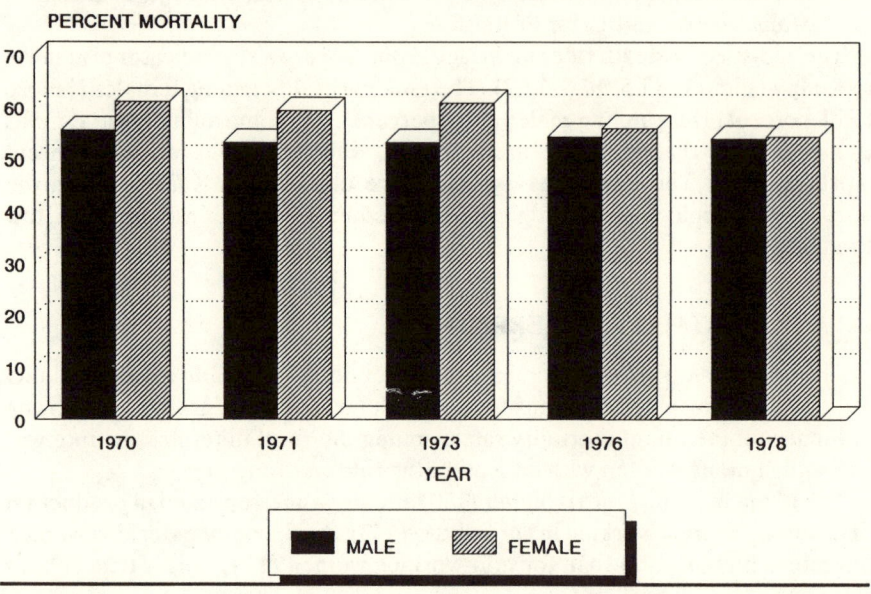

Figure 17.6
Age Specific Death Rates for Urban Children 0–4 Years, 1970–1978.

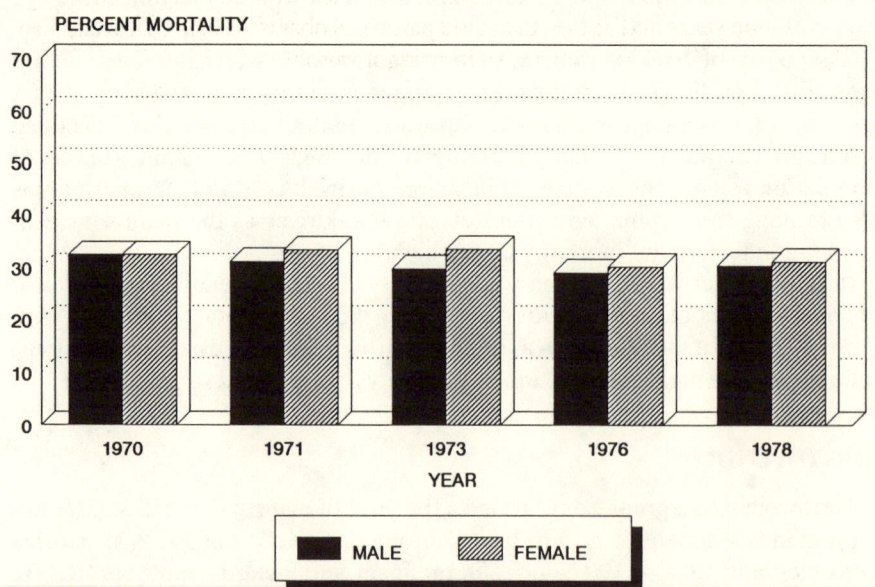

Source (Both Figures): Registrar General of India (1983).

Figure 17.7
Age Specific Death Rates for Indian Children 0–4 Years, 1970–1978.

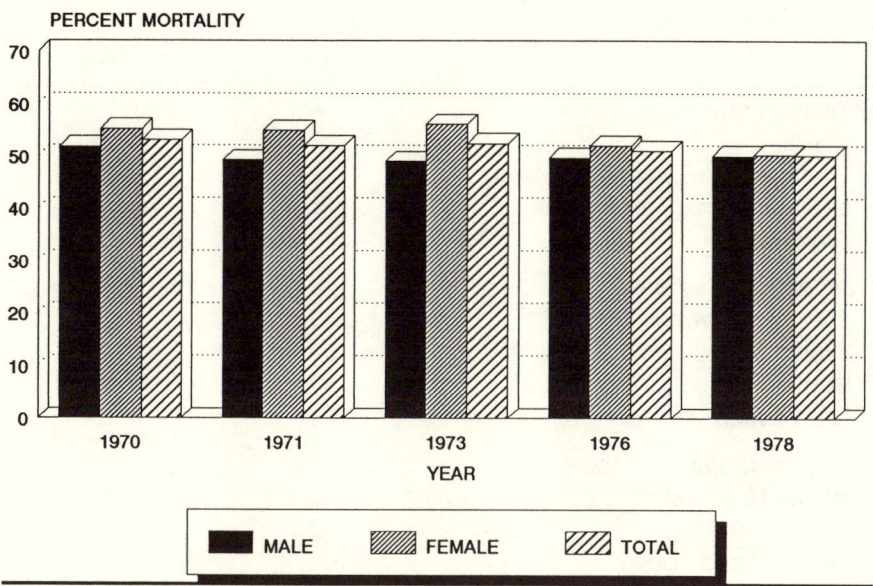

Source: Registrar General of India (1983).

compared to 3.1 kg in higher socioeconomic groups (Ghosh 1977). Chai (1980) reports that 30–40 percent of babies are born with low birthweights. In a survey it was found that about three-fourths (71.8 percent) of the total deaths in the perinatal period were directly or indirectly due to low birthweight. It has also been shown that the mortality rate among infants of 1,000 gms or less birthweight was 85–96 percent; between 1,000 and 1,500 gms, 50–53 percent; between 1,501 and 2,000 gms, 8–31 percent; and between 2,001–2,500 gms as 2.6–20 percent (Sharma 1984).

MAJOR CAUSES OF INFANT AND CHILD MORTALITY IN INDIA

Infant deaths within the first week are caused mostly by maternal and delivery related factors, such as extremes of age, multiparity at short birth intervals, malnutrition, and hard physical work. All these tend to result in a low birthweight baby whose chances of dying are 3 to 4 times that of normal weight babies. Most of the deliveries take place at home, under unhygienic conditions and assisted by untrained persons, resulting in a high death rate due to problems of delivery and subsequent infections, the most prominent among them being neonatal tetanus. Neonatal tetanus, which can be easily prevented by

Table 17.5
Infant Mortality Differentials for India, 1978.

Differentials	Mortality	
	Rural	*Urban*
Education of women		
Illiterat	145	88
Literate, below primary	101	57
Literate, primary and above	71	47
All literates	90	50
Occupation of women		
Farmer, fishermen	143	106
Production and related works	150	129
Workers	142	98
Nonworkers	134	64
Age at marriage of women		
Below 18 years	156	88
18–20 years	132	67
21 years and above	90	46
Source of drinking water		
Tap	112	66
Hand pump	121	81
Well	143	84
Pond/Tank/River	115	106

Source: Registrar General of India (1983).

immunizing pregnant mothers, accounts for 6–10 percent of total infant deaths. This is due to using unclean instruments for cutting the umbilical cord and use of contaminated dressings like ash or cow dung. It may be noted here that in some Indian states deaths due to neonatal tetanus assume alarming proportion; for example, 60 percent of the infant deaths in Uttar Pradesh are due to this single cause.

The main causes of child deaths are tetanus, diarrheal diseases, and respiratory infections. Diarrhea is a major killer, causing 4–5 percent of the deaths in the first year and 30 percent in the age group 1–4 years. It is estimated that children under five years suffer 45,000,000 episodes of diarrhea per year — 1.5 million children under five years die of the disease each year, about 80 percent dying due to dehydration (ICMR 1979; Ghosh 1985). This leads to the startling realization that about 2,500 children die every day due to dehydration from diarrhea.

Figure 17.8
Infant Mortality in Rural Areas of India by Availability of Social Amenities, 1978.

SOCIAL AMENITIES

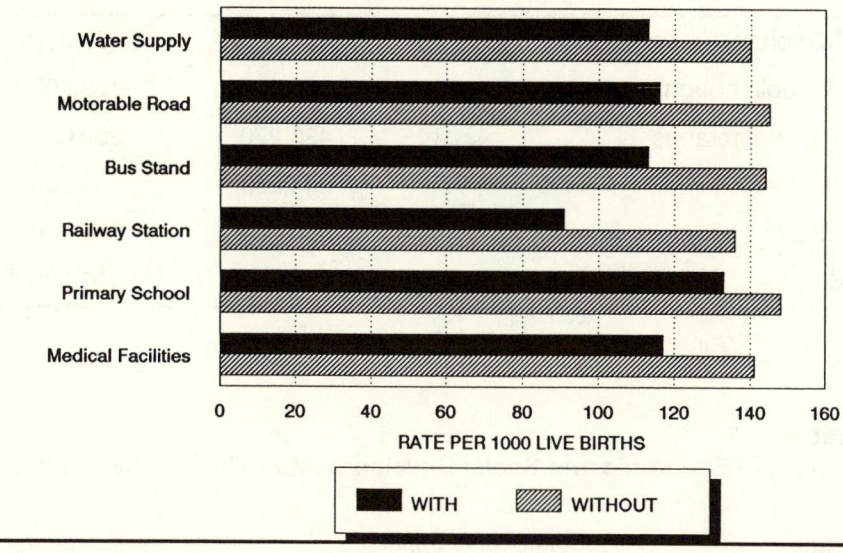

Source: Registrar General of India (1983).

Pneumonia and other respiratory infections also contribute significantly to death in infancy and preschool years, accounting for 25–30 percent of deaths.

Some of the other major diseases contributing to infant and childhood mortality are measles, tuberculosis, whooping cough, and polio (Registrar General of India 1983). It is thus evident that a great deal of mortality and morbidity among the infants and children is preventable by immunization. Data presented in Table 17.6 suggest the magnitude of the problem.

DISCUSSION

From these data the following main points emerge, which need further elaboration.

1. The demographic profile of the people of India has undergone considerable changes since the beginning of this century. The notable changes that have occurred are in curtailing crude birth and death rates and enhancing life expectancy at birth. Literacy levels have also gone up sharply. The fertility rates, however, have declined only marginally. The consequence of all these has been a mammoth increase in the popula-

Table 17.6
Annual Mortality and Morbidity of the Illnesses Preventable by Immunization.

Diseases	Morbidity	Mortality
Pulmonary tuberculosis	4,000,000	400,000
Whoopin cough	3,000,000	150,000
Neonatal tetanus	423,270	250,000
Diphtheria	245,250	5,000
Polio	200,000	2,000
Measles	16,000,000	200,000

Table 17.7
Levels of Economic and Social Development in Three Indian States.

State	Economic Development (% of population below poverty line)	Social Development	
		Literacy (%)	Female Literacy (%)
Kerala	47.0	69.2	64.5
Punjab	15.1	47.7	34.1
Uttar Pradesh	50.1	27.4	14.4

Table 17.8
Birth and Death Rates in Three Indian States.

State	Birth Rate	Death Rate	Infant Mortality	Child Mortality, 1–4 Years
Kerala	26.0	7.2	42	9
Punjab	30.3	9.4	117	12
Uttar Pradesh	39.6	16.3	157	23

Source (Tables 17.6–17.8): Ghosh (1985).

tion and a substantial increase in the population belonging to older age groups. The implications in terms of health of the people are that the country has to invest huge resources in providing health care to this population of 700 million people. It is thus imperative that immediate steps be initiated to reduce fertility rates. The government proposes to reduce the growth rate of 2.24 (1971–1981) to 1.0 by 2000 A.D.

2. The country has also succeeded in reducing infant mortality substantially, but the prevailing rate (114/1,000 live births) also is still very high. Maternal mortality (4.8/1,000 live births) is still very high. It is noteworthy that infant mortality, especially in rural areas, has declined very little since 1970. The major causes of deaths among infants continue to be diarrhea, tetanus, and respiratory infections. All of these are largely preventable by immunization.

There is a general feeling that the infant mortality rate can only be further reduced provided there is economic growth. However, the data available from China, Sri Lanka, and Kerala in our own country strongly suggest that infant mortality of around 50 per 1,000 can also be achieved in low-income nations (for a detailed discussion, see Nag 1983, 1984).

It would be in order, therefore, to examine the Kerala situation in the context of a few select states in India. The two dimensions of development are economic and social. The percentage of population below the poverty line may be considered as a good indicator of economic status, and the level of literacy may be considered as an indicator of social progress (Ghosh 1985). Tables 17.7 and 17.8 give relevant details for three Indian states—Kerala, Punjab, and Uttar Pradesh. Kerala is characterized by high social development and poor economic development, while Punjab exhibits high economic and poor social development. Uttar Pradesh lags behind in both indicators. It is thus evident that rapid social development, even where economic development is low, can improve the health status of the people. Data presented in Table 17.5 and described earlier also support such a contention.

3. The incidence of some communicable and vector-borne diseases, such as malaria, plague, cholera, and polio, has been contained significantly; smallpox has been eradicated. The incidence, however, of others, especially malaria, is still very high. It is true that not many people now die due to these diseases, but still a large number of them are afflicted by them. These diseases thus add enormously to the overall morbidity rates. For example, in 1982 over two million persons were afflicted by malaria in the country (Rural Health Division, Government of India 1983).

4. While several of the old communicable diseases have been contained, the country faces dangers from new communicable diseases such as encephalitis and dengue. The emergence of these diseases has been

shown to be directly related to faulty construction of the irrigation canals and unplanned rapid urbanization.

5. Rapid industrialization with inadequate measures of pollution control and the unsafe disposal of industrial effluents have caused serious occupational health hazards. This includes hazards from silicosis, asbestosis, byssinosis, and pneumoconiosis; in addition, leakage of gases from several chemical industries poses health hazards.

PROBLEMS OF TRANSITION

India is rapidly changing from an agrarian to an industrialized society. At this juncture of transition, the country faces twin problems in providing better health to its people. On the one hand, the menace of old communicable diseases like malaria continues and the threat from newly acquired communicable diseases like encephalitis and dengue is ever mounting. On the other hand, the nation has to divert substantial resources and manpower to combat the so-called diseases of developed countries — cancer, hypertension, diabetes, and coronary disorders, as well as the health hazards caused by industrial facilities.

It may be noted that India is a signatory to the Alma Ata Declaration and has also signed the South East Asian Health charter with the World Health Organization (WHO) for achieving the goal of health for all by 2000 A.D. Consequently, the government has made the decision to promote community-based development and deliver health, nutrition, and family welfare services through the primary health care system. It has also been decided that a set of complementary strategies will be implemented. These include education concerning prevailing health problems and the methods of identifying, preventing, and controlling them; promotion of food supply and proper nutrition, an adequate supply of safe water, and basic sanitation; maternal and child immunization against major infectious diseases; prevention and control of locally endemic diseases; promotion of mental health; and provision of essential drugs (Government of India, Ministry of Health and Family Welfare, 1981, 1982a).

REFERENCES

Agarwal, A., R. Chopra, and K. Sharma. 1982. *State of India's Environment, 1982: A Citizen's Report.* New Delhi: Center for Science and Environment.

Agarwal, A., and S. Narain. 1985. *State of India's Environment, 1984–85: A Second Citizen's Report.* New Delhi: Center for Science and Environment.

Bose, A., D. B. Gupta, and M. K. Premi. 1982. *Social Statistics: Health and Education.* New Delhi: Vikas.

Chai, O. P. 1980. Causes of infant and early childhood deaths and measures of reduction. Paper presented at the WHO Workshop for MCH Officers at State Level. New Delhi: National Institute of Health and Family Welfare.

Chandrashekar, S. 1959. *Infant Mortality in India, 1901–55.* London: Allen & Unwin.

Davis, K. 1951. *The Population of India and Pakistan.* Princeton: Princeton University Press.

Ghosh, S. 1985. Dimensions of morbidity and mortality among children. Paper presented at Workshop on Genetic Epidemiological Approaches to Health Care. New Delhi: National Institute of Health and Family Welfare.

———. 1977. *The Feeding and Care of Infants and Young Children.* New Delhi: Voluntary Health Association of India.

Government of India. 1983. *Annual Report 1982–83.* New Delhi: Ministry of Health and Family Welfare, Nirman Bhawan.

———. 1982a. *Statement on National Health Policy.* New Delhi: Ministry of Health and Family Wefare.

———. 1982b. *India 1982.* New Delhi: Publication Division, Ministry of Information and Broadcasting.

———. 1981. *Health For All by 2000 A.D.* New Delhi: Ministry of Health and Family Welfare. Report of the Working Group.

———. 1946. *What Malaria Costs India.* J. A. Sinton (1935). New Delhi: Health Survey and Development Committee. Report.

Indian Council of Medical Research (ICMR). 1981. *Recommended Dietary Intake for Indians.* New Delhi: Indian Council of Medical Research.

———. 1979. *Diarrheal Diseases in Infants and Children.* New Delhi: Indian Council of Medical Research.

———. 1974. Bulletin 4(6).

Misra, R. P. 1970. *Medical Geography of India.* New Delhi: National Book Trust.

Nag, M. 1984. Fertility differentials in Kerala and West Bengal: Equity-fertility hypothesis as an explanation. *Economic and Political Weekly* 19:33–41.

———. 1983. Impact of social and economic development on mortality: Comparative study of Kerala and West Bengal. *Economic and Political Weekly* 18 (19):877–900.

Registrar General of India. 1983. *Survey on Infant and Child Mortality, 1979.* New Delhi: Ministry of Home Affairs.

———. 1970–78. *Sample System Reports.* New Delhi: Ministry of Home Affairs.

Rural Health Division, Government of India. 1983. *Quarterly Bulletin on Rural Health Statistics in India.* April-June.

Saxena, G. B. 1971. *Indian Population in Transition.* New Delhi: Commercial Publications Bureau.

Sharma, M. 1984. Health profile of India—problems, services and issues. *Journal of Indian Anthropological Society* 19:93–117.

18 AGRICULTURAL RESOURCES, COMMUNITY DEVELOPMENT, AND EARLY CHILDHOOD MORTALITY IN BANGLADESH

Barry Edmonston

The purpose of this chapter is to report on infant and child mortality in Bangladesh and to add to available studies on community mortality (Anderson 1972; Begun 1977; Edmonston 1983b; Edmonston and Andes 1983a; Edmonston and Andes 1983b; Huda 1980; Huda 1982; Miller and Stokes 1978). The assumption underlying this inquiry is that there exists considerable variation in community mortality — in populations of varying mortality levels — and that it is possible and important to understand the broad features related to these variations. This research is exploratory rather than confirmatory, since the aim is to discover and identify general community correlates of infant and child mortality within the context of an ecological perspective.

This research estimates infant and child mortality for 240 communities in Bangladesh, derived from the 1976 Bangladesh Fertility Survey, and then uses these mortality data to examine community correlates calculated from a separate community survey. The community-level data indicate that mortality differentials exist in Bangladesh and that the variations are related to general socioeconomic and environmental conditions as well as to health facilities.

Several important problems exist in the statistical analysis of spatial mortality. It has become clearer in recent years what these statistical problems are and, in some cases, how to address them. A secondary purpose of this chapter is to describe these statistical issues in the context of data analysis.

BANGALDESH BACKGROUND

The nation of Bangladesh has a relatively recent history. Bengali-speaking peoples have been self-identified as a cultural group for many centuries, certainly since the Pala Kings of Bengal in the eighth to twelfth centuries A.D.

Even when unified with greater India under Mogul and British rule, the people of Bengal referred to their land as "Bengla Desh," the country of Bengal, rather than "Bengla Prodesh," the province of Bengal (er Rashid 1977). During two centuries of British rule, Bengal was a key and usually separately administered province of India. Although there was some Bengali sentiment opposed to the partition of Bengal based on religion, the partition of India split the province of Bengal into West Bengal, India, and East Pakistan in 1947. This left about 23 million persons residing in West Bengal and approximately 43 million inhabitants in East Pakistan (Mosley and Hossain 1973; Economic and Social Commission for Asia and the Pacific 1981:10–23).

With two segments separated by fifteen hundred miles of India, the nation of Pakistan occupied a unique geographic position among the world's nations. Both East and West Pakistan were primarily Moslem, but differed markedly in language, history, culture, and economy (Ahmad 1975:91). The union of these two disparate wings of Pakistan persisted until December 16, 1971 when, following almost a year of violence and struggle for independence and more than a month of war which involved India, an instrument of surrender proclaimed Bangladesh an independent nation. The human toll of independence was high: perhaps a million deaths and 10 million refugees (Ahmad 1975:385). Moreover, the civil strife followed closely the diastrous March 1970 cyclone that struck the southern coast of the Bay of Bengal, resulting in the deaths of an estimated 500,000 people (Mosley and Hossain 1973). Rarely has a new nation begun its existence with such a cost of human lives.

Population History

At the time of independence in 1971, Bangladesh had an estimated population of 72 million (Mosley and Hossain 1973). By 1981, the population had increased to an enumerated 91 million people and was growing at an annual rate of 2.7 percent. This population increase reflects continuing high fertility (a crude birth rate of about 45 to 50 per thousand during the 1970s), moderately high mortality (a crude death rate of approximately 15 to 20 per thousand during the 1970s), and neglible net international migration (Stoeckel 1973). In 1985, Bangladesh was a populous nation of some 101 million inhabitants, with a population density of 1,830 persons per square mile on the territory of 55,000 square miles.

Bangladesh is surrounded by India on the west, north, and east, with Burma to the southeast. The Bay of Bengal lies on the southern shore. The most striking geomorphological aspect of Bangladesh is the alluvial lowlands that cover much of the country. These lowlands are the gifts of several great river systems that traverse the land. The great rivers flow in broad braided channels which become sandy or silty islands in low water periods and submerged immense plains during the rainy season. Dacca is the capital city of Bangladesh; Khulna, Bairsal, and Chittagong are the three other large cities.

The earliest estimates of mortality in the region indicate a life expectancy at birth of about twenty-five years in India in the late 1800s (Davis 1951:36). Bengali trends likely follow the general trend for India, with life expectancy at birth increasing only modestly to about thirty-two years in 1941. Mortality trends in Bangladesh in recent decades exhibit a pattern somewhat different from many other developing countries, with life expectancy only increasing to about forty-six years in the 1970s, and probably about forty-eight to forty-nine years in 1985. The trend in infant mortality displays comparable changes, from a rate of about 150 per thousand in 1960, to approximately 157 per thousand in the early 1970s, to probably somewhat lower than 150 per thousand at present (Kabir 1978; Kabir 1982; Kabir and Uddin 1990). Infant and child mortality has remained comparatively high and, as will be seen, reflects varied but high mortality conditions in Bangladesh communities.

Disease Patterns

Diarrheal and communicable diseases, coupled with malnutrition, are the principal health problems for infants and children in Bangladesh. Partly because of food shortages and partly due to inadequate rural incomes, malnutrition of varying degrees afflicts a significant portion of preschool children. Poor water supplies, inadequate sanitation, and scarce medical facilities predispose children — especially the malnourished — to numerous infectious diseases (cholera, dysentery, tuberculosis and upper respiratory tract infections, parasites, and tetanus). Surveys of preventable childhood diseases in Bangladesh are found in McCormack and Curlin (1973) and Edmonston and Bairagi (1981).

DATA AND METHODS

Data Sources

Data reported in this chapter are derived from the household interview and community inventory of the Bangladesh Fertility Survey of 1976. The Bangladesh Fertility Survey (BFS) (1978) was carried out between December 1975 and March 1976 by Bangladesh's Division of Population Control and Family Planning. The BFS is associated with an international series of fertility surveys, the World Fertility Survey (WFS), a pioneering effort to understand better the levels, determinants, and factors associated with fertility.

The BFS used a three-stage area probability sample of Bangladesh. In the first stage, explicit clusters were selected, with 160 primary sampling units in rural areas and 80 primary sampling units in urban areas. In the 160 rural primary sampling units, a community survey was also taken, with questions about health facilities, schools, agricultural programs, commercial and governmental facilities, and transportation conditions. Similar community data on the 80 urban areas have been collected by the authors in 1980 for analysis herein. The second stage yielded a random sample of 6,145 households within the primary sampling units, with 5,866 (95 percent) of the households successfully contacted. The third stage involved interviews with 6,513 ever-married women under fifty years of age (98 percent of the eligible residents in the households). These data are the largest, most recent sample of Bangladeshi households with childhood mortality data. (Some recent contraceptive prevalence surveys in Bangladesh collect fertility information, but the age of death for deceased children is not ascertained in these surveys.)

Data Quality

Data collected in the BFS appear to be acceptable for purposes of studying retrospective infant and child mortality (Edmonston 1983a). Comparisons of fertility data indicate generally complete coverage of births, as reported maternity histories from women (Chidambaram, Cleland, and Verma 1980) and show that the omission of births is probably low in the BFS. The retrospectively reported infant death rate from the BFS for the period 1966–1975 is 155 per thousand, as compared to estimates of 147 to 157 per thousand during 1966 to 1973 (Kabir 1982). Looking at mortality during the first ten years of life from the BFS, the survival data indicate life expectancy at birth of forty-six years for both sexes combined, using OECD Region D (South Asia) model life table (Organization for Economic Cooperation and Development 1982). The previously cited infant mortality estimates and the early 1970s estimates of life expectancy at birth of forty-six years imply a slight underreporting of infant and child death in the maternal birth histories. Recent work by the Committee on Population and Demography (1981) of the National Academy of Sciences reports an infant mortality rate between 130 and 160 per thousand for the mid-1950s to mid-1970s period. This latest estimate is too broad to appraise the completeness of reporting of infant deaths in the BFS retrospective maternity histories.

Additional checks were made on the mortality data that indicate data of adequate quality for analysis of community mortality.

1. The number of deaths per year, 1966 to 1975, was plotted and showed reasonable patterns, including trends coinciding with known national mortality fluctuations.

2. The age pattern of mortality was fit with the Weibull survival distribution and compared to the age pattern of mortality from three other Bangladeshi data sources (Edmonston 1985).

3. Communities experiencing immediate effects of the cyclone of 1970 were examined for consistency with the reported mortality levels.

4. Related analysis on mortality by maternal and family characteristics has produced reasonable results (Edmonston 1983a).

The main concern in this chapter moreover, is community variations in mortality compared to national data, where there are potential differences among communities. In particular, we might suspect that more poorly educated rural communities differentially underreport childhood deaths, thereby reducing the urban-rural mortality differences. To the extent that such biases exist in reports on deceased children, they usually attentuate the substantive findings reported in this research.

Age reporting is poor in Bengali populations (Edmonston and Bairagi 1981) and is confounded by the anthropometric status of the child (Bairagi et al. 1982; Bairagi, Edmonston, and Khan 1987). But, according to unpublished work by Stan Becker in Matlab thana, Bangladesh, maternal birth histories seem to improve age reporting for children; moreover, this chapter relies only on broad age groups for analysis.

Data Processing

Prior to tabulating mortality information for each community or primary sampling unit in the survey, records for each live birth were examined from the mother's maternity history. This was done by taking each woman's interview and establishing a separate record for every live birth reported. With a record for each live birth, data were selected if a child was alive at any time during the ten years prior to the survey, or 1966 to 1975. This yielded records on 25,744 children. Children living during this period, whether eventually dying or not, were then used for the calculation of the community mortality ratios.

Calculation of Mortality Ratios

The basic data for this study are mortality ratios, by age and by sex, for the 240 communities of the Bangladesh Fertility Survey. Mortality ratios were calculated to express the community's mortality relative to the Bangladeshi national average. First, all 25,744 children living during 1966–1975 were used to calculate by sex: (1) the probability of living from birth to age 1, and (2) the probability of living from age 1 to age 3. These age groups were used in order to compare infant mortality (the first year of life) and childhood mortality (the second and third years of life). The survival probabilities obtained from all children in the BFS are as follows:

	Females	Males
Birth to Age 1	.848	.839
Age 1 to Age 3	.905	.911

Second, all 25,744 children were aggregated by sex and year of birth for the 240 communities. The number *actually* alive at age 1 and age 3 was compared to the number *expected* to be alive from the national survival probabilities. This mortality ratio is defined as:

$$\text{Mortality Ratio} = \frac{\text{Born - Actually Dead}}{\text{Born - Expected Dead}}$$

Suppose one hundred females are born in a community; we therefore expect (100) x .848 = 84.8 to survive to age 1, or 100 - 84.8 = 15.2 to die, according to national Bangladeshi survival probabilities. If, in fact, ninety females actually survive to age 1, the mortality conditions are better than national levels, and we have a mortality ratio of (100 - 10) / (100 - 15.2) = 1.06. The mortality ratio centers on the national average, 1.0 by definition, and shows worse conditions when greater than 1.0 and better conditions when less than 1.0. It should also be pointed out that this mortality ratio is substantively easy to interpret; a ratio of 2.0 indicates twice as many children die as would be expected from Bangladesh's national data, and ratio of 0.5 demonstrates that only one-half as many children die as would be expected from national data.

Six mortality ratios were calculated for each of the 240 communities: birth to age 1 and age 1 to age 3, with both age groups for females, males, and both sexes. These six mortality ratios are the response variables for the analysis reported here.

Statistical Issues with Spatial Mortality Data

Two different statistical problems exist with multivariate analysis of spatial mortality. Both problems severely restrict the data interpretation, and neither is easy to solve. First, the specific sample variances for spatial mortality are complex, reflecting the design effects of the sample survey and inherent stochastic error in the death process. Pocock, Cook, and Beresford (1981) consider the appropriate weights for dealing with stochastic variation in death rates. Estimating the appropriate weights for spatial mortality data requires an iterative weighted least squares estimation that has been applied, at present, to only two data sets. In general, we can say that estimation of multivariate equations for spatial mortality with unweighted cases overestimates the regression coefficients and exaggerates the statistical tests.

One should note, in particular, that there are three types of variance involved in the multivariate analysis of spatial mortality: (1) sampling variation of the observed mortality rate around the "true" mortality rate; (2) variance around the underlying "true" rate that is explained by the model; and (3) unexplained variance around the underlying "true" rate. The key point is that there is a variance — number 1 — that the model inherently does not explain and that yet, in standard analysis of variance calculations, is included in the multiple correlation coefficient. Because of the nature of the variance in spatial mortality rates, the standard multiple correlation coefficient has no implicit interpretation in this situation (multiple R is presented in this chapter with the caution that it has limited assistance in comparing the results).

The second difficult statistical issue is spatially correlated error in the mortality data (Cook and Pocock [1983] offer a readable review of this issue). As is well known, multiple regression and other variants of the general linear model make a critical assumption that the cases or observations are independently distributed (Cox and Snell 1981:33–34). Frequently, though, observations are made close in time or space or using the same measuring instrument or observer. For spatially distributed data, we might worry that some unknown or unmeasured covariate is relevant to mortality but, being excluded, leads to an error term in the multivariate model that is spatially correlated. Such spatially correlated errors can lead to serious overestimates of the size and significance of the model. The most frequent clue to problems of spatially correlated errors are spatial clusters in the residuals. Unfortunately, some researchers tend to interpret these regionally clustered patterns as "regional effects," without recognizing the extent to which they derive from spatial autocorrelation.

DETERMINANTS OF COMMUNITY INFANT AND CHILD MORTALITY

Numerous studies provide evidence that socioeconomic conditions and mortality are inversely related at the national (Preston 1976) and subnational levels (Anker and Knowles 1980; Young, Edmonston, and Andes 1982). For purposes here, we focus on those community-level factors that have been implicated as influencing infant and childhood mortality. We ignore important factors for Bangladesh mortality pertaining to the individual child (Edmonston 1983c), mother (Edmonston 1983a), or family.

Age

The exact age of an individual in the early years of life is a relatively powerful predictor of mortality (Edmonston 1982). Most populations display a J-shaped mortality function, with mortality high during the neonatal period, dropping rapidly during the postneonatal period, and then often declining less markedly during the weaning period (Jelliffe and Jelliffe 1978). And since medical, family, and environmental conditions are likely to affect children differentially by age, it is important to examine child mortality within selected age groups.

Sex

Although life expectancy at birth is generally higher for females in most societies, there are numerous examples of higher female mortality during the early childhood years (United Nations 1973). More specifically, even when female infant mortality is lower, the age-specific death rates for age 1 to age 4 are sometimes higher for females. This suggests that mortality investigations examine sexes separately in order to separate sex differences from the influence of other factors.

Family Factors

As the immediate health environment for the child, the family plays a key role in affecting mortality. Several aspects of the family are important for childhood health: various nutritional factors (Latham 1975), housing conditions, sanitation and drinking water, and the health of other family members, especially the mother (Anker and Knowles 1980). For the community analysis reported here, information is not available for diverse variables regarding the family. Nevertheless, a measure of average female education in the community is available, and this measure has emerged as a crucial variable in previous epidemiological analysis.

Medical Facilities

The more available and effective the medical facilities in a community, the lower should be infant and childhood mortality. Other studies have emphasized, however, that medical facilities are embedded in the development process itself (Young, Edmonston, and Andes 1982) and that the existence of a medical facility reflects a process more general than mortality intervention. Moreover, the effectiveness of medical facilities is difficult to measure, even though it is important in the study of mortality. For these reasons, we might expect a negative effect of medical facilities on childhood mortality yet recognize initially that a measure of the existence of medical facilities in a community is only the first step in the study of this variable.

Sanitation

Various infectious diseases, zoonoses, and nutritional conditions vary regionally and are sometimes affected by community health programs. The major aspect of the physical environment in Bangladesh that bears on child health is the quality of water. Our community survey obtained information on the water sources and the disposal of sewage for the community. While it is easy to ask questions about the water supply, it is expensive to test the water supply for a community's residents. Our data rely solely on simple questions from key informants in the communities.

Agricultural Development

Considerable variation often exists in the agricultural development in a nation's villages (Noble 1980). Water and irrigation systems usually vary, the adoptions of new seed varieties is seldom uniform, and newer insecticides and fertilizers are random in their adoption. The mortality data for Bangladeshi communities is relatively unique in that we have comprehensive information available about agricultural development in the rural areas.

EXPLANATORY VARIABLES FOR THE COMMUNITIES

Community conditions are affected by six explanatory variables for the 240 Bangladeshi communities. First, the average years of completed schooling for women in the community is calculated as an indicator of family socioeconomic status. Since there is generally a correlation between family socioeconomic status and childhood mortality, we expect to see lower mortality in communities where females are better educated.

Five other variables were created by Guttman scalogram analysis (Coombs, Coombs, and Lingoes 1978), a cumulative unidimensional scaling technique. These five scales were constructed to indicate several aspects of the community: health resources (particularly medical facilities), general community facilities, access to urban centers, sanitation facilties, and agricultural development. All these scales were calculated from the community inventory of the Bangladesh Fertility Survey and independently collected data. A community survey was taken in 160 of the rural communities and smaller towns at the same time as the 1975–1976 BFS. For the eighty larger urban communities, separate information was collected in 1980 using government data. A potential limitation to this approach is that there are relatively few cases in some of the variable categories. This limitation is balanced to some extent by multivariate analysis relying on explicit categorical explanatory variables. That is, Guttman scalogram analysis is primarily relied upon to select items for the scales and to arrange the order of items for statistical presentation. The coefficients of reproducibility and scalability indicate adequate cumulative scales for the following measures.

The health resources scale includes six items measuring the community's health facilities and personnel. Each item was coded as present in the community if it was within three miles — or walking distance — of the community center. With these six items, the health facilities scale progresses from no facilities (21 communities) to pharmacy (34 communities), government dispensary (26 communities), qualified doctor (30 communities), hospital (17 communities), maternal-child health clinic (7 communities), and health centers (105 communities).

The general community facilities scale is based on the existence of local and government facilities. In increasing order, the community facilities scale goes from no facilities (20 communities) to youth club (30 communities), community center (36 communities), bank (21 communities), government guest house (15 communities), and urban centers with a police force (118 communities).

The urban access scale measures the accessibility to a community of other areas of Bangladesh. It has ten items which form a cumulative scale, although the lowest three and highest three items were collapsed for multivariate analysis after making the scale. The urban access scale, after collapsing the lowest three and highest three categories, progresses from those without newspapers and postal service (39 communities), village radio (29 communities), bus stop (31 communities), paved road (20 communities), telephone service (19 communities), telegraph (13 communities), and launch, steamer, or railroad service (89 communities).

The sanitation conditions scale comprises three variables related to a community's sanitation. Three communities have no sanitary facilties, eight have sanitary latrines, 146 have tubewells, and 83 have available tapwater.

Agricultural development was measured for rural communities in terms of five variables. For multivariate analysis, a dummy variable coding is used for urban communities to reflect the fact that no agricultural development scale exists for the eighty urban centers in the sample. The agricultural development scale progresses from no development variables present (3 communities), chemical fertilizer (7 communities), new seed varieties (20 communities), some insecticides used (42 communities), and at least one visit of a government agricultural officier (62 communities).

RESULTS

Statistical Model

We turn first to a brief review of the statistical technique for assessing the relative importance of community development indicators with infant and childhood mortality. One-way analysis of variance (ANOVA) with several categorical grouping variables is used for multivariate analysis of the community mortality ratios.

There are several reasons for using this type of ANOVA model in this work. First, it is important to consider the impact of each explanatory variable in the case of intercorrelated predictor variables. Intercorrelations occur when the predictor variables are not independently disturbed and there are associations between them. While there is no unique solution to the question of the exact influence attributable to an explanatory variable that is correlated with other explanatory variables, there are valuable conclusions to be drawn from the form of the relationships. A second purpose of this multivariate model is that it is useful for the analysis of categorical explanatory variables. This makes the model suitable for community data with separate, noncontinuous variables, as well as permitting the effects of an explanatory variable to have nonlinear variation. Third, this model is used to see how the effect of a variable changes when other, possibly correlated variables are included in the multivariate analysis. Fourth, ANOVA offers an efficient method for statistical fitting of data with categorical explanatory variables.

The six explanatory variables, including the five scales, are used in the ANOVA model to predict community mortality from birth to age 1 and from age 1 to age 3. Table 18.1 presents the ANOVA equations for mortality during the first year of life, for each sex, and for both sexes, for the 1966 to 1975 period. On the left-hand side are the six explanatory variables and the categories of the variables. The second column shows the number of communities in each category. The third column presents the gross effects, which are the actual category means minus the grand mean. The grand mean for females, males, and both sexes is shown at the bottom of the table. A positive gross effect indicates higher mortality for the category, while a negative gross effect shows lower mortality. In the fourth column are the net effects, the estimates for the effect of that category after holding constant the other explanatory variables in the ANOVA model. Thus, the net effects are the results of the estimation of the ANOVA equation with adjusted deviations of the category from the grand mean.

Note that the multiple correlation coefficient (multple R) is shown for each equation at the bottom of the table. But, as mentioned previously, this has a limited interpretation in this situation because of stochastic error in the response variable. In particular, multiple R has neither a limiting condition of 1.0 nor do we know the probability density function. At best, it offers some general notion of comparative explained variance between the ANOVA equations.

Infant Mortality

We turn now to the results shown in Table 18.1. Looking briefly at each explanatory variable, the association of average female education and infant mortality is not greatly attentuated when all the other variables are entered in the ANOVA equation.

Urban access and community facilities display neither a regular pattern nor sizable coefficients. Likewise, with the exception of the three communities with no sanitation, there is no evidence of a noteworthy association between sanitation facilities and infant mortality.

The category health resources demonstrates a general pattern of higher infant mortality in communities with few or no facilities and lower mortality in communities with three or more facilities. The pattern is not monotone, however, and there are some differences between the influences for females and males. There is the suggestion of about a 15 to 40 percent variation in infant mortality depending upon the health facilities in a community.

Agricultural development, in spite of its theoretical importance for food supplies and economic progress, fails to display a consistent, interpretable pattern. In general, the eighty urban communities with no agriculture have slightly lower infant mortality. Among the 160 rural communities, the only instances of noticeably high or low mortality are categories with few communities.

TABLE 18.1
Community Variation of Infant Mortality, by Sex, for BFS Communities, 1966–1975

	Sample Size	Females		Males		Both Sexes	
		Gross Effects	Net Effects	Gross Effects	Net Effects	Gross Effects	Net Effects
Female Education (in years)							
0– .49	53	.06	.08	.25	.26	.16	.18
.50– .99	66	.13	.11	.06	.09	.09	.10
1.00–1.49	38	−.01	−.02	.02	.06	.03	.04
1.50–1.99	25	−.14	−.14	−.14	−.16	−.14	−.16
2.00–2.99	29	.16	.16	−.14	−.17	.00	−.01
3.00+	29	−.44	−.42	−.36	−.47	−.42	−.47
Urban Access							
0–2, low	39	.03	−.10	.14	.06	.10	−.01
3	29	.16	.07	.02	.11	.09	.10
4	31	.26	.19	.13	.11	.18	.14
5	20	−.12	−.11	−.10	−.09	−.10	−.10
6	19	.09	.08	.01	.11	.05	.09
7	13	−.17	−.16	−.16	−.04	−.17	−.11
8–10, high	89	−.12	−.02	−.07	−.10	−.10	−.05
Community Facilities							
0, none	20	.14	−.08	.23	.01	.19	−.03
1	30	.18	−.11	.03	−.10	.09	−.11
2	36	.08	−.19	.02	−.08	.06	−.13
3	21	−.08	−.24	−.08	−.05	−.08	−.14
4	15	−.17	−.24	.17	.24	.02	.02
5, many	118	−.06	.17	−.06	.03	−.06	.09
Sanitation Facilities							
0, none	3	−.18	−.27	.07	−.14	−.07	−.23
1	8	.20	.04	−.12	−.27	.03	−.12
2	146	.07	.02	.03	−.09	.05	−.03
3, many	83	−.13	−.04	−.05	.18	−.10	.07
Health Resources							
0, non	21	.09	.16	.24	.15	.18	.15
1	34	.26	.26	.09	.03	.15	.11
2	26	.25	.29	.01	.04	.15	.17
3	30	−.08	−.09	.01	−.10	−.02	−.09
4	17	−.07	−.06	−.07	−.11	−.07	−.09
5	7	−.17	−.26	−.36	−.43	−.27	−.34
6, many	105	−.12	−.14	−.05	.02	−.08	−.05
Agricultural Development							
0, low	3	.12	.21	−.26	−.36	−.11	−.11
1	7	.09	−.08	.22	.07	.17	.01
2	20	−.03	.04	−.10	−.19	−.08	−.10
3	42	.00	−.09	.09	.08	.05	.00
4	62	.03	.06	−.01	.05	.01	.06
5, high	26	−.08	−.03	−.08	−.07	−.09	−.07
no agriculture	80	−.06	−.07	−.05	−.03	−.05	−.05
Grand Mean		.98		1.00		.98	
Sample Size	240						
Multiple R		.44		.38		.49	

TABLE 18.2
Community Variation of Early Childhood Mortality (age 1 to age 3 years), by Sex, for BFS Communities, 1966–1975

	Sample Size	Females		Males		Both Sexes	
		Gross Effects	Net Effects	Gross Effects	Net Effects	Gross Effects	Net Effects
Female Education (in years)							
0– .49	53	.01	.02	−.01	−.08	.02	.01
.50– .99	66	.04	.03	.16	.08	.07	.04
1.00–1.49	38	−.05	−.03	.21	.20	.06	.07
1.50–1.99	25	.38	.37	.13	.27	.29	.34
2.00–2.99	29	−.08	−.10	−.19	−.17	−.15	−.16
3.00+	29	−.28	−.30	−.54	−.36	−.37	−.32
Urban Access							
0–2, low	39	.11	.09	.28	.06	.14	.04
3	29	.10	.14	.19	−.08	.13	.04
4	31	−.27	−.37	.22	.01	−.04	−.19
5	20	.13	.06	.02	−.21	.09	−.04
6	19	.09	.07	−.14	−.43	−.03	−.16
7	13	.31	.28	.10	−.09	.27	.20
8–10, high	89	−.08	−.03	−.25	.21	−.15	.05
Community Facilities							
0, none	20	.01	.20	.09	−.01	.04	.08
1	30	.09	.20	.19	−.02	.11	.07
2	36	.06	.03	.38	.16	.15	.03
3	21	−.11	−.23	.08	−.11	−.01	−.16
4	15	.22	.16	−.04	−.21	.13	.01
5, many	118	−.05	−.07	−.19	.00	−.10	−.01
Sanitation Facilities							
0, none	3	−.69	−.68	−.20	−.26	−.38	−.38
1	8	−.28	−.40	.31	.39	−.03	−.07
2	146	.06	.03	.14	.16	.08	.06
3, many	83	−.05	.02	−.27	−.32	−.13	−.09
Health Resources							
0, non	21	−.22	−.39	.31	.06	.00	−.14
1	34	.07	−.03	.00	−.22	.05	−.06
2	26	.14	.07	.36	.25	.23	.19
3	30	.14	.10	.19	.11	.16	.13
4	17	−.07	−.19	.14	.09	.01	−.05
5	7	−.07	−.18	−.30	−.20	−.18	−.22
6, many	105	−.04	.08	−.21	−.04	−.10	−.01
Agricultural Development							
0, low	3	−.94	−.94	.00	.53	−.41	−.21
1	7	−.06	.01	−.34	−.39	−.09	−.07
2	20	−.01	.12	.04	.15	.03	.15
3	42	.07	.00	.16	.15	.10	.06
4	62	−.07	−.11	.01	−.02	−.04	−.08
5, high	26	.19	.28	−.22	−.28	.00	.02
no agriculture	80	−.06	−.02	−.16	−.14	−.11	−.08
Grand Mean		.91		.93		.91	
Sample Size	240						
Multiple R		.32		.32		.33	

Early Childhood Mortality

Table 18.2 presents the ANOVA results for the survival of children from age 1 to age 3. We recapitulate the results briefly. The net effect of average years of female education in a community is lower early childhood mortality with improved education. There is one caution: early childhood mortality for intermediate female education shows higher mortality than communities with less education.

Urban access, community facilities, and sanitation facilities display little consistency in the net effects. There are few instances of noteworthy effects and none that bear interpretation.

Unlike the results shown in Table 18.1, health facilities do not demonstrate an inverse association. The gross effects evidence lower early childhood mortality for communities with four or more facilities, but after taking other factors into account, the net effects are not consistent.

The eighty urban communities with no agriculture have slightly lower mortality, particularly for males, compared to rural communities. There is no apparent association of agricultural development and early childhood mortality.

DISCUSSION

The interpretation of data collected in a multiple purpose survey without a specific focus on community mortality must be treated with some caution. The original intent of the Bangladesh Fertility Survey was to understand the levels and determinants of individual fertility in Bangladesh, and the survey well serves that purpose. Using the maternal birth histories for estimates of community mortality is novel and provides a unique, important source of information for social epidemiological study. The main limitations in this approach are twofold.

1. The original birth data possibly underestimate the overall level of infant and child mortality, with possible differential reporting by community.
2. The small number of deaths in some communities introduces random error into the specific community mortality estimates.

The community inventory provides some useful information about 160 rural communities, which we have supplemented for eighty urban communities, but additional data would be valuable. Thus, interpretations of these data should be considered as an exploratory study of Bangladeshi mortality conditions. Since community mortality data are rare, the Bangladesh Fertility Survey offers a valuable source of mortality information from which several conclusions may be drawn.

The moderate association of average female education with lower mortality corroborates other research on this topic (Brass 1980; Caldwell and Ruzicka 1985). Related community research in Jordan (Edmonston 1983b) and Peru

(Edmonston and Andes 1982) also suggests that communities with better-educated women are likely to have lower mortality. Part of the impact of the mother's education may be associated with the improved economic status of the family; another portion may be because of better nutritional and health knowledge. The results for Bangladesh show that female education probably reflects broader community conditions: the social processes that are significant in improving the education of women are closely connected at the community level.

Achieving an average female education of at least three years, for example, is associated with about 40 percent lower infant mortality for a Bangladesh community, compared to national averages. Reductions in early childhood mortality (for children age 1 to age 3) would be slightly less in communities with an average of three years or more female education. These communities typically display 30 to 40 percent lower mortality than national averages. We thus see that improved female education (or its associated underlying community conditions) has a powerful association with decreased childhood mortality.

We have also seen that provision of health facilities seems to be related to community levels of infant mortality in Bangladesh. Furthermore, both sexes benefit from adequate health facilities, particularly in the first year of life. The nature of health facilities appears to be distinctive, depending upon the age of the child. In the first year of life, health facilities have only a moderate association; in the second and third years of life, health facilities have a modest, mixed relationship with mortality. We conclude, based on these results, that a general improvement in health facilities, with extension of clinic services, would provide a valuable input to lower childhood mortality.

This work fails to show that there is a general association between mortality and various measures of general community development, urban access, and sanitation. What should be concluded from this lack of empirical support for commonly held notions about the determinants of mortality in a high mortality population? Two points seems pertinent. First, the communities under study here experience one of the highest mortality levels currently existing. Infant and child mortality is high, indices of development are low, and there is a much greater homogeneity of communities in rural areas than is typical in most developing nations. It is likely, therefore, that we may be studying a population with communities below the threshold at which general development measures and agricultural development indicators are associated with lower mortality. Second, other studies have demonstrated the impact of maternal and child factors (Swenson 1980; Edmonston 1983a), specific childhood diseases (Chen, Chowdhury, and Huffman 1980), diarrheal diseases (Chen 1980; Oberle et al. 1980), and malnutrition (Chen, Chowdhury, and Huffman 1980) on childhood mortality in Bangladesh. There should be no doubt that, as providers of public health programs, we are aware of measures that could be taken immediately to achieve up to 50 percent reductions in under-five-year-old mortality (Chen et al. 1981). But though these measures might be implemented on a community basis, they do not currently vary by community. Hence, we do not observe community variations in childhood mortality for these conditions since there is, at this moment, little association between these known intermediate determinants of childhood mortality and some of the community measures used in this study. More thorough investigation is needed to understand the conditions and mechanisms by which these community factors might be related to potential, intermediate factors for mortality reduction.

Agricultural development, as measured by an impact of newer technology, also bears no apparent relationship to infant, early childhood, and overall childhood mortality in this community-level study. This is not to say that associations may not exist with specific crops, patterns of agricultural production, or specific farm systems; the aggregate level of data in this study did not focus on these factors. Agricultural patterns of time allocation (Farouk and Ali 1977) and agrarian structure (Chowdhury 1982) deserve future study for their relationship with childhood mortality.

Two general suggestions for factors associated with reduced childhood mortality in Bangladesh communities are evident in this research. First, socioeconomic gains by families and improved status of women — as measured by female education — are related to lower mortality. Second, health facilities with extended programs are especially desirable and are associated with improved mortality of infants and children. It should be emphasized that none of these suggestions conflicts with other development programs in Bangladesh (Islam 1979; Rahim 1978). Indeed, the measures that reduce childhood mortality normally benefit other development goals.

NOTE

Geoffrey Jarvis was indispensible in the first stages of data processing, deriving the community mortality estimates and linking the mortality data with the community inventory information. Diane Haggblom helped as a statistical clerk with descriptive statistics, Guttman scales, and the analysis of variance.

Our thanks to the government of Bangladesh for their official approval to analyze the Bangladesh Fertility Survey and to the International Centre for Diarrheal Disease Research, Bangladesh (formerly the Cholera Research Laboratory) for providing residence and office space during several stays with them. Comments on this work by our colleagues, Radheshyam Bairagi and Frank Young, greatly improved the final draft of this chapter. Finally, we acknowledge an intellectual debt to discussions with Stan Becker, Khawja Huda, and Mohammad Kabir for their insights which sharpened our understanding of Bangladesh community mortality.

REFERENCES

Ahmad, Kamruddin. 1975. *A Socio-Political History of Bengal and the Birth of Bangladesh*. Dacca, Bangladesh: Zahiruddin Mahmud Inside Library.

Anderson, James G. 1972. Causal models of health service systems. *Health Services Research* (Spring) 7:23–42.

Anker, Richard, and James C. Knowles. 1980. An empirical analysis of mortality differentials in Kenya at the macro and micro levels. *Economic Development and Cultural Change* 29 (October):165–85.

Bairagi, Radheshyam, K. M. A. Aziz, M. K. Chowdhury, and B. Edmonston. 1982. Age misstatement for young children in rural Bangladesh. *Demography* 19(4):447–58.

Bairagi, Radheshyam, Barry Edmonston, and A. W. Khan. 1987. Effects of misstatement on the utility of age-dependent anthropometric indicators of nutritional status in rural Bangladesh. *American Journal of Public Health* 77(3):280–82.

Bangladesh Fertility Survey. 1978. *Bangladesh Fertility Survey*. Dacca, Bangladesh.

Begun, James. 1977. A causal model of the health care system: A replication. *Journal of Health and Social Behavior* 18(March):2–9.

Brass, William. 1980. Policies for the reduction of mortality differentials. *Population Bulletin of ECWA* (December) 24:3–28.

Caldwell, John C., and Lado T. Ruzicka. 1985. The determinants of mortality change in South Asia. In *Dynamics of Population and Family Welfare*. K. Srinivasan and S. Kukerji, eds. Bombay, India: Himalaya Publishing House.

Chen, Lincoln C. 1980. Epidemiology and causes of death among children in a rural area of Bangladesh. *International Journal of Epidemiology* 9:25–33.

———. 1973. ed. *Disaster in Bangladesh*. New York: Oxford University Press.

Chen, Lincoln C., J. Chakraborty, A. M. Sardar, and M. D. Yunus. 1981. Estimating and partitioning the mortality impact of several modern medical technologies in basic health services. *Proceedings of the International Population Conference, Manila, 1981*. Liège, Belgium: International Union for the Scientific Study of Population.

Chen, Lincoln C., A. K. M. A. Chowdhury, and S. L. Huffman. 1980. Anthropometric assessment of energy-protein malnutrition and subsequent risk of mortality among preschoolchildren. *American Journal of Clinical Nutrition* 33:1836–45.

Chidambaram, V. C., J. G. Cleland, and Vijay Verma. 1980. Some aspects of WFS data quality: A preliminary assessment. *Comparative Studies* No. 16. London: World Fertility Survey.

Chowdhury, Anwarullah. 1982. *Agrarian Social Relations and Rural Development in Bangladesh*. London: Allanheld, Osmun.

Committee on Population and Demography. 1981. *Estimation of Recent Trends in Fertility and Mortality in Bangladesh*. Report No. 5. Washington, D. C.: National Academy Press.

Cook, Derek G., and Stuart J. Pocock. 1983. Multiple regression for geographical mortality studies, with allowance for spatially correlated errors. *Biometrics* 39:361–71.

Coombs, Clyde, Lolagene Coombs, and James C. Lingoes. 1978. Stochastic cumulative scales. In *Theory Construction and Data Analysis in the Behavioral Sciences*. S. Shye, ed. San Francisco: Jossey-Bass.

Cox, David R., and E. J. Snell. 1981. *Applied Statistics*. London: Chapman & Hall.

Davis, Kingsley. 1951. *The Population of India*. Princeton, N. J.: Princeton University Press.

Economic and Social Commission for Asia and the Pacific. 1981. *Population of Bangladesh*. Country Monograph Series No. 8. New York: United Nations.

Edmonston, Barry. 1985. The age patterns of childhood mortality in Bangladesh: A comparison of data using the Weibull survival function. *Proceedings of the*

American Statistical Assocation, 1985. Washington, D. C.: American Statistical Association.

———. 1983a. Demographic and maternal correlates of infant and child mortality in Bangladesh. *Journal of Biosocial Science* 15 (April):183–92.

———. 1983b. Community variations of infant and child mortality in rural Jordan. *Journal of Developing Areas* 17 (July):473–90.

———. 1983c. A microanalytic stochastic model of human fertility in Bangladesh. *Jamasamkhyra* 1 (June):61–73.

———. 1982. International variations in the age pattern of infant and child mortality. *Proceedings of the American Statistical Association, 1982*. Washington, D. C.: American Statistical Association.

Edmonston, Barry, and Nancy Andes. 1983a. Community variations in infant and child mortality in Peru. *Journal of Epidemiology and Community Health* 37(June):121–26.

———. 1983b. Community variations in infant and child mortality in Peru: A social epidemiological study. In *Infant and Childhood Mortality in the Third World*. Jean Bourgeois-Pichat, ed. Paris: CICRED and World Health Organization.

———. 1982. Variaciones en diferentes comunidades en mortalidad infantil y durante la lactancia en Peru. *Demografia y Economia* 16(4):560–81.

Edmonston, Barry, and Radheshyam Bairagi. 1982. eds. *Infant and Child Mortality in Bangladesh*. Dacca, Bangladesh: Institute for Statistical Research and Training, University of Dacca.

———. 1981. Errors in age reporting in Bengali populations. *Rural Demography* 8(1):63–87.

Edmonston, Barry, William Greene, and Ken Smith. 1981. Multivariate analysis of survival data: An appraisal using Bangladeshi mortality data. *Proceedings of the American Statistical Association, 1981*. Washington, D. C.: American Statistical Association.

er Rashid, Haroun. 1977. *Geography of Bangladesh*. Dacca, Bangladesh: University Press.

Farouk, A., and Muhammad Ali. 1977. *The Hardworking Poor: A Survey of How People Use Their Time in Bangladesh*. Dacca, Bangladesh: Bureau of Economic Research, University of Dacca.

Huda, Khawja. 1982. Effect of community factors on childhood mortality in Bangladesh. In *Infant and Childhood Mortality in Bangladesh*. B. Edmonston and R. Bairagi, eds. Dacca, Bangladesh: Institute of Statistical Research and Training, University of Dacca.

———. 1980. Differentials in child mortality in Bangladesh: An analysis of individual and community factors. Ph.D. diss., Cornell University.

Islam, Nurul. 1979. *Development Planning in Bangladesh: A Study in Political Economy*. Dacca, Bangladesh: University Press.

Jelliffe, D. B., and E. F. Patrice Jelliffe. 1978. Growth and Development. In *Diseases of Children in the Subtropics and Tropics*. 3d ed. D. B. Jelliffe and J. Paget Stanfield, eds. London: Edward Arnold.

Latham, Michael. 1975. Nutrition and infection in national development. *Science* 188, 9(May):561–65.

Kabir, M. 1982. Infant and child mortality in Bangladesh: Estimates from the 1975 Bangadesh fertility survey. In *Infant and Child Mortality in Bangladesh*. B. Edmonston and R. Bairagi, eds. Dacca, Bangladesh: Institute of Statistical Research and Training, University of Dacca.

———. 1978. Estimation of mortality of Bangladesh for the period 1961–1971 from the intercensal survivorship ratios. *Rural Demography* 5(1–2):61–71.

Kabir, M., and M. Uddin. 1990. Estimating mortality and fertility from two census age distributions. *Journal of Official Statistics*.

McCormack, William M., and George T. Curlin. 1973. Infectious diseases: Their spread and control. In *Disaster in Bangladesh*. Lincoln C. Chen, ed. New York: Oxford University Press.

Miller, Michael K., and C. Shannon Stokes. 1978. Health status, health resources and consolidated structural parameters: Implications for public health care policy. *Journal of Health and Social Behavior* 19 (September):267–79.

Mosley, W. Henry, and Monowar Hossain. 1973. Population: Background and prospects. In *Disaster in Bangladesh*. Lincoln Chen, ed. New York: Oxford University Press.

Noble, Allen. 1980. Food production and population growth in Bangladesh. *Asian Profile* 8 (February):53–77.

Oberle, M. W., M. H. Merson, M. S. Islam, A. S. M. M. Rahman, D. H. Huber, and G. Curlin. 1980. Diarrheal disease in Bangladesh: Epidemiology, mortality averted and costs at a rural treatment centre. *International Journal of Epidemiology* 9 (4):341–48.

Organization for Economic Cooperation and Development. 1982. *Mortality in Developing Countries*. vols. 5 and 6. *New Model Life Tables for Use in Developing Countries*. Paris: Organization for Economic Cooperation and Development.

Pocock, Stuart, Derek G. Cook, and Shirley A. A. Beresford. 1981. Regression of area mortality rates on explanatory variables: What weighting is appropriate? *Applied Statistics* 30:286–95.

Preston, Samuel. 1978. Mortality, morbidity, and development. *Population Bulletin of the United Nations Economic Commission for Western Asia* (December) 22:63–75.

———. 1976. *Mortality Patterns in National Populations*. New York: Academic.

Rahim, A. M. A. 1978. Leading Issues in Rural Development. In *Current Issues of Bangladesh Economy*. A. M. A. Rahim, ed. Dacca, Bangladesh: Bangladesh Books International.

Stoeckel, John. 1973. Population: Demographic trends. In *Disaster in Bangladesh*. Lincoln Chen, ed. New York: Oxford University Press.

Swenson, Ingrid. 1980. Relationships between pregnancy status, sex of infants, maternal age and birth order, and neonatal and post-neonatal mortality in Bangladesh. *Social Biology* 28:299–310.

United Nations. 1982. *Model Life Tables for Developing Countries*. Department of International Economic and Social Affairs, Population Studies, No. 77. New York: United Nations.

———. 1973. *The Determinants and Consequences of Population Trends*. vol. 1. New York: United Nations.

Young, Frank, Barry Edmonston, and Nancy Andes. 1982. Community-level determinants of infant and child mortality in Peru. *Social Indicators Research* 4:200–20.

19 THE EDUCATION OF WOMEN AND THE MORTALITY OF CHILDREN IN BANGLADESH

Shirley Lindenbaum

Recent studies critical of the narrow technology-oriented and interventionist approach of some health care programs suggest that broader development efforts, including investment in education for women, may be far more effective (Mosley 1984; Mensch et al. 1985; Zimicki 1986). Several authors in this volume (Swedlund, Malhotra, Andes and Edmonston) also point to a strong association between female education and infant and child mortality in nineteenth-century New England, three regions in India (Kerala, the Punjab, and Uttar Pradesh), and Bangladesh.

The finding that maternal education reduces child mortality has been well documented now in Latin America (Behm 1982; Palloni 1981), Africa (Caldwell 1979; Caldwell and McDonald 1981; Mosley 1984) and Asia (Cochrane, O'Hara, and Leslie 1980; Cochrane, Leslie, and O'Hara 1982; Caldwell and McDonald 1981; D'Souza and Bhuiya 1982; Jain 1984). Most of these studies, using large-scale demographic data, are concerned with establishing the mechanisms by which education can be seen to have its effect. With the effect of maternal education well documented for Bangladesh (D'Souza and Bhuiya 1982; Chowdhury 1982), the following small, closely focused study attempts to catch some of the microdynamics of the puzzle, following an anthropological approach that treats education as an "empty category," its changing meanings defined by informants' recollections and opinions, documented in local records, and demonstrated in the everyday behavior of educated and uneducated people. A simultaneous reading is taken also of broader social currents and historical trends so that local data are interpreted in the context of wider events. The study took place between February and May 1983 in two villages (Shotaki and Shugondhi) of Matlab Upazila, Comilla District, an area of Bangladesh where I had carried out some fieldwork in the past (Lindenbaum 1975, 1981, 1986).

The resident villagers are predominantly Muslim agriculturalists growing rice, jute, oilseed, vegetable crops, and, more recently, wheat and potatoes. Small communities of Hindus provide specialized services as fishermen, barbers, goldsmiths, and shopkeepers. In the context of a rather strict form of *purdah*, women perform the concealed tasks supporting these diverse activities, processing and storing crops, in addition to their better-described labors of cooking, reproduction, and caring for the ill. In recent years, poor women here as in other regions of Bangladesh (McCarthy and Feldman 1983) have begun to work as day laborers and domestic servants in the households of other villagers. With landlessness now approaching 50 percent in the region, some males find wage labor in the city of Dacca or in the smaller towns, some seek short-term employment harvesting crops in other regions of Bangladesh, and some wealthier kin groups send selected family members to the city to establish commercial ventures.

The effectiveness of education in Bangladesh must be seen in the context of recent changes in the political economy of the region. The period of the 1950s and 1960s was a time of marked economic and social transformation. The movement of East Bengal from colonial dependence on Britain to its wider incorporation into capitalist world relations led to the emergence of a small but significant Muslim middle class of traders, shopkeepers, and professionals, who still retained a foot in the village; the sons of less well-to-do village farmers began their search for urban or rural wage employment; and the local prestige system moved from one based on land and aristocratic values to one based on the accumulation of money and social class. At the same time, marriage transactions began to change; the bride's rather than the groom's family became the principal donor of marriage wealth, a change that began among wealthier, urban families in the 1950s, and among the poorer families of Shotaki and Shugondhi in the 1970s (Lindenbaum 1981). The new marriage system rests on a shortage of appropriate — wage-earning — men, rather than on the scarcity of socially desirable women, which was the fundament of the old system. The age of women at marriage began to rise, and as the discussion that follows will show, families began sending their daughters to school to match daughter's education with groom's income as a qualification for marriage.

In the early days of the study, it became apparent that it would not be difficult to record the educational level[1] of most women in the study villages. Unlike such vague or difficult-to-determine information as a woman's age or the specific occupation or location of absent males (sons and brothers), women's educational levels are widely and accurately known. Adults and children recall with accuracy the educational level of their married and now-departed close kin, as well as that of other women in their own and adjacent *baris* (patrilineal family compounds). The one exception was nonelite elderly women, whose educational accomplishments sometimes were unknown or of little interest to others. This gap, however, underscores the significance of education in defining the social identity of contemporary women.

There are many indications that the current value attributed to the education of women is a recent phenomenon, part of larger processes of transformation occurring in the region. One way to trace this apparent change is to examine the history of the local school. One of three high schools in the Union (a group of villages), it is the institution that most educated residents of the two adjacent study villages have attended or currently attend. Begun in 1939 as a private primary school with classes 1 through 5 and upgraded in 1943 to admit students to class 8, it became a high school (up to class 10) in 1945. That year, the government officially recognized the school, and the first group of students – all male – sat for the Secondary School Certificate (SSC) examination, the qualification given upon successful completion of ten years' schooling. Although a few girls from elite families attended the school's primary grades in its early years, the first girl entered class 6 (or high school) in 1953. A second female rose to class 6 in 1954, becoming in 1959 the first woman student to pass the SSC exam. In the early 1950s, then, a significant increase in female school enrollment occurred, with more girls entering primary school and proceeding to the secondary level.

By 1983, the student population consisted of 275 boys and 150 girls in primary school and 249 boys and 94 girls in secondary school, giving a sex ratio of 2.15:1 in the entire school and 1.83:1 in the primary grades. These figures seem comparable to the nationwide trend in which the boy/girl ratio in primary school was 4:1 in 1950 and 1.7:1 by 1980 (Sattar 1982:32). Although the total number of primary school students in Bangladesh in recent years may have declined, since school enrollment has not kept pace with population increase (*Bangladesh Times*, March 20, 1983), the local school data indicate that the number of girls attending school has actually increased. Meanwhile, the first woman began teaching in the primary school in 1976. Married into an elite Shughondi family, she has passed the SSC and Primary Teachers Institute examinations, and her own children attend the school.

Islamic schools provide a second avenue of education in the region. The Shughondi Islamic school (*maktab*) began in 1913, giving instruction in mathematics, Bengali, and Arabic. Since 1939, when the local school opened, students attending early-morning *maktab* study only Arabic, as in other Islamic schools in the area. Not all students attend Islamic schools; about twenty-five boys and twenty-five girls attend the Shugondi *maktab,* while the Shotaki *maktab* has a somewhat smaller enrollment. Some children attend no school at all.

The changing educational experience of women, which began in Bangladesh in the 1950s, has many important consequences. First, although many women still do not attend school, the community of local women can be divided in two: those over age forty who have little or no education and those under forty whose educational experience ranges from primary school to SSC (a graduate of class 10), or even to a B.A. (an additional two years). Although highly educated women (and men) tend to reside in Dacca or some other urban area, the considerable visiting between village and town creates a

Table 19.1
Proportion of Women with Some Formal Education in Shotaki and Shugondhi, 1983.

Age (Years)	Women with No Education	Women with Some Education	Total No. of Women	% with Some Education
60 +	64	11	75	14.7
40–59	141	58	199	29.1
20–39	214	210	424	49.5
10–19	128	192	320	60.0

social universe of village residents that includes a changing mix of educational achievement.

Information about the educational level was obtained for every woman in the two study villages. The mean number of years of schooling in 1983 for women over age sixty was 0.53 (n = 75), for women aged 40–59, 1.25 years (n = 199). For women aged 20–39, however, the mean rises to 2.96 (n = 424).[2] The dramatic increase in women's education may be better expressed in Table 19.1

Although 14 percent of women over age sixty report having had some education, they did not attend school for long, as Table 19.2 illustrates.

The current generation of adult women thus has educational levels that differ vastly from those of past generations. Daughters are more highly educated than their mothers. In the case of 101 mother-daughter pairs, sixty-six daughters at the time of their marriage had an education exceeding that of their mothers, thirty-one had the same education, and four had less. However, of the thirty-one pairs with the same education, twenty-seven had no education, and four had reached the same grade in primary school. Of perhaps greater importance, daughters-in-law are now more educated than their mothers-in-law. Of the 139 co-resident mother/daughter-in-law pairs in the two study villages, seventy-two daughters-in-law have more education, sixty-two the same (of which sixty-one pairs have no education and one pair studied to class 5), and five have less education than their mothers-in-law. This generational feature of women's experience will be discussed later.

In general, women marry husbands who are more educated than themselves, a not-unexpected situation. However, a sample of 298 married couples shows that thirty-nine wives have more education than their husbands, a finding that initially seemed surprising. In most of these cases, however, the husband has a job (*chakri*) and is thus a wage-earner, or he belongs to a family with sufficient land to produce a food surplus. That is, the husband's economic condition is stable, or even favorable, and his family is in a position to acquire more highly educated daughters-in-law for their sons, a strategy that reproduces or raises a family's social status.Thus, in several cases, the more-educated wife is the

Table 19.2
Proportion of Women with Greater Than 5 Years of Formal Education in Shotaki and Shugondhi, 1983.

Age (Years)	Women with < 5 Years Schooling	Women with > 5 Years Schooling	% with > 5 Years Schooling
60+	74	1	1.3
40–59	189	10	5.0
20–39	329	95	22.4
10–19	(school experience for this cohort not yet complete)		

groom's second or third partner, the earlier, uneducated wives having been divorced. Moreover, where the husband/wife educational disparity is greatest, the contribution of the groom's family to marriage costs increases. In one family, a young farmer with no education, whose bride had studied to class 5, contributed more wealth than did his brother who had studied to class 6 and had married a woman with seven years' schooling. Where educational levels are equal, marriage expenses tend to be shared by the two sides, indicating that female education currently has a social value equivalent not to male education but to the economic condition and presently valued social status of the husband and his family.

The changing meaning of education for women in Bangladesh can be demonstrated also by examining the matter from another direction. A small but educationally diverse sample of men and women age forty and over was asked to define the qualities desired in marriage partners and the qualities desirable for members of their own sex, for two periods of time: the past generation and the present.[3] The most frequently mentioned attributes included *bangsha* (hereditary title of the lineage [Chowdhury 1982]), the beauty of the bride (*shundor*, meaning, in particular, the lightness of her skin), the family's social status (*bhadralok*, upperclass, "gentlefolk"), economic condition, and education. Ranked by the number of times each attribute was mentioned, the results show an interesting shift over time.

As Tables 19.3 and 19.4 indicate, men today are less interested in the hereditary status of the bride's family and more interested in her family's economic condition. They are still preoccupied with the bride's beauty. A wife's education, unmentioned for the first period, is now as important as the social and economic status of her family. When women consider the features they desire in a husband, they are now most interested in his employment and economic condition. The groom's education, also unmentioned for the earlier period, is now in third place. (It should also be noted that the qualifications concern women's education and men's *higher* education.) Women are also less interested in the hereditary status of the husband's family and more in its

Table 19.3
Men's Views of Qualities Desired in Marriage Partners in Shotaki and Shugondhi, 1983.

Men's Views of Qualities Desired			
In Wives		**In Husbands**	
Past	*Present*	*Past*	*Present*
1. *Bangsha*	1. Beauty	1. *Bangsha*	1. Employment
2. Beauty	2. Socioeconomic condition	2. Socioeconomic condition	2. Higher Education
3. Socioeconomic condition	3. Education	3. Employment	3. Socioeconomic condition
	4. *Bangsha*	4. Education	4. *Bangsha*

economic condition, which is no longer necessarily tied to *bangsha*. Education has entered into the self-evaluation of a bride, and women's priorities are compatible with the finding that educated women are marrying men with jobs or with sufficient land to farm, even though the husbands may have less education than they do.

Men currently view employment (in wage labor) as the most desirable qualification of husbands, followed by education and economic condition. As to the qualities of wives, women continue to regard their own family's hereditary status as important, but beauty is given less current notice by women than by men. The economic condition of a woman's family is an important feature of a woman's self-evaluation, as is her own education, unmentioned for the past.

Women's education is thus a rapidly moving social counter. Its current meaning differs from that of the recent past, when only young women from elite families went to school. At that time, female education may have more nearly been a proxy for social and economic status. Now, women of the four locally recognized social classes[4] may go to school, although many children from the lowest social categories do not attend, or attend intermittently, since their contribution to household labor is of greater value.[5]

A woman's education currently defines a new aspect of her status at the time of marriage. Whether she marries a more highly educated groom or one with no education, a woman marries into a family considered to be of equal or higher status than her own (isogamic or hypergamic marriages); the family group pursues old strategies of marriage alliance with new social components. Educated women are said to be a lesser financial burden for their families at the time of marriage. Women's education has thus broken loose from an earlier cluster of socioeconomic attributes and is no longer a proxy for hereditary or social status.

Table 19.4
Women's Views of Qualities Desired in Marriage Partners in Shotaki and Shugondhi, 1983.

Women's Views of Qualities Desired			
In Wives		**In Husbands**	
Past	*Present*	*Past*	*Present*
1. *Bangsha*	1. *Bangsha*	1. *Bangsha*	1. Employment
2. Beauty	2. Socioeconomic condition	2. Socioeconomic condition	2. Socioeconomic condition
3. Socioeconomic condition	3. Beauty	3. Employment	3. Higher education
	4. Education		4. *Bangsha*

Education differs in one important aspect from other attributes considered desirable in a bride. In a sense, education belongs to the woman alone. To some degree it reflects upon her family's ability to bear the expense of schooling and the loss of her youthful labor. Unlike the hereditary or social status of her family, however, it describes something specific to the woman herself. Like physical beauty, it contributes to her sense of identity, but unlike beauty, education has a more dynamic effect on the behavior of the educated person and of others toward her, a feature to be considered next.

How Education Changes Women

Ninety people (fifty-one men and thirty-nine women) from all four social classes, with educational experiences ranging from no education to a Master of Commerce, were asked to discuss how education might affect women. Forty-one men and thirty-five women approved of education for women; ten men and four women did not. Those who thought that education was not a virtue were predominantly older males with little or no education. In general, the responses were overwhelmingly favorable.

The perceived effects of education cluster around three main topics: the psychological changes education brings about in women; the economic value accruing from education; and the new status conferred and its implications.

Psychological Effects

As indicated earlier, education is a newly respected attribute of women in general rather than of women in elite families only. Most men now appreciate the self-sufficiency of educated women; they "depend upon themselves," they become "proper persons" (*manush*), they become "brave and smart." Even those who disapprove of women's education stress the behavioral and psychological consequences of schooling, such as that educated girls "choose husbands for themselves and do not depend on their fathers and mothers," their "character becomes bad," or "they do not serve their parents or nurse their husbands well." Those who approve point to the woman's enhanced ability to live harmoniously with her husband and his relatives. Thus, it is said that educated women "become psychologists," their "dealings with their husband's family are admirable," and they "begin to behave in a gentle manner."

Women agree that dealings with their husband's relatives improve and stress that conjugal life is also happier. They comment that they are not too shy to discuss things in their husbands' households, they become "frank" (*mishuk*), and they consider their family life to be "progressive." Educated women also feel themselves to be more intelligent, even that their behavior is "more polite." The perceptions of both men and women thus indicate that the significance of educating women has less to do with the content of school work than with the genesis of manners and the emergence of a sense of companionship in marriage.[6]

Economic Value

As indicated, men and women agree that it costs less for an educated woman's family to arrange a marriage. Once married, men especially note that an educated wife who can read and write appreciates the income and expenditures of her new family and has a better sense of handling financial and domestic affairs. The role of the mother as tutor, saving the expense of an outside instructor, is often mentioned favorably by more-educated people. Less-educated women point to the value of literacy in land disputes; a woman who can read and write has no need to take court documents to outsiders who may not be trustworthy. She can act alone to protect her own and her family's interests. Similarly, an educated woman who receives a letter from her husband need not depend on a literate woman who may convey only part of the text and come between the couple.

Women often suggest that educated women can find employment (*chakri*) in family planning or school teaching and that her income would help to support her parents. This is an interesting recurrent theme, since female employment is recent and rare in the region. Moreover, local women could name only three women who had a job and not all knew the names of all three. Nevertheless, 45 percent of women and 31 percent of men spoke of women finding paid work, by which they do not mean day labor. Of further interest, the data on women's education show that parents, especially in nonelite families, tend to give the highest education to first-born daughters, with subsequent daughters attending school for less time. Thus, the first-born studies to class 10, the second to class 8, and the third to class 5. While higher education is an investment toward a marriage that will reflect upon the entire family, the parents of first-born daughters also actively seek employment for them. It could be said that first-born daughters are becoming "sons" in many poor rural families. This new view of the employability of daughters suggests a *potential* shift in future morbidity and mortality rates in rural areas of children under five, with the better survival of daughters, especially those of educated women (Lindenbaum 1975).

New Status and Its Implications

Educated women are said to take upon themselves the role of family tutor (a task with desirable social as well as economic implications), be better nurses for sick husbands, and are better caretakers for the entire family. Men say that educated women also keep the house cleaner and entertain guests well, and women agree that education improves their standards of housework and household management. Uneducated women note that educated brides acquire good husbands who may take them to foreign parts (*bidesh*), which may mean another country but usually refers to a place beyond the local community, such as Chittagong or Dacca. They note also that educated women "buy soap and saris and eat good food" and that "they and their children enjoy good health," indicating that illiterate women are not mystified about the connections among behavior, economics, and health. Moreover, they add, educated women marry at a later age and do not have to perform exacting agricultural work. This latter point sometimes leads to a discussion of how many years of schooling are needed to provide protection from hard labor. It is generally agreed that young women with secondary schooling to classes 5, 6, or 7 might still be found doing agricultural work, processing crops within the *bari*, but not those with matriculation and beyond. "With education to class 10 or a B.A.," it is said, "you can pay maidservants to work and carry water for you."

MOTHER'S EDUCATION AND THE HEALTH OF CHILDREN

Evidence concerning the psychological and social changes effected by educating women brings us closer to the question of the relationship of mother's education and the mortality of children. Women and men observing the first generation of educated women (other than the small elite of earlier years) point to its liberating effect. Educated women themselves speak of the new tool that makes them self-propelled, of a freedom from dependency and constraint. Others comment on the way education changes women, gives them a desirable "autonomy," and provides them with skills and attributes now considered useful and highly respected. Education transforms a woman in the eyes of others and increases the woman's own self-esteem. Subtle changes in the form and quality of family relationships have thus resulted in the willingness of many men to exchange a dependent wife for one who may be economically more helpful but also more self-assertive. How does this translate into better health for her children?

Some of the answers to this question have been suggested already. Educated women are said to keep themselves, their houses, and children neater and cleaner, an observation which superficially appears to be the case. A focus on sanitation must come, in part, from lessons learned at school. A textbook used in class 3, for instance, has segments on sanitation and hygiene and shows Salam and Mina washing their hands before eating. Mina also washes her plate at a tap and covers her rice and vegetables to keep them free from contamination. The book speaks of the importance of burying rubbish and refuse and of keeping flies away. A group of class 6 children, asked why an emaciated child (pictured in one of their textbooks) seemed in such bad condition, said it was because he was dirty and did not eat good food. Class 3 children also report that they learn about hygiene and cleanliness, a fact confirmed by the female schoolteacher, who indicated that she also inspects children for tidiness and sends home children with skin infections until the condition improves.

Passing children on village paths, it is easy to determine if they attend school. School children are polished clean, they have unsoiled clothes, their skin shines, their hair is combed and glossy. Schoolgirls may be directed to focus more on cleanliness than boys; schoolbooks show Mina performing more hygienic acts than Salam, and schoolgirls report washing their own clothes, while boys indicate that their mothers keep them clean. Moreover, the one school toilet is used by girls, not boys.

Schooling encourages upwardly mobile behavior. The behavioral style of the elite becomes a model for others to imitate, with personal cleanliness perhaps being the easiest to follow, the quality of clothing and nutrition the most difficult. Schoolgirls have the freedom to leave the *bari* every day, where they are exposed to a wider range of people and experiences than those who work at home, or even those who work as maidservants. Given the constraints of *purdah* (the seclusion of women), there is no similar context in which uneducated girls can join as equals with a cross-section of young people from surrounding villages, whose behavior they may intimately observe and follow. Cohorts of girls who travel together through secondary school watch each other with an attentive eye, imitating the smallest fashions in hairstyle and clothing. With schooling completed, they still try to gain news of the higher education, marriage, and fortunes, especially, of their elite companions. Schooling endows girls with prestige, and as the comments of uneducated women indicate, educated girls try hard to emulate the behavior of "gentlefolk." For reasons of status, educated women prefer to wash with tank or tubewell water at home, bypassing public bathing in canals and rivers, and thereby avoiding waters shown to be most contaminated (Khan et al. 1981).

Schooling also presents girls with new sources of authority from whom they seem willing to learn. Of the schoolgirls who visited me almost daily, all said they had access to a radio, even if it was not in their own home. Bengali songs are their passion, but they listen also to broadcasts concerning health and family planning, and some girls in class 6 know what time of day to catch the evening news. The clang of the schoolbell throughout the morning alerts children in different classes to set out for school, drawing them into a time-structured existence.

On many occasions during the study I was struck by the quick conversational replies of young women who had been to school, in contrast to their uneducated mothers or mothers-in-law. Young women with five or six years of education — as well as younger schoolgirls and schoolboys — showed great interest in the research, sometimes crossing the boundaries of one or two *baris* to participate in the discussions. Educated young people were more familiar with an interrogatory style that sometimes puzzles or fatigues their uneducated elders. Moreover, they enjoy the interchange. The experience of schooling, however, goes beyond acquaintance with new conversational styles. Women speak of a newfound consciousness, a sense of cognitive change (*paribartan hoi*) that empowers them to act. "If a girl studies to class 5 she feels there is nothing she cannot do," said one man with five years' education himself. The evidence from Shotaki and Shugondhi thus seems to support Caldwell's (1979) and Levine's (1980) suggestion that classroom participation is a form of assertiveness training, especially for girls who otherwise grow up in contexts that do not encourage them to express their thoughts or feelings.

HEALTH CARE

When children fall ill, what do their families do? A sample of the adults accompanying patients at the Shotaki clinic[7] for diarrheal disease during three weeks in April 1983, shows that, although the admission fee was 20 *taka* (a little less than $1), the facility serves mainly the poor and uneducated. Eighty-eight people were interviewed, seventy-seven women and eleven men, of whom fifty-nine women and ten men were uneducated. The percentage of uneducated women (76.8) thus substantially exceeds the percentage of uneducated women of similar age (over twenty) in the population at large (53.5). (It is also the case that children of the poor and uneducated are more frequently ill.)

When one looks at the diarrheal disease treatment behavior of the forty-seven mothers in the sample with children age five and under, the picture becomes more complicated. When their young children experienced severe diarrhea, sixteen of the thirty-one uneducated mothers, and eleven of the sixteen educated mothers came directly to the clinic and did not seek prior treatment. Thus, roughly half of the uneducated mothers but two-thirds of the educated women sought treatment with oral rehydration solution (ORS) or intravenous saline. This behavior, it might be argued, is the informed choice for medical care in the case of diarrhea. It could also be said that uneducated mothers made more vigorous attempts to find alternative medical care and that their choice of practitioners was weighted in favor of local (largely self-trained) practitioners. The numbers are too small to draw any conclusions. One illuminating way to determine if uneducated and educated mothers pursue different or more effective health care is to consider the following case study.

A young widow in her late twenty's with four children, Khorsheda studied to class 7.[8] Her second eldest child, a boy of about eight, seemed to her to be thin, slow growing, and to suffer from many intermittent fevers. Seeking a variety of cures during March 1983, she began with bespelled water from a local *huzur* (Islamic woman curer), but the water had no visible effect. Next she turned to a local allopath and then to an allopath in the distant town of Munshiganj, both of whom prescribed tonics costing 50 *taka*. Toward the end of March, seeing no improvement, she took her son to a still-more-distant hospital at Munshiganj where, she had heard, MBBS-trained doctors were available. This trip, which was her own idea, required assistance from a variety of kin.

Khorsheda first persuaded her mother-in-law to accompany her, a considerable feat, as we shall see. Since the journey required that she stay away from home for two days, she left her other three children with her mother, whose house she passed on her way to the ferry station. Her older sister's husband's relatives, who lived near the hospital, provided lodging for the party of three. Several days later Khorsheda returned home with the hospital laboratory reports (the child was diagnosed as having several types of worms), worm medicines, and a tonic. As her mother commented caustically, she had succeeded due to the generosity of *certain* kin.

While the journey required a far-flung support system, Khorsheda had conceived of and directed the complex arrangements against considerable odds. Since her husband's untimely death eighteen months earlier, her less-educated mother-in-law had shown little sympathy for the young widow's predicament. She viewed her daughter-in-law as an educated woman who should find employment to support her children and herself. Immediately after her husband's death, Khorsheda began to appreciate the precariousness of her position and asked that a small amount of land and the house in which she resided be legally assigned to her. Her parents-in-law were unsympathetic to this request, and Khorsheda appealed to one of the community's most influential members, a man who is her mother's brother (in somewhat distant kin terms). This man argued her case, and the deceased husband's parents reluctantly granted her a small plot of agricultural land, the house, and the house site in the *bari*. Still, the mother-in-law repeatedly proposed that Khorsheda should leave the village and find a job.

Khorsheda, meantime, tried to find a way to earn a livelihood while living at home with her children. She thought about a sewing machine to make and sell clothes but lacked the money to buy one. She sent a message to her mother's brother (who had meantime moved to Dacca) asking that he visit her on his next trip to Shotaki and continued matching wits with her mother-in-law, whose cooking hearth she shared and who she said had begun giving her children an inadequate amount of food. Fortunately, Khorsheda's mother's house is situated near the local school, and her children were able to visit there for snacks and meals.

This story of tenacity and perseverance describes the behavior of a young woman whose educational experience exceeds that of her mother and her mother-in-law. She has a sense of social geography beyond the limits of the household compound, she knows where good medical care is available and how to gain access to it (cf. Nag 1981). Further, as an educated person she can command the assistance of educated people in better circumstances than herself.

Those who responded to her requests for assistance were all her elders — mother, sister's husband, mother's brother, reluctant mother-in-law. It is significant that the dispute between Khorsheda and her mother-in-law centers around the deployment of family resources between the generations, as Caldwell (1979) might have predicted. Khorsheda successfully orchestrates resources in favor of her children; the mother-in-law views Khorsheda instead as an educated person who should "replace" the wage-earning son she has lost, not someone she is obliged to support. While the dispute is at base an economic one, we also witness the contested terrain now occupied by educated women. We should note also that Khorsheda's activities are directed at "preventive" health measures — nourishing food for the children, an attempt to maintain a standard of healthy growth. Her children, three of whom attend school, are kept tidy and clean. Despite her poor financial position following her husband's death, Khorsheda has a sense of herself as an educated person of a certain social standing, expressing embarrassment when visitors find her in a ragged work sari, processing food grains in her *bari* courtyard.

Khorsheda's story illustrates the predicament facing a young mother who loses the mainstay in a precarious support system. Khorsheda was able to secure help from close and distant kin whom she judged could assist her. Most educated women do not face widowhood so early in married life. Uneducated women, however, do suffer similar deprivation, in that they are frequently "divorced" during the early years of marriage. With the increasing mobility of the male labor force, and in the context of a straitened national economy, some men find it to their advantage to enter into sequential marriages with a number of women, since husbands keep the marriage wealth pledged to them for each union. The predominantly uneducated and poor women who suffer enforced return to their parents' households often have infants they must continue to care for. (One would expect the mortality rates of such infants to be extremely high.) Any family resources they can muster are pledged toward the expenses of another marriage, which they (and their parents) hope will provide a safer haven than the last. Shaikh's (1985) analysis, based on data from Matlab obtained between 1975 and 1979, however, shows that divorce is inversely related to the education of both bride and groom; the lowest divorce rates occur among brides and grooms with secondary education or higher. Thus, educated women have access to networks of support that are acceptable to call upon and that are more likely to stay in place for the duration of their married lives.

Education has a substantial effect not only on the stability of marriage but also on a woman's age at first marriage. As uneducated women at Shotaki observe, educated girls marry later, which may favor the future mother and her children. Before marriage, educated daughters do little strenuous work. Prestige accrues to the family able to keep its daughters at home in apparently unproductive luxury, the rewards of such image management being a well-regarded marital alliance (Lindenbaum 1975:78). A young woman living at home until age nineteen or twenty is thus likely to approach motherhood in a healthier and better-nourished state than an uneducated, harder-working younger person. Having invested in the education of their daughters, even nonelite families give them special attention in the few years prior to marriage. Better-nourished educated women may thus give birth to babies of greater birthweight, a condition judged to be a survival advantage (Khan et al. 1981). They may also experience greater success in breastfeeding, especially if they return home for the birth of the first child, a custom many women aspire to, since they eat and rest better in their own homes.

One further biosocial consequence of education lies in the fact that, as the present study shows, educated women tend to marry into economically "secure" families. In this region, women in economically well-placed families (social class 1 and most of social class 2) light the hearth fire twice a day for two separate food preparations (apart from breakfast), while in some of social class 3 and all of class 4 they light the fire but once a day (late morning). Bacterial contamination of food, an important cause of diarrhea in children (Black et al. 1982), may thus occur more often among the poor and less educated who eat foods following longer periods of storage. School lessons concerning the storage and reheating of cooked food should make an important difference in families where cooking occurs only once a day.

That children of the poor (and presumably less educated) have higher mortality rates than do children of their better-nourished counterparts (Chen, Rahman, and Sarder 1980) may be related to changes in diet during illness. Since it is believed that diarrhea in infants is caused by spoilage of the mother's breast milk, she avoids meat, fish, eggs, and, often, salt, a regimen which, if frequently repeated, would further adversely affect her nutritional state and ability to nourish the infant. In addition, a breastfed child on supplemental food also has its diet changed until the diarrhea stops. In some cases, the mother withdraws breast milk for the duration of the illness and, in most cases, eliminates rice and decreases bread, puffed rice, biscuits, banana, and other supplements. These dietary modifications would seem to have two deleterious effects. Repeated diarrhea episodes lead to a downward spiral in the nutritional status of both mother and child, a constitutional challenge that better-nourished, better-educated women and their children may be in a position to withstand.[9] In addition, the interrupted course of suckling could inhibit the mother's capacity to produce milk, leading to the infant's further nutritional deprivation. Data from the study are insufficient to say whether educated mothers follow a better course of nourishment during illness episodes. The infants admitted to the Shotaki clinic frequently cried for food (as described by their attendants), but it sometimes seemed that it was because the mothers had not prepared well for this unusual and disorienting period away from home. Dietary modifications during illness and the use of supplemental foods are topics that could be investigated more fully.

HEALTH CARE BELIEFS

As described above, the health-seeking behavior and health status of educated and uneducated women differ. The question of health beliefs is another matter. Contrary to what one might expect, the study provides no evidence that education significantly changes the ideas of women about the causes of illness. Rich and poor, educated and uneducated, Muslim and Hindu—women share, on the whole, similar beliefs concerning the origin of illness. It is only among the most-educated women (and men) and only for certain diseases that one finds different notions concerning disease origin. Thus, some fundamental postulates about the workings of the human body and the universe still provide a domain of belief from which the causes of specific illnesses are deduced. In conversations with 206 persons (155 women and fifty-one men) concerning the cause of illness (primarily diarrhea, fever, and scabies) the germ theory was mentioned only twice. One forty-year-old man with a Bachelor of Science degree said that dysentery (but not diarrhea) in a variety of age groups was caused by lack of cleanliness; diarrhea in patients beyond breastfeeding age was due to "irregular eating." In a second exception, a twenty-three-year-old woman with a SSC qualification noted that her one-year-old child suffered from chicken pox, an infectious disorder caused by germs. Dysentery in the same child, however, as well as in a three-year-old sibling, was considered a hereditary disease acquired from the mother. Apart from these two cases, there was general agreement that infant disorders result from spirit attack associated with bad winds and that illness in all age groups stems from various bodily imbalances caused by poor eating habits, hard work, and, occasionally, punishment from God.

CONCLUSION

Just as the sanitation movements (rather than knowledge of the modes of disease transmission) are said to have had more to do with increased survival in the nineteenth century, so the spread of the "manners of hygiene" that results from education has manifold effects on the life chances of Bangladeshi women and their offspring. The cognitive, social, and biological consequences of educating Bangladeshi women may thus be a more effective means of ensuring the survival of children than the introduction of specific medical interventions (Zimicki 1986) or the massive infusion of international aid. That does not mean, however, that maternal education is equally effective in all places at all times. Child mortality differentials by maternal education were found to be greater in the poorest provinces of Kenya (Mosley 1984) and Latin America (Palloni

1981), where the mother lived in poor economic circumstances. A review of studies of the relationship between parental education and child mortality also found that the greatest effects of education occurred in areas with the highest mortality (Cochrane, O'Hara, and Leslie 1980).

As indicated earlier, the effectivness of education in Bangladesh must be seen in the context of recent widespread economic and political change. Education should not be viewed merely as an information "handout," a body of knowledge that transforms the mind and the behavior of the recipient along predictable lines. The present study, for example, found no evidence to indicate that education significantly modified the ideas of women about the causes of illness. Rather, the acceptance of education and its social messages reflects and contributes to the new class structures, ideologies, and family forms emerging in the region. Men now value educational achievement (in both women and men) over a family's hereditary standing when assessing the benefits of a particular marriage."Education" is an index of membership in a class culture that extends beyond the boundaries of the local village and a key to acquiring resources in newly forming systems of distribution.

Female education is thus one strategy by which families increase the prestige and survival chances of the kin group, an older tactic in new garb. The implications of the change are hardly hidden from the women themselves, who see an increasing army of poor village women paid for their day's labor with small portions of food. As one woman said, "I work to eat." Since desirable employment for educated or uneducated women is still rare, most women stay in the countryside. It remains to be seen whether large numbers of educated women will begin to seek employment in the towns and whether this will sever strategic support networks, extinguish their locally appreciated value, and hinder or enhance their ability to increase the survival chances of the next generation.

NOTES

I am grateful to Dr. William B. Greenough, Director, ICDDR, B in 1983, for his invitation to carry out the study and for providing facilities, and to Manisha Chakraborty, ICDDR, B/Matlab health assistant, and Mohammed Elias, a resident of one of the study villages, both of whom assisted in the research. Dr. Stan D'Souza and Susan Zimicki, ICDDR, B Community Studies Research Working Group, both provided support and insightful comments as the study proceeded. Mr. Dil Mohammed, Shotaki Union Council chairman, also took an interest in the research and contributed in many ways to ease living and working conditions in the field. It should be noted that this descriptive study was designed to provide data and hypotheses that could be tested by further epidemiological investigation. The original report thus concluded with a list of questions to be quantified (Lindenbaum, Chakraborty, and Elias 1985).

1. Although I use the word uneducated to refer to those with no formal schooling, I do not mean to deprecate the informal schooling of cultural information transmitted from generation to generation outside the classroom.

2. Women's ages are estimated according to a consensus of data: Matlab census birth registration records, my own data on birth order of a woman among siblings, the number of a mother's pregnancies, her recollection of the *Hartal* (strike) of 1929, and other historical local events. Ages may thus be off in either direction by several years.

3. The sample consisted of twenty individuals.

4. People recognize four social classes based currently on the following criteria: reputation of the *bari* name within the area and the *upazila* (district); number of educated people in the *bari*; amount of land and wealth; whether family members labor for themselves or for others.

5. In addition, although primary school is now free and books are distributed without cost to classes 1 and 2, the poorest children do not have the clothing to permit them to attend school daily, or their families consider a rise in status would not be accepted by the elite and by others (the view of some poor women in the Hindu fishing caste).

6. A phrase suggested by Stephen Kunitz.

7. The Union Council has named the local clinic (a health facility for treating cholera and diarrhea) the Shaitnal Union Council Hospital. The clinic is staffed by four local paramedics, three male and one female.

8. This is not her real name.

9. This nutritional regime may be a cause also of the postpartum condition women call *shutika*, a nutritional anemia experienced by numerous village women.

REFERENCES

Bangladesh Times (1983), March 20.

Behm, Hugo. 1982. Empirical findings on the association between education and child health status: Discussion. *Health Policy and Education* 2:269–73.

Black, R., K. H. Brown, S. Becker, A. R. M. Abdul Alim, and M. J. Merson. 1982. Contamination of weaning foods and transmission of enterotoxigenic *Escherichia coli* diarrhea in children in rural Bangladesh. *Transactions of the Royal Society of Tropical Medicine and Hygiene* 76(2):259–60.

Caldwell, J. C. 1979. Education as a factor in mortality decline: An examination of Nigerian data. *PopulationStudies* 33(3):395–414.

Caldwell, J. C., and P. McDonald. 1981. The influence of maternal education on infant and child mortality. Int. Pop. Conference. Manila. vol. 2. Liège: International Union for the Scientific Study of Population.

Chen, L. C., M. Rahman, and A. M. Sarder. 1980. Epidemiology and causes of death among children in a rural area of Bangladesh. *International Journal of Epidemiology* 9(1)25–33.

Chowdhury, A. K. M. A. 1982. Education and infant survival in rural Bangladesh. *Health Policy and Education* 2:369–74.

Cochrane, S. H., J. Leslie, and D. J. O'Hara. 1982. Parental education and child health: Intracountry evidence. *Health Policy and Education* 2(3/4)213–48.

Cochrane, S. H., D. J. O'Hara, and J. Leslie. 1980. The effects of education on health. *World Bank Staff Working Paper.* no. 556. Washington, D.C.:World Bank.

D'Souza, S., and A. Bhuiya. 1982. Socioeconomic mortality differentials in a rural area of Bangladesh. *Population and Development Review* 8(4):753–69.

Jain, A. 1984. Determinants of regional variations in infant mortality in rural India. Population Council, N.Y.

Khan, M. U., W. H. Mosley, J. Chakraborty, A. M. Sarder, and M. R. Khan. 1981. The relationship of cholera to water source and use in rural Bangladesh. *International Journal of Epidemiology* 10 (1):23–5.

Levine, R. A. 1980. Influences of women's schooling on maternal behavior in the Third World. *Comparative Education Review* 24 (2/2):53–105.

Lindenbaum, S. 1975. The value of women. In *Bengal in the Nineteenth and Twentieth Centuries*. J. R. McLane, ed. Michigan State University, South Asia Series, Occasional Paper 25:75–85.

Lindenbaum, S. 1987. Loaves and fishes in Bangladesh. In *Food and Evolution: Toward a Theory of Human Diets*. M. Harris and E. Ross, eds. Philadelphia: Temple University Press.

———. 1986. Rice and wheat: The meaning of food in Bangladesh. In *Food, Society and Culture*. R. S. Khare and M. S. A. Rao, eds. Durham, N. C.: Carolina Academic Press.

———.1981. Implications for women of changing marriage transactions in Bangladesh. *Comparative Education Review* 12 (11):394–401.

Lindenbaum, S., M. Chakraborty, and M. Elias. 1985. The influence of maternal education on infant and child mortality in Bangladesh. International Center for Diarrheal Disisease Research, Bangladesh. Special Publication no. 23.

McCarthy, F., and S. Feldman. 1983. Rural women discovered: New sources of capital and labour in Bangladesh. *Development and Change* 14:211–36.

Mensch, B., B. Lentzner, and S. H. Preston. 1985. *Socio-Economic Differentials in Child Mortality in Developing Countries.* New York: United Nations.

Mosley, W. H. 1984. Child survival: Research and policy. *Population and Development Review.* Supplement to vol. 10.

Nag, M. 1981. Impact of social development and economic development on mortality: A comparative study of Kerala and West Bengal. Center for Policy Studies. Working Paper no.78.

Palloni, A. 1981. Mortality in Latin America: Emerging patterns. *Population and Development Review.* 7 (4):623–49.

Sattar, E. 1982. *Universal Primary Education in Bangladesh.* Bangladesh: University Press.

Shaikh, M. A. K. 1985. Marriage and marriage dissolution in a rural area of Bangladesh. Canberra: M.A. thesis, Australian National University.

Zimicki, S. 1987. L'Enregistrement des causes de décès par des non-médecins: deux experiences au Bangladesh. In *Mésure et Analyse de la Mortalité, Nouvelles Approaches.* J. Vallin, S. de Souza and A. Palloni, eds. I.N.E.D. Travaux et Documents, Cahier No. 1.19.

CONCLUSION

Alan C. Swedlund and George J. Armelagos

One expressed purpose of this collection is to emphasize the long-term association between the human population and disease. This history is punctuated by two or three, perhaps numerous, major transitions through which many of the world's populations have passed. Humans have lived with infectious disease for the last four million years, and it is reasonable to expect that there have been significant effects on this relationship which are directly attributable to evolutionary processes. What we learn or are reminded of here is that micro-organisms are rapidly evolving, extremely diverse, and quite capable of changing their relationship with their human hosts. We have to temper Haldane's (1949) and others' views about the role of infectious disease in human evolution. It is an anthropocentric view that asserts the importance of human evolution in this dyad. If certain infectious diseases have attenuated over the last several thousands or even hundreds of years, then it is no doubt due to the ubiquity, reproductivity, and variability of the pathogen rather than the host. And, as Svanborg-Eden and Levin suggest and Black implies, the human host is probably best adapted through a general immune system, capable of reacting to a broad range of pathogens, than by any specific adaptation to a particular micro-organism.

Another inference we might make from the long view is that the difference between a pathogen and another micro-organism is subtle and complex. Pathogenicity in the biomedical sense is a function of the virility of the pathogenic organism, the susceptibility of the host, and a large number of intervening environmental factors. Epidemics require a substantial number of these conditions to be met before the outbreak will occur. Diseases like cholera can be widespread and asymptomatic in a population until those conditions are obtained. This history of medicine is, in part, the history of our growth in understanding the ecology of disease and the systemic nature of illness, as Kunitz relates. It is now taken as wisdom, if not profundity, that we are part of an interdependent web of life, that health is a state of adjustment with other organisms and disease, is a state of "failure of adjustment," either short-term or long-term. It has taken western medicine from the mid-nineteenth century to well into the twentieth century to develop this model. Yet, in some ways, it is remarkably similar to the conventional wisdom of traditional societies that have no precise knowledge of the nature of micro-organisms.

Third, taking again the long view, we cannot rule out that certain kinds of adaptations that were appropriate to past evolutionary contexts may not be operative or even problematic today. Does the "thrifty gene" or some polygenic facsimile exist (Weiss and Szathmary herein)? Do such traits lead to degenerative or chronic conditions under certain contemporary regimes? Even more provocatively, are there patterns of behavior or behavioral response that are conditioned by genetic adaptation to past environments (Harrison and Jenner; Harpending, Draper, and Pennington)? Haas, Andes and Edmonston, Lindenbaum, and others represented in this volume might be able to define a model for the explanation of infant mortality that includes maternal age, socioeconomic status, diet, and sanitation, and that they would find perfectly acceptable and that would also account for a majority of the variation in observed infant mortality. Harpending, Draper, and Pennington and perhaps others would quite likely not find that model sufficient, regardless of the R^2. They would likely attribute some residual effect to an as yet unidentified gene(s).

There is a broad range of kinds of transitions identified in the chapters contained here. More difficult to deal with are the hypothesized states or conditions that bound a transition. Several authors deal with topics that raise the conventional dichotomy between traditional and "acculturated" or modernizing societies. Others make various references to a rural $vs.$ urban dichotomy that, in effect, is a similar frame of reference. The steady states we often infer for such comparisons are probably often nonexistent or problematic, at best. A better understanding of the dynamics of these populations is still very much in order. Also, the vague use of such terms as rural, urban, modernizing, and acculturated provides little precision with which to analyze rates or magnitudes of change.

Virtually all of the contributors point, in some way, to the importance of population structure to the understanding of disease in populations in transition. This should not be surprising, as they are overwhelmingly oriented toward epidemiological and demographic research. Rigorous demographic research in indigenous contemporary, historical, and prehistoric populations is still in its infancy. Many times we have heard the refrain that deterministic methods in demography require significant modification when applied to those groups with whom anthropologists and development specialists often work. There is now an extant and growing body of methods designed for these purposes, and we can expect a considerable expansion of our understanding of the dynamics of small populations in the near future.

One of the most common themes or topics cross-cutting these chapters is the issue of infant and early childhood mortality. So much of the cost of disease in transitional populations is borne by infants and children. The various approaches taken and types of populations being described may make a complex set of risks seem even more complex than it is. From a longitudinal perspective, we can see that the interaction of nutrition, feeding practices, and infection have always been prevalent, and infants have been the group at highest risk. Scrimshaw (1978), Johansson (1984), Harpending, Draper, and Pennington (this volume), and others have documented the role of infanticide and child neglect as regulating mechanisms in many societies. However, we must also recognize that the health of children is generally regarded as an indicator of well-being by indigenous peoples and health professionals alike, and most societies express their desire to keep morbidity and mortality of children at an absolute minimum. Transitional groups may pay particularly high costs in the loss of children.

Despite the complexity and variability of this problem, the litany of causative factors and the variables associated with reductions in infant mortality are remarkably similar across time and space. Mosley and Chen (1984) have reviewed a broad range of research among developing populations and present a general review of the proximate and ultimate factors responsible for the infant mortality observed. Their list of proximate causes echoes the diseases and nutritional factors outlined by the authors included here. Most importantly, they address those ultimate factors that create the conditions of malnutrition, disease, and death. The socioeconomic and political forces that lead to poverty, and hence to deprivation of basic needs, are not limited in time and space and remain as perhaps the most difficult problem to address for populations undergoing transition today. Gortmaker (1979), Mosely and Chen (1984), and others increasingly insist that significant efforts to reduce morbidity and mortality must deal with these political and economic factors in order to be truly effective.

The geneticists and immunologists among us have shown through their examples the difficulties with which the human population responds to infectious micro-organisms. Adaptive responses in the ecology of human disease will almost always favor the pathogen over the human host. The technological responses that modern medicine has made are indeed impressive, but as McKeown (1976), Kunitz (1986), and many others have argued, the attenuation of the major infectious diseases in the last 150 years has had more to do with nutrition, hygiene, and public health than the use of antibiotics or other therapeutic or curative measures. This has given us in the western world some optimism that we can indeed control infectious disease, but we cannot be smug or complacent. The rise of antibiotic resistance in many organisms and the appearance of significantly modified or novel pathogens, such as the AIDS virus, make it all too clear that we cannot assume that we have yet entered that phase in Omran's Epidemiological Transition (1971) where infectious disease is no longer a serious problem.

The western world increasingly is turning to the chronic and degenerative diseases as the arena of health concern. So-called traditional or indigenous populations, as they migrate to developed areas or are penetrated by western technology, diet, and economic growth, are also facing an increased incidence of the chronic diseases. As Malhotra notes in his conclusion, the internationalization of industrial development also exposes these populations to new levels of risk from hazardous occupations and toxic materials. His chapter was completed just prior to the incident in Bhopal, India in which an estimated 2,600 people were killed and possibly tens of thousands more injured, making his expressed concern a stark reality.

There is much that remains to be done in order to improve our understanding of the epidemiology of populations undergoing transition. Basic research is still in a relatively immature state, while at the same time there is great need for the application of knowledge to existing problems. The contributors to this volume unanimously agree: human biologists and medical anthropologists increasingly need to become more aware of, and active in, addressing those problems that threaten Third World societies today.

REFERENCES

Baker, P. T., J. M. Hanna, and T. S. Baker, eds. 1986. *The Changing Samoans: Behavior and Health in Transition.* Oxford: Oxford University Press.

Gortmaker, S. L. 1979. Poverty and infant mortality in the United States. *American Sociological Review* 44(2):280–297.

Haldane, J. B. S. 1949. Disease and evolution. Supplement to *La Ricerca Scientifica* 19:68–76.

Johansson, S. R. 1984. Deferred infanticide: Excess female mortality during childhood. In *Infanticide in Animals and Man.* G. Hausfater and S. Hrdy, eds. New York: Aldine.

Kunitz, S. J. 1986. *Mortality since Malthus.* In *The State of Population Theory: Forward from Malthus.* D. Coleman and R. Schofield, eds. Oxford: Blackwell.

McKeown, T. 1976. *The Modern Rise of Population.* New York: Academic.

Mosley, W. H., and L. C. Chen. 1984. An analytical framework for the study of child survival in developing countries. In *Child Survival: Strategies for Research. Supplement to Population and Development Review.* W. H. Mosely and L. C. Chen, eds. 10:25–45.

Omran, A. R. 1971. The epidemiological transition. *Millbank Memorial Fund Quarterly* 49:509–38.

Scrimshaw, S. 1978. Infant mortality and behavior in the regulation of family size. *Population and Development Review* 4:383–403.

CONTRIBUTORS

Armelagos, George J.
Department of Anthropology
University of Florida
Gainesville, FL 32611 USA

Barrett, John A.
Department of Genetics
Downing Street
University of Cambridge
Cambridge, England CB2 3EH

Black, Francis L.
Department of Epidemiology and Public Health
Yale University School of Medicine
New Haven, CT 06510 USA

Draper, Patricia
Department of Human Development and Family Studies
Pennsylvania State University
University Park, PA 16802 USA

Edmonston, Barry
The Urban Institute
2100 M. St.
Washington, DC 20036 USA

Eriksson, A.W.
Institute of Human Genetics
Faculty of Medicine, Free University
P.O. Box 7161
1007 MC Amsterdam
The Netherlands

Fellman, J.O.
Samfundet Folkhalsans Genetisca Institut
00101 Helsinki 10
Finland

Haas, Jere D.
Division of Nutritional Sciences
Cornell University
Ithaca, NY 14853 USA

Harpending, Henry C.
Department of Anthropology
Pennsylvania State University
University Park, PA 16802 USA

Harrison, Geoffrey A.
Department of Biological Anthropology
58 Banbury Rd
Oxford OX2 6QS
England

Jenner, David A.
Department of Biological Anthropology
58 Banbury Rd
Oxford OX2 6QS
England

Jorde, Lynn B.
Department of Human Genetics
University of Utah School of Medicine
Salt Lake City, UT 84132 USA

Kunitz, Stephen J.
Department of Preventive and Community Medicine
Rochester School of Medicine
Rochester, NY 14642 USA

Levin, Bruce R.
Department of Zoology
University of Massachusetts
Amherst, MA 01003 USA

Lindenbaum, Shirley
Graduate Program in Anthropology
City University Center, CUNY
33 W. 42nd St.
New York, NY 10036 USA

Malhotra, K.C.
Anthropometry and Genetics Unit
Indian Statistical Institute
102 Carrackpore Trunk Rd.
Calcutta 700 035
India

Mielke, James H.
Department of Anthropology
Univesity of Kansas
Lawrence, KS 66045 USA

Pennington, Renee
Department of Anthropology
Pennsylvania State University
University Park, PA 16802 USA

Pitkänen, K.
Department of Economic and Social History
University of Helsinki
00100 Helsinki 10
Finland

Roberts, Derek F.
Department of Human Genetics
University of Newcastle Upon Tyne
19 Claremont Place
Newcastle Upon Tyne NE2 4AA
England

Salzano, Francisco M.
Departamento de Genética
Instituto de Biociências, UFRGS
Caixa Postal 1953
90001 Porto Alegre, RS
Brazil

Svanborg-Eden, Catharina
Department of Microbiology
University of Lund
Lund, Sweden

Swedlund, Alan C.
Department of Anthropology
University of Massachusetts
Amherst, MA 01003 USA

Szathmary, Emöke J. E.
Dean of Social Sciences
University of Western Ontario
London, Ont N6A 5C2
Canada

Vargas, Luis A.
Instituto de Investigaciones Antropologicas
Universidad Nacional Autonoma de Mexico
Ciudad Universitaria
Delegacion Covoacan, 04510
Mexico 20, D.F.

Weiss, Kenneth M.
Department of Anthropology
Pennsylvania State University
University Park, PA 16802 USA

INDEX

Acquired immune-deficiency syndrome (AIDS), 56–57
Acute hemorrhagic conjunctivitis, 56
Acute pyelonephritis, disease-mediated selection and, 39
Admixture model, gene frequency and, 23
Agricultural populations: diseases in, 129–31; in Mexico, 147–51; nutritional deficiencies in, 132
Alameda County study, 281
Aleuts, diabetes in, 106–7
Amerindians, diabetes in: broken down by population location, 78–84; Dogrib studies, 91–98; environmental factors and, 90–91, 111; in Eskimos and Aleuts, 77, 106–7; genetic factors and, 85, 111–12; New World syndrome, 105, 114–18; oral glucose tolerance test procedures, 76; in paleo-Indians versus Athabaskans, 106; in the Pima, 77, 85, 86, 89, 90–91, 108, 111–12; prevalence of, 75–77; prevalence of, in Mayan villages, 107; risk factors in contrasting populations, 112–13; role of obesity and, 96–97, 107–8; thrifty gene hypothesis and, 86–90; triglyceride levels and, 113–14

Amerindians, gallstones in: environmental factors and, 111–12; genetic factors and, 111–12; New World syndrome, 105, 114–18; in the Pima, 108, 110, 112; population comparisons of morbidity ratios for, 109; prevalence of, 108–11; risk factors in contrasting populations, 112–13; triglyceride levels and, 113–14
Analysis of variance (ANOVA), one-way, 342–43
Arthez-d'Asson (French Pyrenees), impact of industrialization on, 27–28
Aseptic meningitis, 56
Assault sorcery (*tokabu*), 302, 303–6, 308
Asurini, 59–60, 66
Athabaskans, 77, 106

Bangladesh: background of, 333–34; disease patterns in, 335; Fertility Survey (BFS) of 1976, 335, 336; population demographics, 334–35. *See also* Childhood mortality in Bangladesh; Education of women in Bangladesh
Birthweights: in India, 323, 325. *See also* Neonatal mortality and birthweight